Children and Young People's Nursing

Principles for Practice

Second Edition

Children and Young People's Nursing

Principles for Practice

Second Edition

Edited by

Alyson M. Davies
Swansea University, UK

Ruth E. Davies
Swansea University, UK

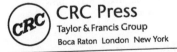

CRC Press
Taylor & Francis Group
Boca Raton London New York

CRC Press is an imprint of the
Taylor & Francis Group, an **informa** business

CRC Press
Taylor & Francis Group
6000 Broken Sound Parkway NW, Suite 300
Boca Raton, FL 33487-2742

© 2017 by Taylor & Francis Group, LLC
CRC Press is an imprint of Taylor & Francis Group, an Informa business

No claim to original U.S. Government works

Printed in Great Britain by Ashford Colour Press Ltd, Gosport, Hampshire
Version Date: 20160322

International Standard Book Number-13: 978-1-4987-3432-5 (Paperback)

Library of Congress Cataloging-in-Publication Data

Names: Davies, Alyson, 1963- , editor. | Davies, Ruth, 1954- , editor.
Title: Children and young people's nursing : principles for practice /
[edited by] Alyson Davies, Ruth Davies.
Description: Second edition. | Boca Raton : Taylor & Francis, 2017. |
Includes bibliographical references and index.
Identifiers: LCCN 2016012713| ISBN 9781498734325 (pbk. : alk. paper) | ISBN
9781498734332 (e-book) | ISBN 9781498734349 (vital book) | ISBN
9781498734356 (epub)
Subjects: | MESH: Pediatric Nursing--methods
Classification: LCC RJ245 | NLM WY 159 | DDC 618.92/00231--dc23
LC record available at http://lccn.loc.gov/2016012713

Visit the Taylor & Francis Web site at
http://www.taylorandfrancis.com

and the CRC Press Web site at
http://www.crcpress.com

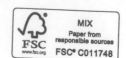

To Tom (17 April 1987–3 August 2006)
and
To Gwilym and Megan

Contents

Foreword

It is critical that advocates and champions of children's rights engage with professionals who are responsible for delivering services for children and young people. In order to give the United Nations Convention on the Rights of the Child (UNCRC) real meaning and bring the articles to life, we must develop an understanding of what is meant by a 'rights-based approach' and examine how practical application can be asserted across our services.

This textbook reflects the commitment of nursing professionals to children's rights and expresses the intrinsic link between children's rights and effective practice leading to positive outcomes. The book challenges boundaries of current practice in children and young people's nursing and encourages a new generation of children's nurses to become critical thinkers.

Wales has a strong track record of recognizing the UNCRC. The National Assembly for Wales can be rightly proud of the legislation that it has passed which promotes and protects children's rights, not least of which is the groundbreaking Rights of Children and Young Persons (Wales) Measure 2011, which requires Welsh ministers to have due regard to the UNCRC in everything they do. Guidance, regulations and policy emanating from the Welsh government have also reflected this commitment, often explicitly. The problem facing child rights advocates lies in determining how to safeguard and enforce children's rights when children may be unable to exercise them of their own will.

The challenge therefore for all professionals working with children and young people is turning this commitment into improvements in the everyday experience of those children and young people accessing services. This book is a valuable contribution.

The themes in the book take us back to the fundamental point that children's needs are distinct and this must be recognized in practice. As Charles Lamb said, 'A child's nature is too serious a thing to admit of its being regarded as a mere appendage of another being'.* If we are to fully recognize Article 24 of the UNCRC, which recognizes the right to enjoy the highest attainable standard of health, children must be at the heart of healthcare planning and delivery, with all considerations and decisions ultimately focused on the child.

Of course, the articles of the UNCRC are indivisible so as well as the central issue of the best interest of the child being at the core of what nurses do, we must also consider the voice of the child in all discussions. A successful model of provision of health services will have voice and choice within the rights-based framework.

Edited by two highly experienced children's nurses who have worked in higher education for a number of years, this book includes submissions from nurse practitioners, researchers and academics, covering issues most pertinent to children's lives today. Chapters on safeguarding, child and adolescent mental health, participation and school nursing, among others, are interspersed with case studies from visionary practitioners. This edition is enhanced by new chapters on neonatal nursing, recognizing and supporting siblings' needs and involving children and young people in research to inform service delivery at home and in hospital.

Children's and young people's nurses have challenging, stimulating and rewarding careers. They play a vital role not only in providing direct care but also in promoting physical health and well-being. This should be on the must-read list of not just undergraduate and postgraduate nursing students but all practitioners who work with children and young people.

Sally Holland
Children's Commissioner for Wales

---

* Charles Lamb (1775–1834): A bachelor's complaint of the behaviour of married people. In E.V. Lucas (ed.) (1912) *Elia and the last essays of Elia,* Chapter 25. Methuen: London. Available at https://ebooks.adelaide.edu.au/l/lamb/charles/elia/book1.25.html.

Preface

In the second edition of this book we have remained true to the spirit of the first by asking contributors from the world of practice and academe to provide chapters based on a rights-based approach to care. We have also remained true to our ideal that 'children and young people are a distinct group of patients and clients with their own particular needs who are entitled to expertly crafted care' (2011, p. xi). Over the last century children and young people's (CYP) nursing has developed its own body of knowledge which enables it to deliver safe, effective and evidence-based care to CYP and their families. There is concern, at the time of writing, that this is under threat following reviews by the Nursing and Midwifery Council and Lord Willis (Shape of Caring Review).* These policy drivers will lead inevitably toward a radical reshaping of the CYP pre-registration undergraduate programme, and it remains to be seen whether this will have an adverse effect on future care delivery within CYP nursing. In the meantime we hope this book will serve to promote and publicize the care CYP nurses presently provide as well as the positive difference they make to CYP and their families.

Throughout this book we explore how CYP rights may be respected and implemented in actual practice across a range of settings. We are mindful of the challenges children and young people face worldwide including war, famine and political unrest, while closer to home austerity measures and inequalities threaten to undermine their right to a healthy, happy and fulfilling life, to be valued, to have their voice heard and have the freedom to make choices. We hope to show that it is possible to achieve all of these ideals if CYP nurses underpin their practice with a rights-based approach to care. Our aim is to give an overview of the roles CYP nurses are presently engaged in and to highlight how complex this can be, involving as it does an in-depth knowledge and understanding of an age range spanning 0–24 years which encompasses very different physical, psychological and emotional stages of development.

This edition is in four parts. In Part 1 the context of CYP nursing is explored. This section examines challenging issues which arise in the delivery of nursing care and analyzes how these may be addressed. In Chapter 1, Jill John and Richard Griffith analyze what is meant by children's rights, and they examine how children can participate in their own healthcare and the challenges this can pose in practice. These are portrayed through the use of case studies which are thought provoking and clearly illustrate practice issues for CYP nurses. The authors critically discuss why and how the CYP nurse must practice inclusive child-centred care and act as an advocate to ensure that children's rights are protected and promoted. CYP rights are central to Catherine Powell's chapter on safeguarding and child protection where she explores the CYP nurse's roles and responsibilities. The difficult topic of child death is addressed and serious case reviews are explored, with messages from the Laming Inquiry and the death of Victoria Climbie being used to provide salient lessons as to why CYP nurses must be proactive in ensuring children are protected. Catherine's chapter is a powerful one and highlights why CYP nurses must have a sound knowledge base as well as a clear understanding of safeguarding and child protection issues in their daily practice.

In Chapter 3, Sally Hore presents real-life cases that show disturbing evidence of how the restraint of CYP in the UK and the US has led to a number of deaths in hospitals, remand centres and care settings. Using examples from practice Sally sets out the CYP nurses' role and responsibilities in restraint, and her guidance has the potential to improve current practice and save lives. Her call for clear national policy and guidelines as well as educational and training programmes is more than warranted. It is clear that far more needs to be done to ensure safe restraint, and Sally rightly questions whether current practice complies with the UN Convention on the Rights of the Child.

In Part 2 it is shown why family-centred care (FCC) must be inclusive of all members of the child's family and not focus solely on the parents. Sue Higham's critique of this concept in Chapter 4 shows why CYP nurses must be 'critical thinkers' and question research findings as well as current practice and in particular their own attitudes toward family members. Utilizing research and recent international trends in family policy as well as family dynamics, Sue reminds us that families come in all shapes and sizes and that we need to

---

* Health Education England (2015) (Chair: Lord Willis) *Raising the bar: Shape of Caring Review: A review of the future education and training of Registered Nurses and Care Assistants*. HEE: London.

respect these differences. The need to engage with and value the contribution fathers make, whether to their child with chronic illness or while their child is hospitalized, is salutary. Likewise, the need for CYP nurses to engage with grandparents reminds us that they too are important family members. The message of this chapter is clear: rather than focusing purely on mothers, CYP nurses need to shift their focus to the whole family which includes fathers, grandparents and others.

Chapter 5 which was specifically commissioned for this second edition addresses the needs of siblings, underlining the need to be inclusive and consider the family as a whole. Maria O'Shea, Mary Hughes, Eileen Savage and Clare O'Brien discuss the needs of siblings who have a brother or sister with long-term health needs through illness or disability. The authors discuss the psychosocial needs of siblings and the imperative to include siblings in family-centred care and to give them the information they need. This involves CYP nurses recognizing the special relationship between siblings, which is significantly challenged by ill health, disability and bereavement, in order to support their emotional and psychological needs at a challenging time for the children and the family. In Chapter 6 Pat Colliety and Vasso Vydelingum explore the need for a culturally sensitive approach to care. Using a rights-based approach they discuss and analyze the challenges and issues affecting CYP from ethnic minorities in the community, at school or in healthcare settings. They explore the use of the terms *culture, race* and *ethnicity*. The implications for practice are discussed while engaging nurses to challenge possible assumptions which may limit the scope of the care delivered through pertinent and thought-provoking case studies.

Part 3 examines care delivery across a range of settings, again illustrating the right of the child and young person to access and receive child-centred services and family-centred care. In Chapter 7 Elisabeth Podsiadly provides a powerful analysis of neonatal nursing. A historical overview is provided, followed by a discussion of prematurity as a global issue and the role of the millennium development goals in the drive toward reducing mortality rates. Neonatal provision in the UK and non-UK countries is examined as well as the educational issues and ethical dilemmas which arise. The key message is that neonatal nursing faces many challenges through service reorganization, the imperative to deliver high-quality FCC, the drive for high-quality education and the need to ensure a consistent approach to qualified in speciality along with a clearly defined career pathway. These important issues must be considered to ensure the delivery of high-quality care for the child and family.

Cathy Taylor and Susan Jones in Chapter 8 give a fascinating overview of the history and development of school nursing and health visiting and identify how both services work together to provide an integrated service for CYP, their families and local communities. They show how this approach can support the child from infancy to early adulthood and ensure optimum health outcomes. Case studies also show how health visitors and school nurses support families and can adapt their working practices to suit local needs. School nursing and health visiting are both presented as another interesting and rewarding career choice open to CYP graduates.

In Chapter 9 Ruth Davies and Marie Bodycombe-James call upon the Children's Community Nurse (CCN) service to be expanded across the UK to reduce the number of children being hospitalized. Tracing the development of this service shows that care at home was normal practice until well into the twentieth century and that the hospitalization of children is a relatively new development. Drawing on her own research with children with conditions such as leukaemia, asthma and diabetes, Marie is able to identify, using their stories, how the CCN supports them and their families, reduces the need for hospitalization and helps them gain a sense of autonomy and independence to self-manage their condition. The case for increasing CCN provision is made on costs and humanitarian grounds, but readers should note that substantial savings could be made to the present cash-strapped National Health Service by increasing present provision which remains well below what constitutes a safe, comprehensive and sustainable service.

Julia Terry and Alyson Davies in Chapter 10 clearly justify their belief that CYP nurses play an important role in supporting CYP with mental health needs, and readers will find their discussion on present mental health policy most helpful. CYP nurses come into daily contact with those who have emotional and behavioural problems as well as panic attacks, agoraphobia and depression, and the case studies based on actual practice are illuminating. The case for CYP nurses developing therapeutic relationships and communicating with patients/clients as well as working with other healthcare professionals and services to provide maximum support and help is made throughout the chapter and should have a positive effect on practice.

Building on the information given in Chapter 10, Alyson Davies and Julia Terry in Chapter 11 discuss a number of complex mental health conditions including suicide, substance abuse, self-harm, anorexia nervosa, autistic spectrum disorder and attention deficit hyperactivity disorder (ADHD). Each of these conditions is discussed in some depth and with due reference to recent international research findings and statistics. CYP nurses are likely to engage with children and young people affected by these disorders in their daily practice, and the case once again is made for CYP nurses to engage in a therapeutic relationship with the affected child and young person and to work closely with other health professionals to give maximum support to the individual patient/client and their family.

In Chapter 12 Katrina McNamara-Goodger identifies that transition from paediatric to adult service within the UK remains problematic for many young people with life-limiting and life-threatening conditions because of the failure to provide an integrated health and social services system of care delivery. Nevertheless, successful transition is possible and Katrina is able to show through the use of the frameworks and case studies how this may be achieved. The chapter is testimony to how careful planning and interdisciplinary working can result in a person-centred approach to care which respects the young person's right to be valued, have their voice heard and make their own choices during transition, and at their end of life care stage too.

Part 4 focuses on the continuing professional development which all CYP nurses must undergo in order to ensure their knowledge remains current and their practice evidence based.

In Chapter 13 the continuing evolution of advanced practice is examined and analyzed. The debates and issues which arise when discussing the role of the Advanced Nurse Practitioner (ANP) generally and also specifically in relation to CYP nursing are explored. There is a tension between those who believe that a generalist approach and preparation is suitable and those who believe that CYP should be cared for by ANPs who are suitably qualified children's nurses, a position now supported by the Royal College of Nursing in their latest guidance. It is shown how these tensions and controversies engender a healthy debate which can only contribute to clarification of the roles and responsibilities as well as the development of ANP in CYP practice.

Joan Livesley and Angela Lee, in a specially commissioned Chapter 14, set out a clear and convincing argument about why service design and delivery should be informed by CYP themselves. They identify that until fairly recently services have been based on adults' and adult professionals' understandings and beliefs about what CYP need rather than consulting with them directly. Many would-be researchers are understandably concerned about the ethical and legal issue of doing research with CYP and should be reassured by the information and advice given in relation to this as well as guidance on some of practicalities of research. Joan and Angela give many examples of exemplary research with CYP and refer to a range of research studies which involve CYP of all ages and from different social and ethnic backgrounds. After reading this chapter it is probable that readers will not only champion more research with CYP but question those who design and implement service without consulting them.

In the final chapter Alyson Davies and Gary Rolfe show how the use of a portfolio will enable the individual CYP nurse to explore their own knowledge and skills base as well as identify their specific knowledge, competencies and skills in relation to children and young people's nursing. The role of the portfolio in the new revalidation process is discussed along with an analysis of maintaining one in practice. We believe CYP nurses are entitled to a career pathway and should be able to think strategically about their own career progression.

While all the chapters relate in some way to a number of career options we believe CYP graduates may find Chapters 8, 9 and 13–15 particularly helpful if they are considering a future career as a school nurse, health visitor, community children's nurse, advanced nurse practitioner or CYP nurse/researcher.

Following in the tradition of our first edition we once again ask readers to critically analyze and debate the core principles and values set out in this book. Finally, while this book shows that CYP nurses are moving forward by taking on new roles and building upon their own research base, we hope that above all else it shows their continuing commitment to a rights-based approach to care, a commitment which follows directly in the footsteps of Eglantyne Jebb, who drafted the first charter on children's rights:

I believe, we should claim certain rights for children and labour for their universal recognition.*

---

* Jebb E. (1923) Available at, http://www.savethechildren.org.uk/about-us/history.

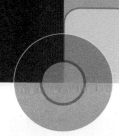

Acknowledgements

Alyson and Ruth would like to gratefully thank:

All the contributors to this book who have given of their time, experience, knowledge and who have written in order to share their knowledge and expertise.

Sally Holland, Children's Commissioner for Wales, for her kindness in taking the time to write an excellent foreword.

The All Wales Community Children's Nurse Forum for their help, kindness and expertise in providing practice exemplars.

Christopher Griffiths, Consultant Nurse Learning Disabilities/Lecturer, Abertawe Bro Morgannwg University Health Board, for his kindness, expertise and help in providing practice exemplars.

Paula Phillips, Community Nurse, Learning Disabilities, Abertawe Bro Morgannwg University Health Board, for her kindness, expertise and help in providing practice exemplars.

Jacquie Taylor, APNP, Kirkcaldy, Scotland, for her kindness, help and expertise in providing practice exemplars.

Mervyn Townley, Consultant Nurse Specialist CAMHS (retired), Aneurin Bevan Health Board, Gwent, for his kindness, expertise and help in providing practice exemplars.

Our families who have shared in and supported us in the process of writing and compiling the book.

Our academic colleagues at the College of Human and Health Sciences, Swansea University, for their support during the writing of this book.

Our colleagues at Taylor & Francis for their patience and who have provided invaluable support and guidance throughout this process.

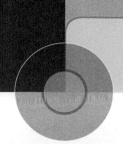

Contributors

Dave Barton PhD, MPhil, BEd, DipN, RGN, RNT
Associate Professor of Nursing (retired)
College of Human and Health Sciences
Swansea University
Swansea, UK

Marie Bodycombe-James RN, RHV, RSCN, DN Cert, PG CertEd, BA, MSc Nursing, Doctorate in Nursing Science
Senior Lecturer, Department of Public Health, Policy and Social
    Sciences, College of Human and Health Sciences
Swansea University
Swansea, UK

Pat Colliety PhD, MA, BSc, PG CEA, RN (Child), RN (Adult), SCPHN
Professional Qualification Lead, School of Health Sciences
Faculty of Health and Medical Sciences
University of Surrey
Surrey, UK

Alyson Davies RGN, RSCN, BSc, MN, PG CertEd
Senior Lecturer in Children and Young People's Nursing
Department of Nursing, College of Human and Health Sciences
Swansea University
Swansea, UK

Ruth Davies RGN, RSCN, RHV, MA, PhD, PG CertEd
Associate Professor and Director of Doctorate in Professional Practice
Department of Nursing, College of Human and Health Sciences
Swansea University
Swansea, UK

Richard Griffith LLM, BN, DipN, PG DLaw, RMN, RNT, CertEd
Senior Lecturer in Health Law, College of Human and
    Health Sciences
Swansea University
Swansea, UK

Sue Higham RSCN, RGN, DPSN, BSc, PG CEA, MA
Lecturer in Children's Nursing
The Open University
Milton Keynes, UK

Sally Holland
Children's Commissioner for Wales
Swansea, UK

Sally Hore BN, MSc Nursing, RN (Child), PG Cert tHE
Senior Lecturer, Children and Young People's Nursing, Department
    of Nursing, College of Human and Health Sciences
Swansea University
Swansea, UK

Mary Hughes PhD, MSc Advanced Practice, BSc, H Dip (Children's Nursing), PG DipT&L, RCN, RGN
Lecturer in Children's Nursing, School of Nursing
Midwifery and Health Systems
University College Dublin
Dublin, Ireland

Jill John BSc, MA, RGN, RSCN, Specialist Community Nurse, PG Cert tHE
Senior Lecturer in Children and Young People's Nursing
Department of Nursing, College of Human and Health Sciences
Swansea University
Swansea, UK

Susan Jones MBE, BSc (Hons), SCPHN (SN), RN
Lead Nurse, School Health Nursing Service
Abertawe Bro Morgannwg University Health Board
Port Talbot, UK

Angela Lee MSc, BSc, PGCE, ENB 415 (Paediatric Intensive Care), RSCN, RGN
Education Development Practitioner, Paediatric Critical Care
Royal Manchester Children's Hospital
Manchester, UK

Joan Livesley PhD, DipN (Lond), BSc, MA, RSCN, RN, RNT
Senior Lecturer, University of Salford (Postgraduate Directorate)
CYP@Salford Research Group
Salford, UK

Katrina McNamara-Goodger RN (General), RN (Child), RHV
Director of Practice and Service Development
Together for Short Lives
Bristol, UK

Clare O'Brien MSc, BNS (Hons), RSCN, H DipSCN, RGN
Lecturer Practitioner, Integrated Children's and General
    Nursing Programme, McAuley School of Nursing and
    Midwifery
University College Cork
Cork, Ireland

Maria O'Shea MSc Advanced Nursing Practice, PG Dip Teaching and Learning, BSc (Hons) Nursing Studies, RCN, RGN, RNT
Lecturer, Integrated Children's and General Nursing Programme
McAuley School of Nursing and Midwifery
University College Cork
Cork, Ireland

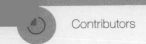

Elisabeth Podsiadly RGN, MSc, BSc Nursing, PGCEA, Advanced Certificate in Perinatal Nursing
Senior Lecturer in Neonatal Nursing, Faculty of Health
Social Care and Education
Kingston University and St. George's University of London
London, UK

Catherine Powell PhD, BNSc (Hons), RGN, RSCN, RHV
Safeguarding Children Consultant and Visiting Academic
University of Southampton
Southampton, UK

Gary Rolfe RMN, BSc, MA, PhD
Emeritus Professor
Swansea University
Swansea, UK

Eileen Savage PhD, Med BNS, RGN, RCN, RM
Professor Chair in Nursing and Head of School
Catherine McAuley School of Nursing and Midwifery
Brookfield Health Sciences Complex
University College Cork
Cork, Ireland

Cathy Taylor RGN, DipN, BSc (Hons) Specialist Community Public Health Nursing (SCPHN) Health Visiting, MSc Nursing, HEA Fellow
Senior Lecturer, Programme Manager of BSc (Hons) Specialist
Community Public Health Nursing (SCPHN), Department of
Public Health, Policy and Social Sciences
Swansea University
Swansea, UK

Julia Terry MSc, BSc (Hons), DipHE, PG CE, SFHEA, RMN
Senior Lecturer, Mental Health Nursing, Department of Nursing
College of Human and Health Sciences
Swansea University
Swansea, UK

Vasso Vydelingum PhD, BSc (Hons), PG DipEd, RN, RHV, DN
Associate Senior Lecturer, School of Health Sciences
Faculty of Health and Medical Sciences
University of Surrey
Surrey, UK

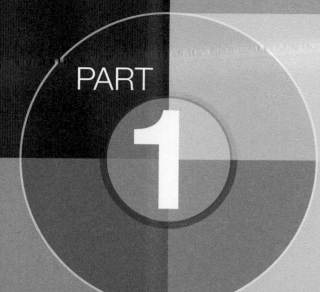

CHILDREN AND YOUNG PEOPLE'S HEALTHCARE IN CONTEXT
A Rights-Based Approach

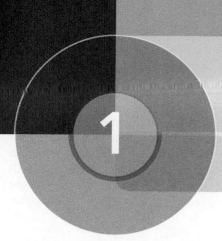

The right for children and young people to participate in their own healthcare

JILL JOHN AND RICHARD GRIFFITH

OVERVIEW

This chapter examines the evidence for children and young people's right to participate in their own healthcare. It begins with a historical overview of children's rights and legislation and then examines the evidence by exploring the following questions:

- How far have we come?
- Where are we now?
- What more can we do?

Case law examples and evidence-based research are examined and examples of frameworks and excellent practice from healthcare and associated allied professions are provided.

INTRODUCTION

There is a growing acceptance in the UK and elsewhere that children and young people should participate more in making decisions about issues that affect them. Increased children and young people's participation has been fuelled by a convergence of new and developing ideas from quite different perspectives, such as the growing children's rights agenda and the new sociology of childhood.

The key benchmark for children's rights is the 1989 United Nations Convention on the Rights of the Child (UNCRC) that the UK ratified in 1991. It is the most extensively ratified human rights treaty in history and was the culmination of six decades of work with Somalia and North America, the only UN member countries to opt out of the charter. The UNCRC provides a framework for the development of national policies and laws to protect the rights of children and young people throughout the world, and is considered by many as being instrumental in the development of more child-friendly policies in Britain (O'Halloran 1999). The main weakness of the convention, however, is that there is no direct method of formal enforcement, and governments are merely directed to undertake all appropriate methods available to them to implement the rights. Member states had to report back to the UN initially 2 years after their ratification and implementation and then every subsequent 5 years, although occasionally the response from the UN committee exceeds this timescale.

Until recently, it has been difficult to reconcile differences between historically held beliefs about children and young people's inability to make decisions and findings from research that contradict these assumptions (Alderson 2007). Children and young people's participation in healthcare decisions is heavily influenced by such assumptions, in particular an identified need for adult guidance and the need to reduce attempts to reason or listen to their views (Flatman 2002; Alderson 2007). The notion of working with children, young people and families in the involvement of their care (physical and otherwise), including the decision-making process, would have been seen as totally inappropriate as little as 30 years ago, when parents and other family members were seen as amateurs who frequently got in the way of professionals trying to do their job (Darbyshire 1994). Indeed the first UK report to the UN committee appeared to reflect a protectionist ideology supporting the view that young children are unable to make decisions themselves, with the emphasis being on parents as the consumers of healthcare which could be argued both marginalizes and objectifies children and young people (Fulton 1996).

HISTORICAL OVERVIEW OF CHILDHOOD AND CHILDREN'S RIGHTS

Until the nineteenth century and the increase of industrialization it could be argued that the notion of childhood was largely an invention (Boyden 1991, cited in James et al. 1999). Rates of fertility and mortality were high owing to the spread of deadly and untreatable infectious disease, including typhoid and cholera. Families therefore had many children because a high percentage of children died under the age of 1 and many more did not live beyond 5 years. It is difficult for historians and others to calculate infant mortality rates as births were not registered until 1837; however, church records before this time showed that funerals always exceeded baptisms. Aries (1962) identified that medieval European children were not segregated from adults and therefore were not thought to require any special needs and frequently were dressed in adult clothing. Aries (1962, p. 48), continuing in his studies, eventually described childhood as 'a nightmare from which we have only recently begun to awaken'. Indeed the further back in history one goes, the more evidence there is of a lower level of child care, including an increased likelihood of children not only being killed but also abandoned, beaten, terrorized and sexually abused by those who were supposed to care for them (deMause 1974, cited in Mayall 1994).

The status of children and childhood as it evolved was marked by the absence of practically all civil rights, with no philosophical or legal recognition to self-determination; this rendered children virtually powerless, having little or no control over their own lives, which many consider a marked characteristic of slavery (Verhellen 1996). For example, early Roman law allowed a father to literally have the power of life or death over a child and this power was frequently upheld. The overwhelming power a father had in law was gradually removed during the nineteenth century by Talfourd's Act, the Custody of Infants Act 1839 and the Matrimonial Causes Act 1857. Yet, children were still seen to be in the custody of their parents, who retained considerable power over them. For example, parents could demand that a child in care be handed back when he or she was old enough to earn a wage (*Barnardo v McHugh* [1891]).

However, the twentieth century brought changes in family life associated with both industrial and urban expansion; childhood was gradually seen as a separate period of human life and children became central figures within the family (Boyden 1991, cited in James et al. 1999). Hygiene and public health were a defining feature of 'modern childhood', alongside the development of compulsory education. Impressive improvements were made in both the UK and other developed countries in the areas of health and physical development of children owing to higher standards of living and advances in sanitation and nutrition. Because of this, children have been attributed with certain qualities or disabilities and interest in them has grown considerably. However, socioeconomic inequalities in health still exist in developed societies today, including the UK, and sadly some of these have changed little in recent years. Public Health Wales (2012) indicates a clear link between poor social and economic circumstances and the health and well-being that may be lifelong.

KEY POINT

It has taken centuries to recognize children as important beings in their own right.

REFLECTION POINT

Why do you think that it has taken centuries to recognize children as important beings in their own right? Take a few moments to think of two reasons why children held little importance within the family before the twentieth century.

HOW FAR HAVE WE COME?

Some consider that current-day perception of childhood has changed little and is essentially a preparation for 'adulthood', with a particular onus on guiding, educating, developing and sustaining the physical and moral well-being of children and young people through social institutions that include the family, school, health and welfare agencies. All too frequently, however, these agencies speak for children and young people on the basis that they are incapable of thinking 'like adults' until a certain developmental age is reached (Alderson 2007).

This view of regarding children and young people as 'future adults' instead of 'current or present persons' leads to the knowledge and beliefs of children and young people being either disregarded as irrelevant or totally ignored as a means of understanding their actions, concerns and needs (James and Prout 1990; Mayall 1996). There is an unquestionably growing counterview to this among both academics and professionals, in that children and young people are social actors in themselves and not just subjects of social processes and structures (James and Prout 1990). The emerging sociology of childhood indicates the importance of children and young people actively constructing their own lives by, for example, participating in and negotiating their own healthcare, education and social welfare by utilizing skills that often go unrecognized (Mayall 2002). However, the approaches adopted for children's rights and adults' beliefs regarding this concept in the UK undoubtedly have their origins in the evolution of the child and childhood with an indication that this history continues to influence current attitudes toward children and young people in society and contemporary healthcare practice (Lowden 2002).

Overall, the 54 articles in the convention can be broadly divided into three types of rights:

1. Provision
2. Protection
3. Participation

With participation regarded as the younger sibling of provision and protection it has been identified by the UN Committee on the Rights of the Child as a central underlying principle which must be considered in respect of all other rights; however, it is also one of the provisions sadly most widely violated and disregarded in every sphere of children's lives (Shier 2001).

PROVISION

Article 24 of the UN convention indicates that children and young people have the right to

[the] highest attainable standard of health and to the facilities for the treatment of illness and rehabilitation of health.

The first named concern in the article is

... to diminish infant and child mortality.

Children and young people's right to good healthcare is enshrined in various UK policy, law and public documents, including, most importantly, the UNCRC and the 1989 and 2004 Children Acts. Alderson (2002) indicates that Article 24 of the convention balances local with global attainment and indicates how inspirational some children's rights are. She argues that children and young people's right to be healthy is often unrealistic and unattainable, although the convention clearly indicates the right to every type of healthcare available to them within their own culture. This is unquestionably variable and inequitable even in the UK where we have free health care at the point of delivery let alone worldwide in countries that have no identified healthcare systems.

AREA OF CONCERN IN THE UK

Inequalities in health in the UK have been identified for more than 30 years in both research and policy. They are linked to social exclusion and poverty, which can include unemployment, homelessness and family breakdown, all significant factors for poor health and premature death. Infant mortality figures (deaths per 1000 infants under 1 year), which are an acknowledged robust indicator of public health, are also a major statistic for comparing child health from one nation with that of another. In most parts of the UK, the figures are falling and are roughly half of what they were in the 1950s; however, despite this, there are currently 4.2 deaths per 1000 infants (Office of National Statistics 2012) which is higher than almost all northern European countries, particularly Scandinavia, although considerably better than 11/1000 in 1981. One identified reason for the difference is the continuing amount of children and families living in poverty which has remained around 30% for the last 30 years (Department of Health 2007); with Wales 1% higher than the UK it remains the highest of the UK countries (Welsh Government 2011a) and more than half of families living in poverty are in households where at least one person works. However, the Royal College of Paediatrics and Child Health (2012) has identified that significant progress has been made in improving the health and well-being of children and young people over the last 5 years.

Some children and young people, however, still fail to receive the highest standards of healthcare attainable – a right of all children as set out in Article 24 of the UNCRC.

PROTECTION

Article 19 clearly identifies the need for

> legislative, administrative, social and educational actions to protect children from all types of violence including neglect and abuse.

Theorists of child development, in particular John Bowlby's work in the 1950s, identified that a lack of attachment in early life to main carers could lead to poor parenting in the next generation (Gross 2015). His work attracted and influenced the medical professions' interest in child abuse, with Kempe's (1962) writings on the 'battered child' syndrome more than 40 years ago opening a long and continuous debate on the subject. The decades since have seen a gradual increase in knowledge and expertise in child abuse as well as, of course, in both the public's and government's increasing concern. Vastly improved changes by protection in law came eventually in the form of the 1989 Children Act after a period of considerable debate, activity and consultation with a range of groups, except children and young people. It brought together for the first time both public and private law and sought to establish a new basis for intervention in family life in cases of child abuse, with one of the key principles underpinning the legislation being that the 'child's welfare should be paramount'. It opens with a 'Welfare Check List' (Section 1.1) and in Part 3 defines the 'child in need' which automatically includes children with disabilities (physically and mentally) as well as those likely to suffer or suffered from significant harm. It also clearly indicates the need to take the ascertainable wishes and feelings of children and young people into account as well as their physical and emotional needs.

AREA OF CONCERN IN THE UK

The UK is repeatedly criticized by the UN Inspection Committee for not legislating against the hitting of children and young people by their parents/guardians, and worryingly is the only country that was a member of the EU prior to 1997 not to do so. The judgment in *A v United Kingdom* [1998] contained a promise from the UK government to change its legislation as the defence of reasonable chastisement was unclear and allowed the severe beating of a child in UK law. However, the government has consistently refused to completely prohibit parental use of physical punishment as the government sees it as an unwarranted intrusion in family life.

In 2014–2015 the National Assembly of Wales formulated the Violence against Women, Domestic Abuse and Sexual Violence Bill (Wales) (National Assembly for Wales 2015b). A Welsh assembly member, Julie Morgan, proposed an amendment to the bill to remove the defence of 'reasonable punishment' (National Assembly for Wales 2015a). If accepted and passed this would have made it illegal for parents in Wales to smack their children. The Welsh Labour Government opposed the measure and ruled out any change (BBC 2015). The bill was passed into law without the amendment. Thus a prime opportunity to protect children and their rights was lost.

PARTICIPATION

The principle of the child's right to participate in decision making is indicated in Article 12 of the convention in that the child who is capable of forming his or her own views has the right to

> express those views freely in all matters affecting the child, the views of the child being given due weight in accordance with the age and maturity of the child.

This has been identified by the Committee on the Rights of the Child as a central underlying principle which must be considered with regard to all other rights (Lansdown 2001).

PRINCIPLE FOR PRACTICE

Participation is the keystone of the arch which is the UNCRC. Without the active participation of children and young people in the promotion of their rights to a good childhood, none will be achieved effectively (Badham 2002, cited in Willow 2002).

Acceptance of this principle appears to be evident with the UK through an increase in participation in activities involving children and young people at both the local and government level.

Why is participation so important?

This has been expressed in several ways, often grouped into legal, political or social reasons (Children and Young People's Unit 2001; Willow 2002; see Box 1.1).

For many, a child's or young person's participation is a value or rights-based principle much like democracy and is not something that has to be justified by either evidence or proof that it works (Sinclair 2004). This should not diminish, however, the need to monitor or evaluate to ensure the widest representation of children and young people in a variety of settings and circumstances.

LEGAL RIGHTS

The United Nations (1989) Convention on the Rights of the Child is a universally agreed set of standards that set minimum entitlements and freedoms that should be respected by governments. It is founded on respect for the dignity and worth of each child, regardless of race, colour, gender, language, religion, opinions, origins, wealth, birth status or ability up to the age of 18 years.

Although the UK ratified the convention some 20 years ago, its 54 articles do not have a direct effect on domestic law and children and young people cannot take action in court against them. The convention's articles act only as a yardstick against which the government's treatment of children and young people is audited on a 5-yearly basis by the UN.

Unless incorporated into UK domestic law, the rights set out in the convention do not have the weight of law, they are not legal rights and children and young people cannot rely on them to insist that they be allowed to participate in their healthcare. However, Wales has become the first country to give the UNCRC a legal base within the legislation of the Rights of Children and Young Persons (Wales) Measure 2011 (WG 2011b). This confers normative legal status on the convention in Wales which it does not have elsewhere in the UK (Croke and Williams 2015).

A legal right is defined as an interest recognized and protected by law (Kennedy and Grubb 2002). All other rights, argues Bentham, are 'merely nonsense upon stilts', as once these worthy values are held up to scrutiny by the law they are quickly found to have no legal remedy attached to them (Tait 1883).

BOX 1.1: Rationale for children's participation in decision making

- To uphold children and young people's rights
- To fulfil legal responsibilities (UNCRC; Children Act 1989)
- To improve services
- To improve decision making
- To enhance democratic processes
- To promote children and young people's protection
- To enhance children and young people's skills
- To empower and enhance self-esteem

Source: Sinclair, R., Franklin, A., *Young People's Participation*, Department of Health, London, 2000.

In the UK, legal rights are bestowed on people by placing obligations, called legal duties, on others. Under the Human Rights Act 1998 the state has a legal duty to ensure that it has laws and policies in place to ensure, for example, that one person does not violate the human rights of another.

LEGAL RIGHT TO PARTICIPATE IN HEALTHCARE

CONSENT

Consent to examination and treatment is an area of law that relies on a child/young person's ability to decide rather than an arbitrary age limit. It is an essential element of the lawfulness of treatment and upholds the ethical principle of autonomy or self-determination by allowing a person to decide whether to have an examination or treatment. For the nurse it provides a defence to criminal assault and the tort or civil wrong of trespass to the person (*F v West Berkshire HA* [1990]).

NATURE OF CONSENT

Consent is a state of mind in which a person agrees to the touching of his or her body as part of an examination or treatment (*Sidaway v Bethlem Royal Hospital* [1985]). It has both a clinical and legal purpose:
- The clinical purpose recognizes that the success of treatment depends very often on the cooperation of the child/young person.
- The legal purpose is to underpin the propriety of the treatment and furnish a defence to the crime and tort of trespass.

For capable adults the law is clearer and recognizes the right to self-determination that includes the right to consent to or refuse medical treatment even if this would lead to their death.

Children reach the age of majority or adulthood at 18; however, until that time although the courts acknowledge that no child under 18 is wholly autonomous, they do recognize the right of children/young people to decide whether they wish to participate in their healthcare by allowing them to consent to examination and treatment as they develop and mature with age.

CONSENT AND CHILDREN

Kennedy and Grubb (2000) argue that children pass through three developmental stages on their journey to becoming a fully autonomous adult:

- The child of tender years
- The Gillick-competent child
- Children aged 16–17 years

Consent to treatment for a child of tender years is provided by a person with parental responsibility for the child, usually a parent. However, the decision of the parent must be in the best interests of the welfare of the child and can be overridden by a court exercising its inherent jurisdiction to act in the child's best interests.

CHILDREN OF TENDER YEARS AND PARENTAL RESPONSIBILITY

The concept of parental responsibility replaced the notion of parental rights.

Parental responsibility is defined as all the rights, duties, powers, responsibilities and authority which by law a parent of a child has in relation to the child and its property (Children Act 1989, Section 2). These are not defined or specified in the act. In essence it empowers a person to make most decisions in a child's life including consenting to medical treatment on the child's behalf. A child of tender years must rely on a person with parental responsibility to make decisions about his or her healthcare (Box 1.2).

DELEGATION OF PARENTAL RESPONSIBILITY

The Children Act 1989, Section 2(9) (Office of Public Sector Information 1989) allows a person with parental responsibility to arrange for someone else to exercise it on their behalf. This delegation need not be in writing and allows carers such as schools, nannies and child minders to make delegated decisions on behalf of a person with parental responsibility for the child or young person.

BOX 1.2: Who has parental responsibility for a child?

PARENTAL RESPONSIBILITY

- Parental responsibility is defined as the rights, duties, powers, and responsibility and authority, which by law a parent has in relation to a child (Children Act 1989, Section 3; Office of Public Sector Information 1989).
- Mother
    - Mother has automatic parental responsibility upon the birth of the child (Children Act 1989, Sections 2(1) and (2); Office of Public Sector Information 1989).
- Father
    - Father has parental responsibility if he was married to the child's mother at the time of the birth (Children Act 1989, Section 2(1)) or
    - If he subsequently married the mother of his child (Children Act 1989, Section 2(3); Family Law Reform Act 1987, Section 1; Office of Public Sector Information 1987) or
    - If he became registered as the father of the child after December 2003 (Children Act 1989, Section 4(1)(a)) or
    - He and the child's mother make a parental responsibility agreement (Children Act 1989, Section 4(1)(b)) that is made and recorded in the form prescribed by the lord chancellor or
    - The court on his application orders that he shall have parental responsibility (Children Act 1989, Section 4(1)(c)) or
    - He obtains a residence order (Children Act 1989, Section 12, read with Section 4) or
    - He is appointed as the child's guardian and the appointment takes effect (Children Act 1989, Section 5)
- Acquired parental responsibility can be removed only by a court.

OTHERS WHO CAN ACQUIRE PARENTAL RESPONSIBILITY

- A person in possession of a residence order which could include the father of the child (Children Act 1989, Section 12)
- A person appointed as the child's guardian; once the appointment takes effect this could include the father of the child (Children Act 1989, Section 5)
- A person, other than a police officer, who is in possession of an emergency protection order (Children Act 1989, Section 44(4)(c))
- A person who has adopted a child (Adoption Act 1976, Section 12; Adoption and Children Act 2002, Section 46; Office of Public Sector Information 1976, 2002)
- A step-parent with the agreement of the parent(s) with parental responsibility or by order of the court (Children Act 1989, Section 4A)

A LOCAL AUTHORITY MAY ADDITIONALLY ACQUIRE PARENTAL RESPONSIBILITY

- By obtaining a care order (Children Act 1989, Section 31)
- By obtaining a freeing for adoption order (Adoption Act 1976, Section 18) or a placement order (Adoption and Children Act 2002, Section 21; Office of Public Sector Information 2002)

For example, a nurse may visit a young child to find her in the care of her grandmother. As long as the nurse is satisfied that the grandmother is acting with the authority of a person with parental responsibility such as the child's mother she may accept the grandmother's consent as permission to treat the child.

CARERS

The Children Act 1989 (Office of Public Sector Information 1989) allows those who have care for a child/young person but not parental responsibility to do what is reasonable in all the circumstances to promote or safeguard the child's welfare (Children Act 1989, Section 3(5); Office of Public Sector Information 1989). In terms of medical treatment, what is reasonable would generally require the consent of a person with parental responsibility unless it was an emergency or the treatment was trivial. In a medical emergency situation, abandonment of the child or child protection cases, medical staff can proceed without the consent of the child or parent if it is deemed in the child's 'best interests', although others named as *de facto* carers, e.g. teachers, can assume all duties, powers and responsibilities of a parent if required under these circumstances.

EXTENT OF PARENTAL RESPONSIBILITY

Although the Children Act 1989 (Office of Public Sector Information 1989) does not describe the duties placed on parents, the courts have outlined what parental responsibility means in practice. Parents have a duty to care for their children. It is an offence under the Children and Young Persons Act 1933, Section 1 (Office of Public Sector Information 1933) to assault, ill-treat, neglect or abandon a child under the age of 16. It is one of the rare situations in law where the offence may be committed by omission as well as by action. That is, what a parent fails to do for his or her child is as relevant as what he or she does to the child if it results in neglect or ill treatment. This duty is not restricted to parents. Those who have responsibility for the care of a child are also bound by the same duty. It can be seen that parents are bound by a duty of care to their child and can be prosecuted if they fail to exercise that duty properly.

Although a person with parental responsibility can generally make decisions independently, the freedom of each to act alone is not unfettered.

CASE LAW EXAMPLE

The court held in *Re J* [2000] that there are a small group of important decisions made on behalf of a child that should not be carried out or arranged by one parent alone, although they have parental responsibility under the Children Act 1989. These include (*Re B (A Child)* [2003]):

- Sterilization of a child
- The change of a child's surname
- Circumcision of a child
- A hotly disputed immunization

BEST INTERESTS OF THE CHILD

The parent's right to make healthcare decisions about his or her child is not absolute. Parents' rights exist only for the benefit of the child and must be exercised in the child's best interests. The courts exercise a supervisory role over parental decision making and can overrule a decision that they consider as not being in the best interests of the welfare of the child (Children Act 1989, Section 1).

Under the private law provisions of the Children Act 1989, Section 8, the courts also have the power to settle disputes between two or more people with parental responsibility.

Private law is not a question of child protection and so the threshold criterion of significant harm does not have to be engaged for the court to have jurisdiction.

As long as there is a dispute between people regarding an issue of parental responsibility for a child the court can intervene to settle the issue.

The orders available to the court are:

- A residence order, which settles with whom a child should live and bestows parental responsibility on that person when necessary.
- A contact order, which settles contact arrangements with a child; contact can be as widely interpreted as the court sees fit and ranges from telephone and email contact to visits and holidays.
- A prohibited steps order, which prohibits an action without the permission of the court.
- A specific issues order, which allows the court to settle a specific issue in relation to the parental responsibility of a child.

Prohibited steps and specific issues orders are also used by the courts to settle issues concerning a child's healthcare.

PRINCIPLE FOR PRACTICE

Children and young people are not the property of their parents/carers. Parents/carers have a responsibility for them that continues until such time as the children/young people reach 18 years or are adopted.

In *J (A Minor) (Prohibited Steps Order: Circumcision)* [2000] the English mother of a 5-year-old boy was granted a prohibited steps order preventing his Muslim father from making arrangements to have him circumcised without a court order because ritual circumcision was an irreversible operation which was not medically necessary, had physical and psychological risks and in such cases the consent of both parents was essential.

Authorizing treatment against the wishes of a child's parents is reserved for the most serious cases. In *A&D v B&E* [2003] the High Court accepted that, in general, there is wide scope for parental objection to medical intervention. The court considers medical interventions as existing on a scale. At one end are obvious cases where parental objection would have no value in child welfare terms, e.g. urgent life-saving treatment such as a blood transfusion.

CASE LAW EXAMPLE

In *Camden LBC v R (A Minor) (Blood Transfusion)* [1993] a child's parents refused to allow him to have a blood transfusion for the treatment of B-cell lymphoblastic leukaemia owing to their religious beliefs. The court found that, where the life of a child was at risk and it was essential to act urgently, the private law requirements of the Children Act 1989, Section 8 could be used to seek a specific issue order. This procedure allows the matter to be brought before a High Court judge who could order the treatment without delay and without transferring parental responsibility.

At the other end of the scale are cases where there is genuine scope for debate and the views of the parents are important. These would not raise questions of neglect or abuse that would trigger child protection proceedings. Although a National Health Service (NHS) trust can obtain leave to apply for a specific issues order (Children Act 1989, Section 8), it is unlikely that leave would be granted in the face of unified parental opposition to this type of treatment.

In *Re B (A Child)* [2003] the Court of Appeal held that although it was prepared to settle a dispute between two parents on the issue of childhood immunizations, it would not do so when the dispute was between a parent and the health authorities.

BEST INTERESTS TEST

The test for determining the best interests of a child has developed over a period of time as new cases have been brought to court for judgment. In one of the earliest cases the court limited its consideration of best interest to the life expectancy of the child.

CASE LAW EXAMPLE

In *Re B (A Minor) (Wardship: Medical Treatment)* [1981] a child born with Down's syndrome needed urgent surgery for an intestinal blockage. The parents took the view that it would be kinder to let the child die than to allow her to grow up as a physically and mentally handicapped person. The judge held that the surgery was straightforward and that, as the child was expected to live 20–30 years, surgery was in her best interests.

Some 10 years later the court refined the determination of best interest to include pain and suffering. In *J (A Minor) (Child in Care: Medical Treatment)* [1993], a profoundly brain-damaged child with a very short life expectancy was not thought to be benefiting from treatment and both the parents and medical team sought an order allowing them to curtail treatment.

In the child's interest the official solicitor argued that an absolutist test applied that, in the case of a child, everything should be done to preserve the child's life right to the bitter end and a court was never justified in denying consent to treatment to save life.

The court held that the absolutist test never applied. The denial of treatment to prolong life could only be sanctioned when it was in the best interests of the patient and the test applicable was that of the child's best interests in those circumstances and that was based on an assessment of the child's quality of life and his or her future pain and suffering in relation to the life-saving treatment.

When those with parental responsibility strongly oppose the giving or withholding of treatment by a health professional to a child, the matter will need to be referred to the court for a decision unless it is an emergency (*Glass v United Kingdom* [2004]). Failing to seek the court's approval for a plan of care in these circumstances would be a breach of the child's right to respect for a private and family life under Article 8 of the European Convention on Human Rights (Council of Europe 1950).

AUTONOMY AND CHILDREN AND YOUNG PEOPLE

GILLICK-COMPETENT CHILD

The argument that a child/young person should have the right to make decisions about his or her healthcare becomes more compelling as the child matures toward adulthood. The matter of whether a child under 16 has the decision-making capacity to consent to examination and treatment was decided by the House of Lords in *Gillick v West Norfolk and Wisbech AHA* [1986]. In this case a mother objected to Department of Health advice that doctors could give contraceptive advice and treatment to children under 16 without parental consent. The court held that a child under 16 had the legal capacity to consent to examination and treatment if they had 'sufficient maturity and intelligence to understand the nature and implications of that treatment'.

TEST FOR GILLICK COMPETENCE

Nurses must apply the rule in *Gillick* when determining whether a child/young person under 16 has capacity to consent to examination and treatment.

When determining whether a child has sufficient maturity and intelligence to make a decision nurses will need to take account of

> the understanding and intelligence of the child/young person, their chronological, emotional and mental age, their intellectual development and their ability to reach a decision by appraising the advice about treatment in considering the nature, consequences and implications of that treatment.
>
> *Gillick v West Norfolk and Wisbech AHA [1986] per Lord Scarman*

The aim of the rule in *Gillick* is to reflect the transition of a child to adulthood. Legal capacity to make decisions is conditional on the child gradually acquiring the maturity and intelligence to be able to make treatment decisions. The degree of maturity and intelligence needed depends on the gravity of the decision. A relatively young child would have sufficient maturity and intelligence to be capable of consenting to a plaster on a small cut.

Equally, a child who had the capacity to consent to dental treatment or the repair of broken bones may lack capacity to consent to more serious treatment (*Re R (A Minor) (Wardship Consent to Treatment)* [1992]).

CASE LAW EXAMPLE

In *Re L (Medical Treatment: Gillick Competence)* [1998] a critically injured 14-year-old Jehovah's Witness had refused to consent to life-saving medical treatment because it would involve blood transfusions. The court found that, despite her maturity, L was still a child and her beliefs had been developed through her sheltered upbringing within the Jehovah's Witness community. She knew that she would die without treatment but had not been informed of the likely nature of her death. She was not Gillick competent and it was in her best interests for the treatment to be carried out.

Indeed, to date, the courts have never found a child under 16 who wished to refuse life-saving treatment to be Gillick competent. Decision-making capacity therefore does not simply arrive with puberty; it depends on the maturity and intelligence of the child and the seriousness of the treatment decision to be made.

For example, a nurse giving contraceptive advice and treatment to a child will realize that there is much to be understood by the child if he or she is to have capacity to consent. The nurse would need to be satisfied that not only was the advice understood but also the child had sufficient maturity to understand what was involved.

This would include:

- Moral and family questions such as the future relationship with parents
- Longer-term problems associated with the emotion of pregnancy or its termination
- The health risks associated with sexual intercourse at a young age

A nurse must be satisfied that a child/young person has fully understood the nature and consequences of treatment before he or she can accept their consent or refusal of treatment. It is for the nurse to decide whether or not a child is Gillick competent and able to consent to treatment. However, the power to decide must not be used as a license to disregard the wishes of parents whenever the nurse finds it convenient to do so. Those who behave in such a way would be failing to discharge their professional responsibilities and could expect to be disciplined by their professional body (*Gillick v West Norfolk and Wisbech AHA* [1986]).

KEY POINTS

- Assessing Gillick competence of children and young people is complex and not just chronologically age related.
- When a child or young person is considered Gillick competent, then the consent is as effective as that of an adult. This consent cannot be overruled by a parent.

FRASER GUIDELINES TO ASSESS COMPETENCY

Giving contraceptive advice and treatment to a child under 16 years gives rise to a concern that a practitioner may be accused of procuring sexual intercourse with a child under 16 years, a criminal offence under the Sexual Offences Act (Office of Public Sector Information 2003). To protect nurses from such accusations Lord Fraser in *Gillick* issued guidance to ensure that contraceptive advice and treatment was given only on clinical grounds. There might be exceptional cases when in the interests of the child's welfare a nurse might give contraceptive advice and treatment without the permission or even knowledge of the parents. You must be satisfied that:

- The girl understood the advice
- You could not persuade her to tell or allow you to tell her parents
- She was likely to have sexual intercourse with or without contraceptive treatment
- Unless she received such advice or treatment her physical or mental health was likely to suffer
- Her best interests required such advice or treatment without the knowledge or consent of her parents

It is essential that this guidance is followed in practice to avoid any possibility of criminal conduct.

The defence offered by Lord Fraser's guidance has been extended by the Sexual Offences Act 2003, Section 13 (Office for Public Sector Information 2003). This provides a defence against aiding, abetting or counselling a sexual offence if the purpose is to:

- Protect the child/young person from sexually transmitted infection
- Protect the physical safety of the child/young person
- Protect the child from becoming pregnant
- Promote the child/young person's emotional well-being by the giving of advice unless the purpose is to obtain sexual gratification or to cause or encourage the relevant sexual act

In *R (Axon) v Secretary of State for Health* [2006] the court held that there was no reason why the rule in *Gillick* should not apply to other proposed treatment and advice.

The approach of a health professional to a young person seeking advice and treatment on sexual issues without notifying his or her parents should be in accordance with Lord Fraser's guidelines. There was no infringement of the rights of a young person's parents if a health professional was permitted to withhold information relating to the advice or treatment of the young person on sexual matters.

LEGAL ISSUES IN RELATION TO PROTECTION AND SEXUAL ACTIVITY

It has long been public policy to protect children/young people from being subjected to sexual activity while they are in what is considered to be a vulnerable stage of their development.

The age of consent for all sexual activity was amended by the Sexual Offences Act 2003. Both boys and girls over 16 can now engage in heterosexual and homosexual activity with persons over 16. It is an offence to engage in sexual activity with a person under this age regardless of the age of the offender. Such an activity can range from kissing to sexual intercourse.

However, a person over 18 in a position of trust commits an offence if they engage in sexual activity with a person below that age. The Sexual Offences Act 2003 defines a position of trust as including people who normally have power or authority in a child/young person's life. These include:

- Education staff
- Staff in young offender institutions
- Staff in accommodation provided by local authorities and voluntary organizations
- Staff in hospitals, independent clinics, care homes, residential care homes and private hospitals

It also includes people providing individual services such as court welfare officers and care or supervision order supervisors.

CHILDREN OF 16 AND 17 YEARS OLD

The assessment of the capacity of a 16- or 17-year-old child to consent to treatment would be in accordance with the provisions of the Mental Capacity Act 2005 and its code of practice. Children and young people who have attained the age of 16 years have a right to consent to examination and treatment under the Family Law Reform Act 1969, Section 8 (Office of Public Sector Information 1969). It provides that:

1. The consent of a minor who has attained the age of 16 years to any surgical, medical or dental treatment which, in the absence of consent, would constitute a trespass to his person shall be as effective as it would be if he were of full age; and where a minor has by virtue of this section given an effective consent to any treatment it shall not be necessary to obtain any consent for it from his parent or guardian.
2. In this section 'surgical, medical or dental treatment' includes any procedure undertaken for the purposes of diagnosis, and this section applies to any procedure (including, in particular, the administration of an anaesthetic) which is ancillary to any treatment as it applies to that treatment.

This allows a child of 16 or 17 years to consent to examination and treatment as if they were of full age, that is, an adult. When such consent is given, it is as effective as that of an adult. It cannot be overruled by the child's parent or guardian.

The courts have adopted a very narrow construction of the provisions of Section 8 of the 1969 act. A child to whom the provisions apply can consent only to treatment or examinations which are therapeutic or diagnostic (*Re W (A Minor) (Medical Treatment Court's Jurisdiction)* [1992]). It does not allow consent for the donation of organs or blood. Even the giving of blood samples is excluded (separate provision is made for these under Section 21(2) of the Family Law Reform Act 1969).

KEY POINT

Refusal of medical treatment for all children and young people under 18 will be overturned in the courts.

Contraceptive advice and treatment is considered a legitimate and beneficial treatment under Section 5 of the National Health Service Act 1977 (Office of Public Sector Information 1977) and Section 41 of the National Health Service (Scotland) Act 1978 (Office of Public Sector Information 1978). Children who have attained 16 years can consent to contraceptive advice and treatment including termination of pregnancy.

SO WHERE ARE WE NOW?

The process so far has been painfully slow, although several authors identify that there have been some isolated efforts to enable children and young people to participate in decision making over many years (Neill 1962; Holt 1975; Hoyles 1989). It has in fact been the UK's ratification of the UN convention that has provided a powerful stimulus to discussion of the issue, creating not only an unprecedented high profile but also a growing body of literature devoted to the topic (Shier 2001).

Children and young people are one of the most governed groups by both the state and society and are also some of the highest users of state services including health, education and social services; thus, they are a primary focus for state intervention. This leads to them being frequently viewed as the entry route into social change with no exception when New Labour (2007) came into power in the UK and introduced major policy initiatives to tackle 'social exclusion'. Under this banner, considerable government funds and commitments were expended on children and young people in recent years. Yet this has been reversed in this time of fiscal austerity where there is a disproportionate impact on children and young people, their quality of life and the services they access (Main and Bradshaw 2014; Croke and Williams 2015). Children and young people may have been central to policy agendas but their views have not always been. Most initiatives were and are designed, delivered and evaluated by adults. Although intended to be protective toward children and young people, they frequently leave the adult–child power relations untouched. Yet participation is arguably central to policy agendas, in particular social exclusion, and with children and young people traditionally having limited input to local and national policies the need for greater social participation in ways that meet their wishes and felt need is crucial to their enhanced participation in decision making (Hill et al. 2004).

Participation in practice has undoubtedly been given great impetus in recent years, in particular, with the commitment to children and young people's participation by the constituent governments of the British Isles (Sinclair 2004). However, the government's contribution has to be seen in light of the UN committee reviewing the UK government's implementation of the UNCRC; although the committee has recognized the increased encouragement by the government for consultation and participation by children and young people, the indication is that there is still more to do especially in ensuring that participation leads to change.

YOUTH PARLIAMENTS: AN EXAMPLE OF GOOD PRACTICE

This is one example of the implementation of children's rights at the government level, consisting of democratically elected members between 11 and 18 years old. Formed in 2000, it now consists of 600 members who are elected to represent the views of young people in their area to government and service providers. Endorsed by the three main political parties, more than half a million young people vote in the elections each year, which are held in 90% of constituencies. Members meet regularly to hold debates and plan campaigns at venues that include the House of Lords, House of Commons and the British Museum and have recently included topics such as:

- Voting at 16
- Living wage
- Mental health issues
- Work experience
- Exam resits in math and English

Source: http://www.ukyouthparliament.org.uk/campaigns/

EVIDENCE OF PARTICIPATION POLICY IN THE UK

- Department of Health (2001) – *Seeking Consent: Working with Children*
- Children and Young People's Unit (2001) – *Learning to Listen: Core Principles for the Involvement of Children and Young People*
- Children and Young People's Unit (2003) – 'Action Plan for Children's and Young People's Participation'
- Department of Education and Skills (2002) – *Listening to Learn: An Action Plan for the Involvement of Children and Young People*
- Department of Health (2002) – *Listening, Hearing and Responding: Department of Health Action Plan – Core Principles for the Involvement of Children and Young People*
- Department of Health (2004) – *The National Service Framework for Children, Young People and Maternity Services*
- Welsh Assembly Government (2005a) – *The National Service Framework for Children, Young People and Maternity Services*
- HM Treasury (2007) – 'Aiming High for Young People: A Ten Year Strategy for Positive Outcomes'
- Department of Education and Skills (2006) – 'Care Matters: Transforming the Lives of Children and Young People in Care'
- Department for Children, Schools and Families (2008) – 'Young People Leading Change'
- In 2010 the coalition government formed; a key participation document from it is
- Liberal Democrats (2009) – 'Free to Be Young' (agreed to be adopted by the coalition government)

Source: UK Government, *National Citizen Service*, HMSO, London, 2010.

FROM POLICY TO PRACTICE

Until recent years there had been no systematic monitoring of health processes for 'looked after children' and evidence from localized studies indicated the neglect of routine immunizations and screening, lack of appropriate care for acute and chronic health conditions and failure to diagnose other health (particularly mental) problems in this group (Hall and Elliman 2006). The comparative controlled study carried out by Williams et al. (2001) aimed to assess the health needs and provision of healthcare to school-age children in local authority care. Health needs in the context of this study included mental, emotional and physical health, health education and health promotion. A total of 142 children aged 5–16 in local authority care and 119 control children matched by sex and age were studied. The results showed clearly that looked after children were more likely to:

- Experience frequent changes in their general practitioner
- Have incomplete immunization status
- Have inadequate dental care
- Suffer from anxieties and difficulties in relationships with others
- Wet the bed
- Smoke
- Use illegal drugs
- Receive less health education

However, the overall conclusion of the findings of this study were not dissimilar to those of the afore-mentioned uncontrolled observational studies in that, although there was no clear evidence that the physical health of these children and young people suffered significantly, the overall healthcare of children and young people who had been established in care for more than 6 months was significantly worse than for children and young people living in their own homes, particularly in regard to emotional and behavioural health and health promotion.

EXAMPLES OF POLICY: SOCIAL EXCLUSION

The Department of Health (2002) identified eight key priorities for tackling social exclusion and poverty as being the need to improve the life chances of 'looked after children' through expenditure and education. Both England (Quality Protects) and Wales (Children First) had provided considerable monies since 1999 to improve the health, education and welfare of looked after children and they were identified within the National Service Frameworks (Department of Health 2004; Welsh Assembly Government 2005a) as 'children and young people with special circumstances'.

LEGISLATIVE CHANGES

CHILDREN ACT 2004

The legislation that emerged from the children's bill was the end result of the government green paper *Every Child Matters* (HM Government 2004) published alongside the Victoria Climbié Inquiry (Laming Report) (Department of Health and the Home Office 2003), which summed up the findings of the very public inquiry into the tragic death of Victoria Climbié at the hands of her paternal aunt and her aunt's partner. It proposed changes in legislation to minimize risk for all children and young people and a legislative spine for improving children's lives. It identified five outcomes of 'well-being':

1. Be healthy
2. Be safe
3. Enjoy and achieve
4. Make a positive contribution
5. Achieve economic well-being.

The main aims included:

- Integrated services – the need to encourage integrated planning, commissioning and delivery of services
- Safeguarding – the need for a radical overhaul of child protection procedures to protect vulnerable children

- Information sharing – the promotion of interagency cooperation by the facilitation of legislation that will support information sharing
- Workforce reform – the need for suitable trained staff and the need for multidisciplinary teams with lead professionals

CHANGES IN POLICY IN WALES

The Welsh Assembly Government has established participation as a core value of devolved government in Wales in that 'children and young people are to be treated as valued members of the community whose voices are heard and needs considered across the range of policy making'. It established seven core aims for all its activities for children and young people in its framework for partnership (Welsh Assembly Government 2000).

SEVEN CORE AIMS

- Flying start in life
- Comprehensive range of education and learning opportunities
- Enjoy the best possible health and free from abuse, victimization and exploitation
- Have access to play, leisure, sporting and cultural activities
- Listened to and treated with respect
- Have a safe home and a community that supports emotional and physical well-being
- Are not disadvantaged by poverty

EXAMPLE OF GOOD PRACTICE: FUNKY DRAGON INTERACTIVE WEBSITE

To facilitate participation, the Welsh Assembly Government helped to set up, and funds, the Children and Young People's Assembly for Wales (known as the Funky Dragon). The Funky Dragon is a peer-led organization made up of a grand council of representatives from local children and young people's fora and national and local peer-led groups. It ensures that the views of children and young people aged 0–25 are heard and taken into account in the decision-making process, particularly by the Welsh Assembly Government (http://www.funkydragon.org/en/).

EVIDENCE OF RIGHTS/PARTICIPATION POLICY IN WALES

- Welsh Assembly Government (2000) – *Framework for Partnership with Children and Young People*; seven core aims identified
- House of Commons (2001) – 'Children's Commissioner for Wales Bill'; first in UK
- Welsh Assembly Government (2002) – Participation of children via an interactive website (www.funkydragon.org)
- Welsh Assembly Government (2004) – *Children and Young People: Rights to Action*
- Welsh Assembly Government (2008a) – *Rights in Action*
- Welsh Assembly Government (2008b) – 'Children and Young People's Wellbeing Monitor'
- Welsh Assembly Government (2009) – *Getting It Right*
- Welsh Government (2011a) – 'Children and Young People's Wellbeing Monitor'
- Welsh Government (2011b) – 'Rights of Children and Young Persons Measure'

CHILDREN'S COMMISSIONERS

Norway was the first country to appoint a children's commissioner, called an 'ombudsman', in 1981 to safeguard children and young people's rights. Following the agreement of the UN on the UNCRC, other countries began to follow suit; first Sweden, then others in Europe and the rest of the world.

Frequently described as 'watchdogs' and 'champions' for children and young people they are high-profile independent bodies established to monitor, promote and safeguard children and young people's human rights (Children's Rights Alliance for England 2004). Within the UK, the campaign began in the early 1990s and, gradually, more than 130 organizations in the UK supported the campaign for children's commissioners urged on by the fact that when, in 1995, the UK government presented its initial report to the UN committee it was highly criticized for failing to support children and young people's human rights through an independent mechanism.

Devolved countries encouraged progress and, in 2001, Peter Clarke took up the post of children's commissioner, the first appointment of such a post in the UK. This came sooner in Wales than in the rest of the UK because of the results of the inquiry by Waterhouse et al. (1999) into child abuse in children's homes in North Wales. The Care Standards Act 2000 (Office of Public Sector Information 2000) created a children's commissioner post for Wales following a key recommendation of Waterhouse et al. The report indicated findings that when the children and young people in care had complained about being abused and ill-treated, they had not been listened to. Initially, the post was there to mainly protect children and young people in care, but this was amended by the Children's Commissioner for Wales Bill in late 2000 to give the post holder more powers to protect the rights of all children and young people. Appointments of other children's commissioners in the UK followed soon afterwards, with Northern Ireland in 2003, Scotland in 2004 (also the Irish Republic) and eventually England in 2005, although this post is still not as independent as the others but has responsibilities over policies that affect children and young people in England and Wales such as youth crime and asylum.

These posts not only significantly raise the profile of children and young people but also have a critical role in raising children's awareness about their rights. The success of these posts to some degree relies on their independence from government.

England	Anne Longfield
	http://www.childrenscommissioner.gov.uk/
Wales	Sally Holland
	https://www.childcomwales.org.uk/
Scotland	Tam Bailie
	http://www.cypcs.org.uk/
Northern Ireland	Koulla Yiasouma
	http://www.niccy.org/

EXAMPLE OF PARTICIPATION: EVALUATION OF THE COMMISSIONER'S ROLE

This took place over a 3-year period and was published in December 2008. It involved children and young people from the start. They were on the initial panel to appoint a researcher prior to forming a steering group to look at planning and designing the research methods; in year 2, they were involved with data collection, and in year 3 in the analysis and writing up. The adults were facilitators and the report is full of individual pages of their experience through the research journey (Swansea University, University of Central Lancashire, Save the Children 2008).

One of the 13 recommendations was to

ensure that all organisations providing services for children and young people consider that staff are well informed about the role of the commissioner.

Towler, cited in Swansea University, University of Central Lancashire, Save the Children 2008

KEY POINT

Children's commissioners are frequently described as watchdogs or champions for children and young people and are independent from any government organization.

Children's rights is a curriculum topic in the undergraduate programme in children and young people's nursing in Welsh universities to clearly identify the UNCRC (United Nations 1989); also included are three main areas of rights – provision, protection and participation – in relation to children and young people's health and how they apply to the holistic nursing of children, young people and their families.

NATIONAL SERVICE FRAMEWORK FOR CHILDREN, YOUNG PEOPLE AND MATERNITY SERVICES

This blueprint (Department of Health 2004; Welsh Assembly Government 2005a) clearly sets out and defines standards for the universal services (in England and Wales) which all children and young people should receive including not only optimum health and well-being but also a programme for sustained improvement in children's health. It is a joint policy initiative across both the NHS and local government and supports the Welsh Assembly Government's seven core aims for children and young people and includes them from conception to the age of 18. The National Service Framework was already in the early stages of development when Wanless (2003) was released, but it recommends the proposed extensions to other areas of the NHS. Undeniably there has been involvement of both children and families in the development of the framework (especially in Wales), reflecting the intent shown in the second report to the UN Committee on the Rights of the Child (Department for Children, Schools and Families 1999) to 'promote the voice of the child'.

> ### EXAMPLE OF IMPLEMENTING POLICY IN PRACTICE: SELF-ASSESSMENT AUDIT TOOL
>
> The Welsh Assembly Government (2004) published *Children and Young People: Rights to Action*, which set out that all government policies would deliver children's rights based on the UNCRC; however, the framework used to help make this happen is the National Service Framework through the planning processes of local children and young people's partnerships. Those responsible for the key actions will use a self-assessment audit tool (SAAT) to measure their own progress and this information is used along with other statistics to write their children and young people's plan (CYPP). There are already systems in place to check how well those responsible for the key actions are doing and to make sure that what is entered into the SAAT is correct. The Welsh Assembly Government will then look at the results for the SAAT to identify whether they correspond with the local authority CYPP.

NURSING PRACTICE

Within healthcare, however, the convention represents a shift from a 'highly paternalistic' and medically dominated view to a children's rights–based approach that endorses the child and young person's right to express his or her views and opinions in all matters that affect them. To enable them to do this, however, they require the appropriate information to be given by the appropriately trained professionals. Effective training for healthcare professionals would address common attitudes and prejudices about children's rights and would promote greater respect for the autonomy of children and young people (Lowden 2002). The planning of children's services was made mandatory in 1996 and the second report to the UN committee (Department for Children, Schools and Families 1999) by the UK did at long last include the importance of this as a critical mechanism for improving a broad range of services for children in need and their families.

All health professionals should understand the imperative to work for child- and family-friendly services as an integral part of the philosophy of 'family-centred care' (Casey 1988, cited in Sidey and Widdas 2005; Smith and Coleman 2010). This phrase has become the touchstone for children and young people's nursing practice in the UK, where the needs of the child and young person are considered within the context of the family unit and effective care depends on negotiation and partnership. Although family-centred care gives a welcome emphasis to the nursing relationship in practice, it has its shortcomings, none the least because it gives little consideration to the very difficult professional, ethical, political and rights-based issues that occur in the nursing of children and young people (Samwell 2000, cited in Sidey and Widdas 2005; Smith and Coleman 2010).

A qualitative study by Noyes (2000) goes some way to demonstrate this. A sample of 18 young 'ventilator-dependent' people was purposely selected to reflect age, gender, ethnicity, level of need and location with the aim of describing young people's views (and those of their parents) of their health, social care and education by conducting in-depth interviews. The findings (which are impossible to discuss at great length) are summarized under the relevant articles of the UNCRC and commence with a clear breach of Articles 4 and 42 in failing both to implement the convention effectively and to inform the young people and their parents of their rights. It continues with the failure to uphold Articles 12 and 13 following the identification that some of these young people did not have access to an adequate communication system (if non-verbal); when they did have access, they frequently did not have contact with the people who understood it, so their ability to freely express their views was particularly restricted. In addition, there was evidence of them not always being offered the full protection of both the Children Act (1989) and the patient's charter (Department of Health 1991, 1996). A particular finding on analysis of the in-depth interviews with these young people was an overwhelming agreement of the need for them to be placed at the centre of decision making and subsequently allowed to be in charge of their own lives. This led the researcher to seriously question the appropriateness and effectiveness of the health services offered to these young people who had (when enabled) been highly critical of some of the aspects of their care.

WHAT MORE CAN WE DO?

Children, as minors in law, have neither autonomy nor the right to make choices or decisions on their own behalf, and only too frequently responsibility for such decisions and for their welfare has traditionally been vested with those adults who care for them (Lansdown 2001). Children's rights activists Shakespeare and Watson (1998), in agreement, indicate that the different perspectives on children's rights can result in services being developed, for example, for a child or young person that are determined by other people, particularly professionals and especially for very young and disabled children (cited in Noyes 2000). The need to allow children and young people to participate in matters that affect them is in recognition not only that they are individuals who have opinions and views of their own, but also that these cannot always be represented necessarily by parents or professionals (Sinclair 1996). Payne (1995) also adds with caution that professions such as nursing can be dangerous and restricted places, giving an example of how children who are disabled are frequently treated as an 'object' of concern or care and not, unfortunately, as a citizen with rights.

Consumer participation is now a major component of contemporary health and nursing policy, with the importance emphasized of partnership working with nurses, midwives and health visitors. The NHS plan (Department of Health 2000) clearly identified for the first time that patients should have a real say in the NHS, and subsequent documents indicated that this included consumers becoming empowered participants. However, there was limited mention of children and young people's services in the initial plan. It could be argued that consumer participation at the individual level is familiar territory to children and young people's nurses because of the long history of practicing family-centred care (Smith and Coleman 2010). However, it is considered by many that, to date, healthcare staff and parents may have been overcautious in their assessment of children and young people's ability to understand and contribute their opinions and feelings around healthcare decisions (Foley et al. 2001). Although parents may have realistic expectations of their child's ability, children and young people need to know that nurses and doctors will respect their views and opinions as well (Alderson and Montgomery 1996). In fact, overall, they consider that there should be no need for young people's rights to conflict with the values of the healthcare professional, but that health professionals need in fact their own code of ethics, to incorporate respect for these rights. Bricher (2000) identifies the importance of reflection and rights and indicates that it is imperative that nurses on both an individual and organizational level reflect on their practice to identify just where children and young people's nursing practice is addressing a rights-based approach.

The education of children and young people's nurses to a minimum of degree level (since 2002 in Wales and from 2013 in England) indeed is a step in the right direction for them to examine and understand what is required to enable a rights-based approach to the nursing of children, young people and their families. Advanced nurse practitioners and consultant nurse posts that require education to at the least master's level are still in their infancy in children and young people's nursing; however, these highly educated nurses should be able to push the boundaries forward both strategically and in nursing practice and challenge the paternalistic attitudes that persist within healthcare.

PRINCIPLE FOR PRACTICE

Children and young people need to know that their views will be respected by nurses and doctors.

AUTONOMY, CONSENT AND THE NEED FOR CHILDREN'S NURSES TO BE ADVOCATES

Although both the courts and parliament allow children and young people to make treatment decisions for themselves as they mature, no child/young person under 18 years is a wholly autonomous being (*Re M (A Child) (Refusal of Medical Treatment)* [1999]). There is nothing compelling a nurse to take consent from an obviously Gillick-competent child. The nurse may, if he or she so chooses, take the consent from a person with parental responsibility. Similarly, if a child/young person under 18 refuses medical examination or treatment, then the law does allow others to consent even if the child/young person has capacity. Lord Donaldson summed up the position thus:

> I now prefer the analogy of the legal 'flak jacket' which protects you from claims by the litigious whether you acquire it from your patient, who may be a minor over the age of 16 or a 'Gillick-competent' child under that age, or from another person having parental responsibilities which include a right to consent to treatment of the minor.

Anyone who gives you a flak jacket (i.e. consent) may take it back, but you only need one and so long as you continue to have one you have the legal right to proceed.

Re W (A Minor) (Medical Treatment Court's Jurisdiction) [1992] (Lord Donaldson MR at 641)

When a child/young person with capacity consents to medical examination or treatment, it cannot be overruled by a parent. However, when the same child/young person refuses to consent then you can obtain it from another person with parental responsibility who has the right to consent to treatment on the child's or young person's behalf.

> **KEY POINT**
>
> An exception to this rule exists under the Mental Health Act 1983, Section 131 (Department of Health 1983), in which a child aged 16 or over can consent or refuse informal admission to a psychiatric hospital.

However, to grant autonomy to children and young people to consent to treatment without that of their parents (for whatever reason) and not grant the same autonomy to refuse treatment is a blatant disregard for the concept and of course for children's rights (Bijesterveld 2000). This is clearly indicated in the case of *Re M (A Child) (Refusal of Medical Treatment)* [1999], when a 15½-year-old had her decision to refuse a heart transplant overruled by the High Court, failing to make any commitment to children's right to 'autonomy' and limited itself to allowing her views to be heard. A lack of respect for autonomy of the child serves to undermine not only their self-esteem and confidence but also their capacity to develop decision-making skills and the opportunity to actually make them (Foley et al. 2001; Flatman 2002).

This strong tendency toward judicial paternalism emerged and manifested itself in the 1990s and still (according to many children's rights promoters) continues despite clear standards within the UNCRC to the contrary (Flatman 2002). The trouble with consent law is that it appears to be 'all or nothing' and, although we have discussed the rights of competent children, it fails to address the rights of non-competent children or adults (Alderson and Morrow 2004). So what is the way forward to allow children and young people to participate in the decision-making process of their care, and when relevant to give informed consent? The answers are manifold and are currently being addressed by policy makers, educationalists and children's charities alike. One example is the Department of Health (2001) in its publication *Seeking Consent: Working with Children*, which clearly indicates the need for children and young people's nurses to ensure that they have evidence in their plans of care of actual involvement of children, young people and their families. Also increasingly health boards and trusts have amended consent forms (only used for surgery and invasive procedures) to include the signature of the child/young person to indicate that they have at least been involved in the decision making after appropriate information has been given. This is not an attempt to exclude parents in the decision making but to allow the child to participate appropriately.

The regulatory body for nursing, midwifery and health visiting (Nursing and Midwifery Council 2015, pp. 4–5) also clearly indicates the importance of consent and advocacy in its amended code of professional conduct:

3.4 Act as an advocate for the vulnerable, challenging poor practice and discriminatory attitudes and behaviour relating to their care
4.1 Balance the need to act in the best interests of people at all times with the requirement to respect a person's right to accept or refuse treatment
4.2 Make sure that you get properly informed consent and document it before carrying out any action

This clearly demonstrates to registered nurses that, once they are on the professional register, they are responsible and accountable for implementing rights to all client groups by adopting their professional body's code of conduct.

ADVOCACY IN THE PROMOTION OF PARTICIPATION IN HEALTHCARE

The requirement therefore for children's nurses to act as advocates for the child, young person and his or her family is imperative. It is described by many as ensuring that patients and their families are informed of all rights and subsequently have all the necessary information to make informed decisions, and then supporting them in those decisions while also safeguarding their best interests. Bennett (1999) indicates that true advocacy in nursing practice represents an expressed need by the patient and not a perceived need by the nurse. However, there are broadly three types of advocacy, none of which is necessarily dependent on health professionals:

1. Independent advocacy – Increased services are now available through government schemes and local councils.
2. Collective advocacy – This comes in the form of groups and charities that represent children and young people, including the National Society for the Prevention of Cruelty to Children, Barnardo's and Action for Sick Children.
3. Self advocacy – Promoting the child/young person's ability to make his or her views known.

EXAMPLE OF IMPLEMENTING POLICY IN PRACTICE: INCREASED COLLECTIVE AND INDEPENDENT ADVOCACY SERVICES IN WALES

A task force examined advocacy services for children and young people in Wales and delivered its recommendations in 2005 (Welsh Assembly Government 2005b). This included a tiered model of advocacy delivery across health, education and social care settings. This was intended to streamline processes and encourage greater collaboration among providers, in line with the aims of the Children Act 2004 (Office of Public Sector Information 2004), to improve outcomes for vulnerable children and young people and to ensure more effective use of resources. The task force proposed a collaborative regional model for delivery of children and young people's advocacy services, which should allow greater independence for advocacy providers from service commissioners.

Funding of more than £1.2 million has been given to key children's advocacy providers in Wales: Barnardo's, Tros Gynnal, Voices from Care and the National Youth Advocacy Service. Funding has also been given to local authorities through the Children First programme, to extend advocacy services to children in need.

The Welsh Assembly Government is reviewing arrangements for children and young people to complain about any health service as currently a complaint can only be made against treatment given in a hospital. However, development of advocacy services for children and young people offers considerable support for them as discussed below.

FURTHER ADVOCACY DEVELOPMENT IN WALES: THE NEW SERVICE FRAMEWORK FOR THE FUTURE PROVISION OF ADVOCACY SERVICES FOR CHILDREN IN WALES

This will provide a locally or regionally commissioned service covering health, social care services and education with a particular focus on providing support to assist vulnerable children and young people and is currently being rolled out.

But what more can children and young people's nurses do to advocate for children and young people in healthcare? Critics of the UNCRC suggest that, in fact, it is inherently paternalistic and is closely related to upholding 'positive rights', which generally impose a duty that requires another to do something for you and are founded on the ethical principle of beneficence – 'doing good to another'. Charles-Edwards (2000) identified that advocacy in healthcare should be about promoting negative rights as well as positive, which, for example, would be the child's right to contribute his or her viewpoint and participate in decisions even if the healthcare professionals think that the child is wrong, thus highlighting the difference between advocacy and acting in the child's best interests. So nurses and other healthcare workers need to work toward:

- Ensuring that families are aware of all available health services
- Ensuring that families are informed adequately regarding treatments and procedures
- Encouraging and/or supporting existing healthcare practices
- Ensuring all rights are protected

EXAMPLE OF GOOD PRACTICE

Community children's nurses who are educated to degree level and hold a specialist practice award frequently work closely with children with severe and life-threatening disabilities and are aware of these children's qualities of life (as small as they may be) and frequently act as advocates for the child and family in helping others to understand this perspective.

PRINCIPLE FOR PRACTICE

Advocacy in children's nursing, however, should be about promoting negative rights as well as positive rights.

The UNCRC (United Nations 1989) clearly sets out three levels that respect all children in regard to participation rights and include the right

1. To be informed
2. To form and express views
3. To influence a decision

The fourth level goes beyond the UNCRC and includes the sharing of power and responsibility for decision making. This is actually what is addressed in Gillick, although most children and many adults prefer to stop at stage 3 and share the decision making with people close to them (Alderson and Montgomery 1996; Royal College of Paediatrics and Child Health 2000; British Medical Association 2001). In regard to other models of participation, one has been uniquely influential: Roger Hart's 'ladder of participation', which first appeared in 1992 (cited in Shier 2001) and has been reproduced many times since (Figure 1.1). It was adapted from Arnstein's (1969) 'ladder of citizen participation', and Arnstein originally suggested that different levels of control and participation could be compared with rungs on a ladder. However, the influence of Hart's model was confirmed by research conducted by Save the Children in 1995 when Barn and Franklin (1996) carried out a survey of organizations throughout the UK that included questions on what models and theories had been the most helpful in regard to participation; Hart's was one of the two most frequently mentioned, the other being the theories of Paulo Freire (cited in Shier 2001). Their work is based on general principles such as empowerment and respect for young people rather than specific models and theories. The steps on Hart's ladder describe the degree to which children are in control of the process, up to the eighth level where children initiate the process and invite adults to join them in the decision making.

However, there are many criticisms of Hart, including that the ladder is too idealistic and hierarchical with the objective in striving for the top rung. But what this and other models do is highlight the need to understand and distinguish different levels of empowerment afforded to children and young people. This is somewhat controversial for many people working with and around young people. Essentially, the debate is which of these levels of participation is actually the most meaningful?

Hart's ladder was not constructed to be utilized in a healthcare context and was developed initially for use with 'common children' in society. The Royal College of Paediatrics and Child Health (1997) distinguished four levels of participation:

1. Informing children
2. Listening to them
3. Taking account of their views so they can influence decisions
4. Respecting the competent child as the main decider about proposed healthcare interventions

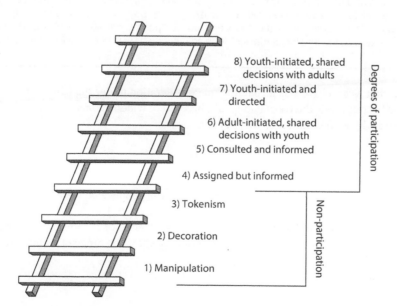

Figure 1.1 Hart's ladder of participation. (Adapted from Hart RA, *Children's participation: from tokenism to citizenship*, Innocenti Essays No. 4, UNICEF International Child Development Centre, Florence, 1992.)

Today they consider it as an ongoing process that should be ethical, safe, meaningful for all and most importantly flexible to suit all those who are involved in how much they want. This includes children and young people as well as carers and families alike (Royal College of Paediatrics and Child Health 2015).

Many believe that shared decision making is most beneficial to both young people and adults. Others believe that young people are most empowered when they are making decisions without the influence of adults. Most often, this does not exclude adults but reduces their role to that of support.

CASE STUDY

Members of the young people's executive at Oxford Radcliffe (known as YiPpEe for short) are children and young people who either have been in hospital themselves or have a sibling who has. They meet and work with adults, giving them ideas about what children and young people want and need in hospital. Some recent projects that they have been involved in include:

- Reviewing food quality and developing menus
- Creating an information booklet for children and young people in hospital
- Making children's rights clearer and more obvious to adults and young people
- Discussing the importance of privacy and dignity for children and young people

---

BEST INTERESTS

DISABLED CHILDREN

When the issue of consent for a disabled child/young person reaches the court, it is nearly always in regard to life-saving treatment and the judge has to rule on the basis of what is in the best interests of the child/young person. Parental consent might be valid if it does not go against the child's or young person's rights as, for a disabled child/young person, it is less likely that their views will be sought, although the principle of an expert to represent them is explicit in the UN convention. It is commonly assumed that a disabled child does not have quality of life and decisions are often influenced by this perception in terms of the best interests of the child (Campbell 2002). The child and young person's welfare is of paramount consideration and historically doctors were judged to know best; however, the courts now take a much more holistic approach to best interests that goes beyond the clinical needs of the child/young person.

CASE LAW EXAMPLE

In *An NHS Trust v MB and Mr & Mrs B* [2006] an NHS trust sought a declaration that it should be lawful in M's best interests to withdraw all forms of ventilation from a seriously ill young boy but his parents objected. M had not been able to breathe unaided since before his first birthday and required positive pressure ventilation. The trust considered that his quality of life was so low and the burdens of living so great that it was unethical to continue artificially to keep him alive.

The court said that M's welfare was its paramount consideration under the Children Act 1989, Section 1. In considering his best interests the court had to take account of wider welfare issues.

It was probable and had to be assumed that M continued to:

- See
- Hear
- Feel touch
- Have an awareness of his surroundings, in particular of the people who were closest to him, namely his family
- Have the normal thoughts and thought processes of a small child of 18 months, with the proviso that because he had never left hospital he had not experienced the same range of stimuli and experiences as a more normal 18-month-old
- Have age-appropriate cognition, a relationship of value with his family, and other pleasures from sight, touch and sound

Those benefits were precious and real and the routine discomfort, distress and pain that M suffered did not outweigh those benefits.

It was therefore not in M's best interests to discontinue ventilation with the inevitable result that he would die. However, it would not be in M's best interests to undergo procedures that went beyond maintaining ventilation such as cardiopulmonary resuscitation or the administration of intravenous antibiotics.

The law appears at times to be contradictory where disabled children are concerned, with an absence of clear guidance (Rowse 2007). Unfortunately, the convention is not widely used in making healthcare decisions, but gradually the Human Rights Act 1998 (from October 2000 in the UK; Office of Public Sector Information 1998) has changed the position of children and young people in being involved in their own healthcare decisions, and health professionals such as children's nurses can act to ensure that this happens.

Law that allows treatment to be forced upon non-competent children and young people appears to assume that they have no understanding worth considering and in fact is at times in conflict with the best interests of the child/young person. It needs work toward providing clearer frameworks comprehensible to professionals, parents, children and young people alike, with the focus of responsibility being on adults to demonstrate that the child/young person is incompetent rather than the child/young person needing to pass a test of competence that many adults would fail (Lowden 2002).

HOW DOES THE UN COMMITTEE THINK WE ARE FARING?

CONCLUDING OBSERVATIONS OF THE COMMITTEE ON THE RIGHTS OF THE CHILD: UNITED KINGDOM OF GREAT BRITAIN AND NORTHERN IRELAND

The UN Committee on the Rights of the Child examined the UK government in September 2008 to see how well it was protecting children's human rights since the last reporting period, and information was provided by the four UK governments. Since considering this evidence, and in some cases visiting the country concerned, the committee has made 124 concluding observations (recommendations) of where the government must do more to put the UNCRC fully into practice in the UK. The four countries, however, are at different points of development and have different priorities. All four have dedicated departments for children and young people and ministers with special responsibilities for policies affecting them as well as their own commissioners. Although all four recognize the challenge ahead of them and have their own plans, there has been a move forward in some areas:

- Article 22: Refugee children and young people will now enjoy the same status as others in the UK.
- Article 37c: Young people in custody will no longer be detained with adults under any circumstances.

The recognition is that, although it is important to take forward their own policies to meet local needs that achieve the goals set out, collaborative working is essential, as is having clearly defined joint targets to tackle child poverty and plans to enable children and young people to participate in decision making on issues that affect their lives. Therefore a joint commitment from all four nations of the UK has been made to take action in response to the UN committee and has been clearly laid out in the document *Working Together, Achieving More* (Department for Children, Schools and Families 2009a); some examples follow.

RESPONSIVE POLICY IN THE UK

ENGLAND

- Department for Children, Schools and Families (2007) – *The Children's Plan*
- Department for Children, Schools and Families (2009b) – *The Children's Plan Two Years On: A Progress Report*
- Department for Children, Schools and Families (2009c) – *UNCRC: Priorities for Action*

In October 2009 England published an update to the children's plan (Department for Children, Schools and Families 2009b) which sets out priorities for taking forward the UN committee's recommendations. The English plan *UNCRC: Priorities for Action* (Department for Children, Schools and Families 2009c) was published alongside the above document.

WALES

- Welsh Assembly Government (2009) – *Getting It Right*

A 5-year rolling action plan for Wales setting out key priorities and actions to be undertaken by the Welsh Assembly Government in response to the concluding observations of the UN Committee on the Rights of the Child (United Nations Committee on the Rights of the Child 2008). It has 16 priorities that will be focused on and will be a living document. It will be subject to regular review and updating to ensure that it keeps abreast of new developments in policy and strategy and remains relevant and timely. Two examples of these include:

1. Tackle poverty for children and young people in Wales – new legislation to address this major issue and local plans will be stronger and give more support.
2. Increase awareness of the UNCRC with both children and adults.

SCOTLAND

- Scottish Government (2009) – *Do the Right Thing*

Launched in September the Scottish government's response to the concluding observations of the UN committee sets out 21 priority areas of action.

NORTHERN IRELAND

As of 2009, Northern Ireland is still developing additional actions for inclusion in its existing children and young people's strategy action plan which are yet to be identified.

REPORT OF THE UNITED KINGDOM CHILDREN'S COMMISSIONERS (UNITED NATIONS COMMITTEE ON THE RIGHTS OF THE CHILD) (2014)

This is a joint report by the four United Kingdom children's commissioners for the UN Committee on the Rights of the Child's examination of the UK's Fifth Periodic Report under the UNCRC. It evidences the commitment to work together to improve the lives of children and young people in England, Northern Ireland, Scotland and Wales. The views and experiences of children inform the work of all the commissioners.

They are concerned that the UK state party's response to the global economic downturn, including the imposition of austerity measures and changes to the welfare system, has resulted in a failure to protect the most disadvantaged children and those in especially vulnerable groups from child poverty, preventing the realization of their rights under Articles 26 and 27 of the UNCRC. The best interests of children were not central to the development of these policies and children's views were not sought.

REGIONAL CHANGES PRIOR TO ABOVE REPORT

The Rights of Children and Young Persons (Wales) Measure 2011 (Welsh Government 2011b) places a duty on the Welsh ministers to have due regard to the UNCRC when exercising their functions. The measure requires a children's rights scheme which sets out the arrangements by which the government will comply with their duty. The scheme, however, does not contain a timetable, quantifiable goals or an implementation and monitoring mechanism. A child rights impact assessment (CRIA) is fundamental to realizing due regard; while a number of CRIAs have been carried out by the Welsh government, their quality and transparency have been inconsistent.

While these are positive developments, they fall well short of incorporation of the convention and they have not been mirrored in England or Northern Ireland. In Northern Ireland there has been little progress since 2008. Few policies or pieces of legislation refer to the UNCRC, and only a very limited number of CRIAs have been conducted. However, the development of a new children's strategy from 2016, alongside child rights indicators, offers the opportunity to consider incorporation of the UNCRC and implementation of the general measures.

In England there has been no legislative movement toward incorporation of the convention, only a ministerial commitment under the 2010–2015 government to 'give due consideration to the UNCRC articles when making new policy and legislation'.

However, the roles of the children's commissioner for England (CCE) and Scotland's commissioner for children and young people (SCCYP) have been strengthened since 2008: the remit of CCE now centres upon the promotion and protection of children's rights with particular regards to Article 11 (UNCRC 1989) in relation to combating the illicit transfer and non-return of children abroad. The SCCYP has been given additional powers by the Children and Young People (Scotland) Act 2014, which introduces an individual investigation mechanism through which children can seek an investigation into alleged violations of their rights.

CONCLUSION

The UNCRC has made great progress in promoting children and young people's rights by providing a benchmark for the implementation of these rights throughout the world. The convention's value, however, has been limited by the failure of many countries, including the UK, to incorporate its provisions into domestic law. Children and young people cannot enforce the rights guaranteed by the convention in a British court, and the UK government does not regard the criticisms of its performance by the UN Committee on the Rights of the Child as a reason to make the convention legally enforceable. Despite this, there is no doubt that the UNCRC has influenced governments toward increased participation by children and young people in policy planning and giving them a voice through the children's commissioners. Some would argue participation in their own healthcare by children and young people remains little changed since the seminal case of *Gillick* in the late 1980s. Children and young people's nurses always work in a climate of consent with their young patients to encourage participation by taking the time to explain procedures and the reasons for treatment. This clinical function of consent is every bit as important as its legal function. Healthcare delivery is far more efficient and effective with the cooperation of the child and young person, and this is more likely to occur when the child/young person knows what the procedure is and why it needs to be performed. We have seen that a child and young person's legal right to express his or her autonomy has developed through a protective common law structure that always has someone available to step in should a child's or young person's refusal of treatment be contrary to their best interests. This paternalistic approach effectively restricts a child's or young person's participation in making choices about their healthcare; either the child/young person agrees to treatment or someone else makes the decision for them. Competence is the key to autonomy, so a competent child or young person should be free to make choices about his or her healthcare regardless of what others consider to be in their best interests. Until the licensed paternalism of health professionals is curtailed and the UK enshrines the articles of the UNCRC in law, children and young people will not be free to fully participate in their healthcare. The Royal College of Paediatrics and Child Health (2012) clearly indicates that children and young people are key stakeholders of the NHS and their interests must be at the centre of health and local government services. With child-centred care (CCC) increasingly challenging the concept of family-centred care (FCC), it is clearly defined as meaning that children and young people's interests need to be the centre of not only our thinking but also practice (Carter et al. 2014). This surely indicates that to achieve this inclusion of children and young people as active participants in their care is imperative. Let us be clear about what participation is. It is about doing and being involved which requires meaningful involvement in decision-making processes (Kellet 2011, cited in Carter et al. 2014). Hopefully we can move forward and address the shortfalls that we still currently have in relation to children and young people participating in their healthcare.

SUMMARY OF PRINCIPLES FOR HEALTHCARE PRACTICE TO INCREASE INVOLVEMENT AND PARTICIPATION OF CHILDREN AND YOUNG PEOPLE

Child health services need to promote the best interest of the child/young person first and foremost. This includes ensuring engagement is carried out in a safe way that does not place children and young people at risk.

- Engagement of children and young people in health services must be at all levels and embedded into the culture and day-to-day practice of health professionals and organizations.
- Health professionals need to continually share learning and good practice and work in partnership with others.
- Engagement with children and young people must be meaningful and non-tokenistic. This means listening, being clear about the purpose, and feeding back to children and young people about changes made as a result of engagement.
- There must be a wide range of approaches to participation because there is no one way of engaging with children and young people. Any approach should recognize diversity and the different perspectives that children and young people may have.

Source: Royal College of Paediatrics and Child Health, *Involving Children and Young People in Health Services*, RCPCH, London, 2012.

REFERENCES

A v United Kingdom [1998] 2 FLR 959.

A&D v B&E [2003] EWHC 1376 (FAM).

Alderson P (2002) Young children's health care rights and consent. In Franklin B (ed.) *The new handbook of children's rights: comparative policy and practice*. London: Routledge.

Alderson P (2007) Competent children? Minors' consent to health care treatment and research. *Social Science & Medicine* 65: 2272–83.

Alderson P, Montgomery J (1996) Children may be able to make their own decisions. *British Medical Journal*, 315: 50.

Alderson P, Morrow V (2004) *Ethics, social research and consulting with children and young people*. London: Barnardo's.

Aries P (1962) *Centuries of childhood*. London: Jonathan Cape.

Arnstein S (1969) A ladder of citizen participation. *Journal of the American Planning Association* 35: 216–24.

Barn G, Franklin A (1996) Article 12: issues in developing children's participation rights. In Verhellen E (ed.) *Monitoring children's rights*. Leiden: Martinus Nijhoff.

Barnardo v McHugh [1891] AC 388 (CA).

BBC (2015) AMs vote against banning smacking children in Wales. Available at http://www.bbc.co.uk/news/uk-wales-31697730.

Bennett O (1999) Advocacy in nursing. *Nursing Standard* 14(11): 40–1.

Bijesterveld P (2000) Competent to refuse. *Paediatric Nursing* 12: 33–5.

Bricher G (2000) Children in the hospital: issues of power and vulnerability. *Pediatric Nursing* 26(3): 277–81.

British Medical Association (2001) *Consent, rights, and choices in healthcare, children and young people*. London: BMA Publishing.

Camden LBC v R (A Minor) (Blood Transfusion) [1993] 2 FLR 757.

Campbell A (2002) Informed choice for adolescents. *Paediatric Nursing* 13(10): 41–2.

Carter B, Bray L, Dickinson A, Edwards M, Ford K (2014) *Child-centred nursing, promoting critical thinking*. London: Sage.

Charles-Edwards I (2000) Children's nursing and advocacy: are we in a muddle? *Paediatric Nursing* 13(2): 12–16.

Children and Young People's Unit (2001) *Learning to listen: core principles for the involvement of children and young people*. London: CYPU.

Children and Young People's Unit (2003) Action plan for children's and young people's participation. Available at www.allchildrenni.gov.uk.

Children's Rights Alliance for England (2004) *The case for a children's rights commissioner for England*. London: CRAE.

Council of Europe (1950) European Convention on Fundamental Human Rights and Freedoms. Rome: Council of Europe. Available at http://conventions.coe.int/treaty/Commun/QueVoulezVous.asp?NT=005&CL=ENG.

Croke R, Williams J (eds.) (2015) *Report to the United Nations Committee on the Rights of the Child*. Wales: Wales UNCRC Monitoring Group.

Darbyshire P (1994) *Living with a sick child in hospital*. London: Chapman & Hall.

Department for Children, Schools and Families (1999) UK 2nd report. Report to the UN Committee on the Rights of the Child. London: HMSO. Available at www.gov.uk.

Department for Children, Schools and Families (2007) *The children's plan*. London: DCSF. Available at http://publications.dcsf.gov.uk/default.aspx?PageFunction=productdetails&PageMode=publications&ProductId=DCSF-01099-2009.

Department for Children, Schools and Families (2008) *Young People leading Change*. Available at www.gov.uk.

Department for Children, Schools and Families (2009a) *Working together, achieving more*. London: DCSF.

Department for Children, Schools and Families (2009b) *The children's plan two years on: a progress report*. London: DCSF. Available at http://publications.dcsf.gov.uk/default.aspx?PageFunction=productdetails&PageMode=publications&ProductId=DCSF-01099-2009.

Department for Children, Schools and Families (2009c) *UNCRC: priorities for action*. London: DSCF. Available at http://publications.dcsf.gov.uk/default.aspx?PageFunction=productdetails&PageMode=publications&ProductId=DCSF-01099-2009.

Department of Education and Skills (2002) *Listening to learn: an action plan for the involvement of children and young people.* Available at www.dcsf.gov.uk.

Department of Education and Skills (2006) *Care Matters: Transforming the lives of Children and Young People in Care.* Available at www.education.gov.uk.

Department of Health (1983) *The Mental Health Act.* London: DH.

Department of Health (1991) *The patient's charter.* London: HMSO.

Department of Health (1996) *The patient's charter: services for children and young people.* London: HMSO.

Department of Health (2000) *The NHS plan.* London: HMSO.

Department of Health (2001) *Seeking consent: working with children.* London: DH.

Department of Health (2002) *Listening, hearing and responding: Department of Health action plan – core principles for the involvement of children and young people.* London: DH.

Department of Health (2004) *The National Service Framework for children, young people and maternity services.* London: DH.

Department of Health (2007) Annual report. Available at www.doh.gov.uk.

Department of Health and the Home Office (2003) *The Victoria Climbié Inquiry: report of an inquiry by Lord Laming.* London: HMSO.

F v West Berkshire HA [1990] 2 A.C. 1 (HL).

Flatman D (2002) Consulting children: are we listening? *Paediatric Nursing* 14(7): 28–31.

Foley P, Roche J, Tucker T (eds.) (2001) *Children in society: contemporary theory, policy and practice.* Basingstoke: Palgrave.

Fulton Y (1996) Children's rights and the role of the nurse. *Paediatric Nursing* 8, 29–31.

Gillick v West Norfolk and Wisbech AHA [1986] AC 112 (HL).

Glass v United Kingdom [2004] 1 FLR 1019.

Gross RD (2015) *Psychology: the science of mind and behaviour.* 7th ed. London: Hodder Arnold.

Hall D, Elliman D (eds.) (2006) *Health for all children.* 5th ed. Oxford: Oxford University Press.

Hill M, Davis J, Prout A, Tisdall K (2004) Moving the participation agenda forward. *Children and Society* 18: 77–96.

HM Government (2004) *Every child matters: change for children.* London: Department for Education and Skills.

HM Treasury (2007) *Aiming high for Young People: A ten year strategy for positive outcomes.* Available at www.hm-treasury.gov.uk.

Holt J (1975) *Escape from childhood, the needs and rights of children.* Harmondsworth: Penguin.

House of Commons (2001) Children's Commissioner for Wales Bill. London: HMSO. Available at http://www.parliament.the-stationery-office.co.uk/pa/cm200001/cmbills/003/2001003.htm.

Hoyles M (1989) *The politics of childhood.* London: Journeyman.

J (A Minor) (Child in Care: Medical Treatment) [1993] Fam 15.

J (A Minor) (Prohibited Steps Order: Circumcision) [2000] 1 FLR 571.

James A, Jenks G, Prout A (1999) *Theorising childhood.* London: Policy Press.

James A, Prout A (eds.) (1990) *Constructing and reconstructing childhood.* Basingstoke: Falmer Press.

Kempe CH (1962) The battered child syndrome. *JAMA* 181: 17–24.

Kennedy I, Grubb A (2000) *Medical law: text and materials.* 3rd ed. London: LexisNexis.

Kennedy I, Grubb A (2002) *Principles of medical law.* Oxford: Oxford University Press.

Lansdown G (2001) *Promoting children's participation in democratic decision making.* Florence: UNICEF.

Liberal Democrats (2009) *Free to be young.* Available at www.libdems.org.uk.

Lowden J (2002) Children's rights: a decade of dispute. *Journal of Advanced Nursing* 37(1): 100–7.

Main G, Bradshaw J (2014) *Child poverty and social exclusion: final report of 2012 PSE study.* York: University of York, Poverty and Social Exclusion in the UK. Available at http://www.poverty.ac.uk/sites/default/files/attachments/PSE-Child-poverty-and-exclusion-final-report-2014.pdf.

Mayall B (ed.) (1994) *Children's childhoods: observed and experienced.* London: Falmer Press.

Mayall B (1996) *Children, health and social order.* Milton Keynes: Open University Press.

Mayall B (2002) *Towards a sociology of childhood. Thinking from children's lives.* Buckinghamshire: Open University Press.

Mental Capacity Act (2005) Available at http://www.legislation.gov.uk/ukpga/2005/9/contents.

National Assembly for Wales (2008) *The National Service Framework for the Future Provision of advocacy services for children in Wales.* Cardiff: NAW.

National Assembly for Wales (2015a) *Violence against Women, Domestic Abuse and Sexual Violence (Wales) Bill.* Notice of amendments. Tabled 24 February 2015. Available at http://www.senedd.assembly.wales/documents/s37042/Notice%20of%20amendments%2024%20February%202015.pdf.

National Assembly for Wales (2015b) *Violence against Women, Domestic Abuse and Sexual Violence (Wales) Bill.* Cardiff: Welsh Government. Available at http://www.senedd.assembly.wales/documents/s37622/Violence%20against%20Women%20Domestic%20Abuse%20and%20Sexual%20Violence%20Wales%20Bill%20as%20passed.pdf.

Neill AS (1962) *Summerhill.* Harmondsworth: Penguin.

New Labour (2007) Available at www.bbc.co.uk (accessed 5 February 2017).

An NHS Trust v MB and Mr & Mrs B [2006] EWHC 507.

Noyes J (2000) Are nurses respecting and upholding the human rights of children and young people in their care? *Paediatric Nursing* 12(2): 23–7.

Nursing and Midwifery Council (2015) *Code of professional conduct.* London: NMC.

Office of National Statistics (2012) *Statistical bulletin: deaths registered in England and wales, 2012.* Newport: ONS. Available at http://www.ons.gov.uk/ons/rel/vsob1/death-reg-sum-tables/2012/sb-deaths-first-release--2012.html.

Office of Public Sector Information (1933) The Children and Young Persons Act. Available at http://www.opsi.gov.uk/RevisedStatutes/Acts/ukpga/1933/cukpga_19330012_en_1.

Office of Public Sector Information (1969) The Family Law Reform Act. Available at http://www.opsi.gov.uk/RevisedStatutes/Acts/ukpga/1969/cukpga_19690046_en_1.

Office of Public Sector Information (1976) The Adoption Act. Available at http://www.opsi.gov.uk/RevisedStatutes/Acts/ukpga/1976/cukpga_19760036_en_1.

Office of Public Sector Information (1977) The National Health Service Act. Available at http://www.opsi.gov.uk/RevisedStatutes/Acts/ukpga/1977/cukpga_19770049_en_1.

Office of Public Sector Information (1978) The National Health Service Act (Scotland). Edinburgh: Local Government Boundary Commission for Scotland. Available at http://www.statutelaw.gov.uk/content.

Office of Public Sector Information (1987) The Family Law Reform Act. Available at http://www.statutelaw.gov.uk/leg.

Office of Public Sector Information (1989) The Children Act. Available at http://www.opsi.gov.uk/acts/acts1989/ukpga_19890041_en_1.

Office of Public Sector Information (1998) The Human Rights Act. Available at http://www.opsi.gov.uk/acts/acts1998/ukpga_19980042_en_1.

Office of Public Sector Information (2000) The Care Standards Act. Available at http://www.opsi.gov.uk/acts/acts2000/ukpga_20000014_en_1.

Office of Public Sector Information (2002) The Adoption and Children Act. Available at http://www.opsi.gov.uk/acts/acts2002/ukpga_20020038_en_1.

Office of Public Sector Information (2003) The Sexual Offences Act. Available at http://www.opsi.gov.uk/acts/acts2003/ukpga_20030042_en_1.

Office of Public Sector Information (2004) The Children Act. Available at http://www.opsi.gov.uk/acts/acts2004/ukpga_20040031_en_1.

O'Halloran K (1999) *The welfare of the child: the principle and the law. A study of the meaning, role, and functions of the principle as it has evolved within the family law of England and Wales.* Aldershot: Ashgate Arena.

Payne M (1995) Children's rights and needs. *Health Visitor* 68(10): 412–14.

Public Health Wales (2012) Deprivation and inequalities 'What are the impacts'? Available at http://www.wales.nhs.uk/sitesplus/888/page/43764.

R (Axon) v Secretary of State for Health [2006] EWHC 37.

Re B (A Child) [2003] EWCA Civ 1148 (CA).

Re B (A Minor) (Wardship: Medical Treatment) [1981] 1 WLR 1421.

Re J [2000] 1 FLR 571 (Fam).

Re L (Medical Treatment: Gillick Competence) [1998] 2 FLR 810.

Re M (A Child) (Refusal of Medical Treatment) [1999] 2 FLR 1097 (CA).

Re R (A Minor) (Wardship Consent to Treatment) [1992] 1 FLR 190.

Re W (A Minor) (Medical Treatment Court's Jurisdiction) [1992] 3 WLR 758.

Rowse V (2007) Consent in severely disabled children: informed or an infringement of their rights? *Journal of Child Health Care* 11(1): 70–8.

Royal College of Paediatrics and Child Health (1997) *Withholding or withdrawing life saving treatment in children: a framework for practice.* London: RCPCH.

Royal College of Paediatrics and Child Health (2000) Guidelines for the ethical conduct of medical research involving children. *Archives of Disease in Childhood* 82: 177–82.

Royal College of Paediatrics and Child Health (2012) *Involving children and young people in health services.* London: RCPCH.

Royal College of Paediatrics and Child Health (2015) *Public Health: Getting it right for Children and Young People.* London: RCPCH.

Scottish Government (2009) *Do the right thing.* A response by the Scottish government to the 2008 concluding observations from the UN Committee on the Rights of the Child. Edinburgh: Scottish Government.

Shakespeare T, Watson N (1998) *Theoretical perspectives of research with disabled children.* London: Jessica Kingsley.

Shier H (2001) Pathways to participation: openings, opportunities and obligations. *Children and Society* 15: 107–17.

Sidaway v Bethlem Royal Hospital [1985] AC 871.

Sidey A, Widdas D (eds.) (2005) *Textbook of children's community nursing.* 2nd ed. Edinburgh: Elsevier.

Sinclair R (ed.) (1996) Special issue on research with children. *Children and Society* 10(2): editorial.

Sinclair R (2004) Participation in practice: making it meaningful and sustainable. *Children and Society* 18: 106–18.

Sinclair R, Franklin A (2000) *Young people's participation.* London: Department of Health.

Smith L, Coleman V (eds.) (2010) *Child and family centred health care: concepts, theory and practice.* 2nd ed. Basingstoke: Palgrave Macmillan.

Swansea University, University of Central Lancashire, Save the Children (2008) *Evaluating the children's commissioner for Wales.* Cardiff: Children's Commissioner.

Tait W (1883) *The works of Jeremy Bentham.* Vol. 3. Edinburgh: Edinburgh University Press.

United Nations (1989) Convention on the rights of the child adopted under General Assembly resolution 44/25. Geneva: UN.

United Nations Committee on the Rights of the Child (2008) Consideration of reports submitted by states parties under Article 44 of the convention. Concluding observations of the Committee on the Rights of the Child: United Kingdom of Great Britain and Northern Ireland. Geneva: UN.

Verhellen E (ed.) (1996) *Monitoring children's rights.* The Hague: Martinus Nijhoff.

Wanless D (2003) *The review of health and social care in Wales.* Cardiff: Welsh Assembly Government.

Waterhouse R, Clough M, Le Fleming M (1999) *Lost in care: report of the tribunal inquiry into the abuse of children in care in the former county councils of Gwynedd and Clwyd since 1974.* London: Stationery Office.

Welsh Assembly Government (2000) *Framework for partnership with children and young people.* Cardiff: WAG.

Welsh Assembly Government (2002) *Participation of children via an interactive.* Available at www.funkydragon.org.

Welsh Assembly Government (2004) *Children and young people: rights to action.* Cardiff: WAG.

Welsh Assembly Government (2005a) *The National Service Framework for children, young people and maternity services.* Cardiff: WAG.

Welsh Assembly Government (2005b) A study of advocacy services for children and young people in Wales. Cardiff: WAG. Available at http://wales.gov.uk/caec/publications/childrenandyoungpeople/advocacystudy/advocacyen.pdf?lang=en.

Welsh Assembly Government (2008a) *Rights in action.* Cardiff: WAG.

Welsh Assembly Government (2008b) Children and young people's wellbeing monitor for Wales. Cardiff: WAG.

Welsh Assembly Government (2009) *Getting it right.* Cardiff: WAG.

Welsh Government (2011a) Children and young people's wellbeing monitor for Wales. Cardiff: WG.

Welsh Government (2011b) Rights of Children and Young Persons (Wales) Measure 2011. Cardiff: WG.

Williams J, Jackson S, Maddocks A, et al. (2001) Case–control study of the health of those looked after by local authorities. *Archives of Disease in Childhood* 85: 280–5.

Willow C (2002) The state of children's rights in 2002. *Childright* 187: 120–9.

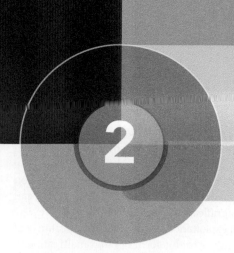

2

Safeguarding and child protection

CATHERINE POWELL

OVERVIEW

This chapter is concerned with one of the most challenging and emotive aspects of child health care, that of child maltreatment. Underpinned by a children's rights perspective, the chapter introduces the professional roles and responsibilities of children and young people's nurses in safeguarding and promoting the welfare of children. It seeks to influence a positive and proactive approach, helping practitioners to feel confident and supported in their roles and able to recognize that safeguarding is primarily concerned with helping and supporting parents in the provision of safe and effective care for their children.

INTRODUCTION

Safeguarding and child protection are first and foremost everyone's responsibility: this includes children and young people themselves, their parents, their families and their communities. However, it is clearly also the remit of those whose professional lives bring them into contact with children. Ensuring children and young people are safe from harm is challenging work, but it can be incredibly rewarding to know that you have helped to protect a child from an abusive or neglectful situation. As a children and young people's nurse or another practitioner working in the field of children and young people's health care, you are ideally placed to recognize situations where children may be at risk of or suffering from harm. This is in part because of your skills in child health and development, but also because your experiences of diverse patterns of family life will help you to recognize when a child's demeanour, behaviour or physical signs do not appear to fit within the spectrum of what might be considered 'normal'. This chapter, which has been extensively revised and updated for the second edition of this book, aims to provide you with the knowledge, confidence and ability to successfully and proactively safeguard and promote the welfare of children and young people in line with your professional code of conduct and statutory and professional guidance (Royal College of Paediatrics and Child Health 2014; Nursing and Midwifery Council 2015; HM Government 2015a).*

REFLECTION POINTS

- How did you feel when you read the opening lines of this chapter?
- How confident are you about your role in protecting children and young people?
- What sources of advice and support for safeguarding children/young people are available to you in your current role?

---

* Unless stated otherwise, the references to statutory guidance are those for England.

The chapter sets out how the United Nations Convention on the Rights of the Child (UNCRC) 1989 has influenced and supported the development of legislation, policy and guidance that keep the focus firmly on children's best interests and their right to be safe and protected. It then provides some definitions of key terms, including what is meant by *safeguarding, child protection, child maltreatment* and *significant harm*. The challenges of measuring the prevalence of maltreatment are also discussed. The chapter next focuses on the principles for practice that help to maximize the nursing contribution to safeguarding and child protection within the multi-agency arena. There is an overview of the provision of assessment-based 'early help' that can promote children's well-being and safety and diminish the risk of significant harm, followed by a brief review of the key categories of child maltreatment, including child sexual exploitation (CSE) and the importance of children and young people's nurses better recognizing and responding to this form of child maltreatment. The case of Victoria Climbié is outlined as providing seminal learning that has cast long shadows forward in changing policy for children and improving practice.

The chapter closes with an overview of the purpose of serious case review (SCR) and the statutory child death review process. The contents of the chapter provide a logical structure that links theory, policy and nursing practice with the ultimate aim of informing and improving practice to benefit the children, young people and families in our care. While written primarily for children and young people's nurses, this chapter is also relevant to the wider group of nursing practitioners who work with children, young people and their families. As such, it recognizes both the range of provision and the powerful potential of a large and diverse workforce (Powell 2016). However, although knowledge and understanding of the subject matter are the keys to success, it is also important to recognize the emotional burden of safeguarding and child protection work, and therefore the need to ensure robust clinical supervision and support. The chapter closes by giving some links to additional sources of information and support.

CHILDREN AND THEIR RIGHT TO PROTECTION

The UNCRC (United Nations 1989) (see also Chapter 1) establishes the irrefutable rights of children and young people and outlines the actions and responsibilities of governments in ensuring that services for children are offered in a child-centred, rights-based framework. The UN convention has been ratified by every country in the world but two: South Sudan and the US. (Somalia, who had not been in a position to sign up previously, ratified the convention in January 2015.)

The UN convention proposes both welfare rights (such as food, health care, housing and education) and protective rights (e.g. from child maltreatment) which are embodied in a series of clauses known as 'Articles'. There is a strong emphasis on ensuring that children and young people have a healthy and safe development into adulthood, together with the provision of extra support for parents and services to meet the needs of children in 'special circumstances'. This group includes children who are disabled, children in the care system and children who are refugees. In essence, the UN convention aims to ensure the best outcomes for children and young people everywhere and provides a mandate for governments to achieve this. The right to freedom from child maltreatment is one of the protective rights and is enshrined in Article 19, which states:

State parties shall take all appropriate legislative, administrative, social and educational measures to protect the child from all forms of physical or mental violence, injury or abuse, neglect or negligent treatment, maltreatment or exploitation, including sexual abuse, while in the care of parent(s), legal guardian(s) or any other person who has care of the child.

Such protective measures should, as appropriate, include effective procedures for the establishment of social programmes to provide necessary support for the child, and for those who have care of the child, as well as for other forms of prevention and for identification, reporting, referral, investigation, treatment and follow up of instances of child maltreatment described heretofore, and, as appropriate, for judicial involvement.

United Nations 1989, Article 19

The four countries of the UK (England, Wales, Scotland and Northern Ireland) have adopted the legal definition of a child as being an individual who has not yet reached the age of 18 years. This is in line with the convention and is the definition used within all of the UK's safeguarding guidance, policy and legislation (All Wales Child Protection Procedures Review Group 2008; HM Government 2015a; Office of the First Minister and Deputy First Minister Northern Ireland 2009; Scottish Government 2014; Welsh Assembly Government 2007). The fact that childhood legally ends at 18 years of age can present a challenge for ensuring the safety and well-being of older children using child health services because young people over the age of 16 years generally begin to choose to access, or to make the transition to, health care in a range of adult-centric settings. It is therefore essential that an awareness of safeguarding and child protection practice and professional responsibilities in keeping children safe reaches those working in 'adult' settings who are likely to encounter 16- and 17-year-olds in the course of their practice. A notable exception is found in Child and Adolescent Mental Health Services (CAMHS), which provide services up until the age of 18 years. This rests on an explicit requirement to ensure that young people under this age who require inpatient care are not admitted to adult mental health facilities because of the risk of harm in that environment (Office of the Children's Commissioner/Young Minds 2007). The case for adolescent units for all institutional health care has, of course, been made, but the provision for older children outside of CAMHS is scanty and reflects adolescents as a 'forgotten group' in health service provision (Kennedy 2010: 38).

In addition to their responsibilities to safeguard and promote the welfare of 16- and 17-year-olds, adult nursing practitioners may also find themselves in a situation where they have to take action because of concerns that arise in relation to children and young people whose parents or carers are the primary service user. An example may be those practicing in urgent care settings who are providing care for adults who present with alcohol misuse, acute mental health problems or injuries arising from suspected domestic violence. Clearly, where the adults have responsibilities as parents these problems may be impacting their ability to provide safe care for their children, and as such it is pertinent for the practitioner to make an informed assessment of the risks and refer to statutory agencies accordingly. Ensuring that safeguarding children and young people is seen as everyone's responsibility, and being in a position to support and supervise practice, is arguably a vital component of the role of children's leads and children's champions across all health care organizations.

REFLECTION POINTS

- Think about the organization in which you practice. Is there 24/7 access to a practitioner with the qualifications and skills to support and advise on all aspects of the care of children and young people, including safeguarding?
- Are you aware of how you can link to services that provide adult mental health or substance misuse care?

It is also important to clarify the situation for unborn children. Although unborn children are not legally defined as children (see, for example, the Children Act 1989), their needs for safety and protection from harm must still be considered in cases where there is concern about the expectant parents' ability to ensure their future safety and well-being. Identifying and responding to such concerns is primarily the responsibility of the midwife and others providing care in the antenatal period, but it is also pertinent to note that in some cases the 'parent to be' may be a child themselves, even if they are living independently from their own parent or, indeed, married.

CHILDHOOD: A GOLDEN AGE?

It is helpful for all practitioners to have an understanding of the nature of contemporary childhood and an appreciation that this is not necessarily reflective of the positive, creative, loving and caring experiences that we would all aspire to, or have been lucky enough to experience. Although readers are encouraged to access the wider literature on the topic, a very brief overview is given here.

The existence of childhood as a separate and distinct chronological stage to adulthood has raised some interesting debates; these embrace the notion of children's rights and the role of parents and the state in ensuring that children and young people have the best possible upbringing (see, for example, the seminal work of Archard 2004). The deliberations about the nature of contemporary childhood often highlight the *oppression* of children through a lack of human rights afforded to others; this is important because it has been linked to their vulnerability to child maltreatment. Examples of the oppression of children include their disenfranchisement, their lack of a say in issues that concern them and the continued use and legality of corporal punishment (i.e. hitting) and other forms of negative chastisement in many societies, including the UK (visit the Children Are Unbeatable! Alliance website for more information). Continuing evidence of children as an oppressed group includes the expectations held by adults of subservience and children's segregation or their exclusion from certain activities or environments. Conversely, those familiar with the child-friendly environment that is close to Great Ormond Street Hospital for Children will, like me, take delight in noting that the entrance to the play park in Coram Fields has a notice stating that 'no adult can enter without a child'.

REFLECTION POINTS

- Think about the language used by adults, including children and young people's nurses, in relation to children and young people.
- How often do we hear small human beings (i.e. infants) being described as 'it'; is this term applied to any other groups in our society?
- What do you think about the negative connotation of the word *childish*?
- What messages about children are portrayed by notices on corner shops or other establishments banning unaccompanied children?
- Are school days the 'best days of your life'?

CASE STUDY

Jodie, a bright and able 10-year-old girl, often misses school and is beginning to fall behind with her learning; last term her recorded attendance demonstrated a drop from 87% to 62%. Many of these absences are recorded as being 'unauthorized'. Jodie's mother, June, is known to suffer from depression and anxiety, and in the past the police have notified agencies (health, social care and education) of some quite serious incidents of domestic abuse. Jodie's stepfather is thought to have a dependency on alcohol, and both parents smoke heavily. The family live in a privately rented house in a run-down area of the city. The landlord is supposed to be undertaking some repairs to tackle a damp issue, but the family has waited for this to happen for some time now. The school nurse visits the home to make an assessment of any health issues that may be preventing her from attending school. An education welfare officer is also in attendance. Jodie is noticed to be thin and unhappy, but anxious to please. She is suffering from wheeziness and uses an inhaler. It seems that June has been relying on her to be the main carer of her 17-month-old half-sibling, Tyron; this includes taking a key role in feeding, changing and bathing routines. Jodie explains that although she loves her baby brother, she is missing her friends and worries about what her teachers will say when she returns to school. The toddler, who appears somewhat grubby and underoccupied, looks to Jodie for comfort in the presence of the two professionals.

REFLECTION POINTS

- What are the key health care needs for each member of this family and how can they best be met?
- How might children like Jodie and Tyron be supported in achieving a good childhood?
- What do positive outcomes of professional intervention look like?

The Children's Society (2014) *Good Childhood* report compares the well-being of children in the UK with those from other westernized countries in Europe and North America. The report provides evidence that children in the UK do not fare well when compared to the experiences of other children in most of these other countries. Children's lower levels of self-reported well-being were found to be clearly correlated with poverty and deprivation, with the impact of economic recession reported to be acutely felt by many children. Protective factors, contributing to a more positive self-reported well-being in childhood, included being active and having access to a computer for social interactions. Importantly, children and young people whose parents offered praise for them doing well, and supported them when they felt upset, reported happier childhoods. Higher levels of well-being were also found in children who said that they were given autonomy and choice. Participative research with children can go some way in ensuring that their voice is heard and that policies are responsive to their needs and experiences.

Children and young people's nurses have been instrumental in tackling some of the traditions of children's oppression, for example by inclusion of children's participation in the design and delivery of services, but there remains more to do. In essence, an understanding of how to influence policies affecting health, long since a cornerstone of health visiting practice (Cowley and Frost 2006), is important for all those on health and social care professional registers who seek to maximize the health and well-being of their client group. This means being able to use the evidence to support changes in health and welfare provision that will benefit children, young people and their families now and in the years to come.

PARENTS

Parents ultimately have the primary role and responsibility to ensure that their children are safe and well cared for, and this is recognized in the UNCRC (1989) in reference to 'those who have care of the child' (see above). However, parenting is widely recognized to be one of the most challenging roles that anyone does, quite probably with the least preparation. Children and young people's nurses, and other health care practitioners who work with families, will recognize that good parenting means providing children with a consistent, warm and loving relationship. It also involves ensuring that their health and welfare needs are met, they are kept safe and protected from harm, they have stimulation and opportunities to learn, and they have the boundaries, stability and consistency that best support their developmental needs into adulthood.

An understanding of the components of good parenting is important in successfully safeguarding children because it can help children and young people's nurses to support parents in providing optimal care for their children within the constraints of their personal, social and economic circumstances. It also provides practitioners with a benchmark for their assessment of family strengths and deficits, including any risk of harm to children and young people. Referring parents to sources of early help and support within universal and targeted provision is an important protective element of safeguarding and child protection practice and one that a range of child health practitioners are well placed to contribute to (see, for example, the *Healthy Child Programme*, Department of Health, Department for Children, Schools and Families 2009a, 2009b). In supporting parents, it is essential to ensure that fathers (including 'absent' fathers) are engaged in the delivery of health care to their children. This is an area that continues to be subject to innovation and improvement following concerns that fathers are often excluded. For example, the work of the National Society for the Prevention of Cruelty to Children (NSPCC) supports Dad's Project, which helps practitioners consider fathers' involvement in pregnancy and the first year of their child's life (Hogg 2014).

REFLECTION POINTS

- How do parents learn how to parent?
- What might 'good parenting' look like?
- At what point should agencies intervene when parenting is thought to be inadequate?
- Do you routinely engage with fathers and how do you ensure that information on their children's health needs is fed back to them, especially in situations where they are absent?

PROMOTING CHILD AND FAMILY-CENTRED CARE

Children and young people's nurses have done much to promote the notion of 'family-centred' care, and this has undoubtedly improved the health care experiences of children and young people over the past 25 years or so and is rightly celebrated within this book. However, as I have previously noted, 'child and family-centred care' may be a more appropriate concept because there is the ever-present danger that in engaging with some families, children and young people's nurses may be drawn to the pressing needs and difficulties of parents, with the risk of failing to fully consider the child's perspective on their experiences and also their views (Powell 2007). Ensuring that the needs and experiences of the child are central to care is particularly important where there are emergent concerns about the possibility of fabricated or induced illness, as well as other forms of maltreatment.

SAFEGUARDING AND CHILD PROTECTION

The terms *safeguarding* and *child protection* are often used interchangeably, with the latter term having something of a revival since the publication of the first edition of this text (see, for example, Munro 2011).

However, *safeguarding* is best seen as an umbrella term that both encompasses child protection and embraces wider activity to support the well-being of children. This can be illustrated by the increasing emphasis on the provision of preventative and early help services to families. According to statutory guidance, safeguarding is defined as

> protecting children from maltreatment; preventing impairment of children's health or development; ensuring that children are growing up in circumstances consistent with the provision of safe and effective care and taking action to enable all children to have the best life chances.

> *HM Government 2015a: 92*

Other countries of the UK, and indeed those with a similar tradition of child welfare (e.g. Australia), take a similar stance. The overarching aim of safeguarding work is to make sure children and young people are able to reach their potential and enter adulthood successfully, and that parents are supported as having the key responsibility to ensure that this happens. Recognizing and responding to children and young people who are at risk of or suffering from child maltreatment and ensuring their protection is an important element of safeguarding practice.

REFLECTION POINT

How does your professional role help to ensure that children and young people enter adulthood successfully?

CHILD MALTREATMENT

Child maltreatment (sometimes referred to as 'child abuse and neglect') is a challenging concept to define simply because what is, and is not, considered to be harmful to a child or young person is often subjective, and will vary over time and between individuals according to their knowledge, beliefs and values (Corby et al. 2012). Statutory guidance (HM Government 2015a) recognizes that child maltreatment may reflect acts of commission as well as omission (i.e. neglect). The World Health Organization's definition provides a succinct and inclusive depiction:

> Child abuse or maltreatment consists of all forms of physical and/or emotional ill-treatment, sexual abuse, neglect or negligent treatment or commercial, or other exploitation, resulting in actual or potential harm to the child's health, survival, development or dignity in the context of a relationship of responsibility, trust or power.

> *Butchart et al. 2006: 59*

While statutory guidance and child protection planning similarly reflect 'categories' of maltreatment, i.e. physical, emotional, sexual abuse or neglect, the reality is that these forms of maltreatment overlap and may co-exist. Child maltreatment is largely perpetrated by parents or carers and others known to the child, including other children. Stranger danger, a source of anxiety to many parents, is by comparison a rare event; indeed it is quite possible that the impact of children being 'wrapped in cotton wool' has led to significantly more harm to children's health and development within populations. Children and young people's nurses will, however, also be aware from the extensive media coverage and ongoing reviews of the existence of so-called 'celebrity abuse'. This includes the alleged abuse perpetrated in hospital settings by the late Jimmy Savile. At the time of writing, institutions were reviewing their policies and procedures concerning hospital visits and engagements by those in the public domain (Gray and Watt 2013; Lampard 2014).

SIGNIFICANT HARM

The concept of 'significant harm', introduced by the Children Act 1989 (England and Wales), is important because it is considered to be the threshold for statutory intervention in family life (i.e. child protection proceedings). When making judgments, lead statutory agencies (children's social care and police) will work with their inter-agency partners, including health representatives, to consider the nature of the harm, the impact on the health and development, any special needs, the parenting capacity to meet the needs of the child and the context of the family and environment. In reality most cases requiring child protection proceedings will reflect a context of concern, rather than necessarily a single easily identifiable incident. The provision of health services to children provides an important 'window of opportunity' for prevention, early help and rescue.

REFLECTION POINTS

- Which of the following scenarios could indicate the possibility of child maltreatment?
  - An expectant mother is smoking small quantities of cannabis.
  - Timothy's father often tells him that he was not wanted; Timothy has Down's syndrome.
  - A mother lashes out at her four-year-old, who has wet the bed for the third time in three nights. She leaves a small bruise on his back.
  - Sally, who is HIV positive, is refusing to allow her baby to be tested.
  - Rosie and John who are 10 and 8 years old are often home before their mother in the evenings.
  - Jim, aged 12 years, is missing school because he has to help care for his disabled father.
  - Tyler, aged 2 years, has sustained a fractured femur. There appears to be no history of how it happened.
  - Joshua, aged 5 years, never seems to be appropriately dressed in cold weather.
  - Usha, aged 14 years, is sleeping with her 19-year-old boyfriend.
  - The parents of Sam, who has cystic fibrosis, have rejected conventional medicine and are treating her with homeopathy.
  - Abdul, aged 14 months, travels unrestrained in his parents' car. They report that they cannot afford a car seat.
  - A father insists on tucking in his 7-year-old stepdaughter; he says it is their 'special time'.
  - Jenna, who is 8 years old, lies awake at night hearing her parents arguing loudly.
- What else would you need to know? In all these cases further information needs to be gathered. The focus of decision making, however, must always be on the impact on, and perspective of, the child (adapted from Powell 2007).

PREVALENCE

It is difficult to say with certainty how many children and young people suffer from child maltreatment in the course of their childhood; it may be a largely hidden problem and identification and response rests on recognition of the issues by professionals and society alike. Corby et al. (2012) suggest that a complete picture of the scale of child maltreatment is unlikely to be established; albeit there are some data sets which can help to inform an understanding. Over the last few years, the NSPCC has led the production of an annual report that draws together a range of data that provides an indication of the safety and well-being of children in the UK (Jütte et al. 2015). The latest report is signalling some welcome improvements in younger children's lived experiences. However, there is still much to do. The report also notes that almost one in five children aged 11–17 years that were surveyed reported experiencing maltreatment while growing up.

Child fatality in the context of maltreatment also appears to be declining in the UK (Sidebotham et al. 2012; Jütte et al. 2015). While such deaths are rare, they may be pivotal in determining policy and practice (see Box 2.1). Although not all deaths from maltreatment will be in the public eye, the number of such deaths is approximately one per week, and while each death represents a terrible tragedy, this is the lowest number since the early 1980s (Jütte et al. 2015). Research that has considered the learning from maltreatment deaths has found that the risks are highest in infancy, but there is also a peak in adolescence, due to risk taking or suicide among young people who had been abused or neglected in their earlier childhood (Brandon et al. 2014). Again, we need to consider how well this age group are cared for by child health services and whether more could be done to meet their particular needs.

The first part of this chapter considered the UN convention and its place in informing safeguarding children policy and legislation, and provided key definitions and an overview of the current understanding of the prevalence of child maltreatment in the UK. A children's rights perspective aids an understanding of the need to consider the lived experiences of children and to ensure that they are listened to, and above all have a right to grow up free from abuse and neglect. A summary of key points thus far is provided below. The second part of the chapter sets out some of the key principles for practice, including ensuring a sound knowledge base to help to identify children who are at risk of or suffering from child maltreatment and to prevent, recognize and respond accordingly.

- Safeguarding children is 'everyone's responsibility'; this includes those whose primary clients are adults.
- The UN Convention on the Rights of the Child (United Nations 1989) explicitly promotes the rights of children to protection from harm, as well as outlining the welfare rights that support healthy development into adulthood.
- Safeguarding children guidance and legislation apply throughout childhood, i.e. until an individual has reached the age of 18 years.
- Although unborn babies are not included in the legal definition of 'a child', it may be necessary to consider safeguarding needs and plan accordingly.
- Protecting children and young people from maltreatment is part of safeguarding, but safeguarding children is a broader concept.
- Child maltreatment is largely perpetrated by parents or carers or others known to the child, including other children.
- There are signs of some improvements in the safety and well-being of children and young people, including fewer deaths from maltreatment. However, there remains much to achieve.

PRINCIPLES FOR PRACTICE

Successful safeguarding children practice balances support for parents, and parenting, with the centrality of the child or young person, their needs and their *right* to be protected from harm. This is a message that has also been shared by Laming (2009), who in reporting on progress on safeguarding and child protection practice post Climbié has eloquently suggested four principles of good practice, which are as follows:

- Put yourself in the place of the child and consider first and foremost how the situation must feel for them.
- Be aware of how easy it is to find yourself justifying and reassuring yourself that all is well, rather than taking a more objective consideration of what has occurred.
- Recognize that sympathy for the parents can lead to your expectations of their parenting being set too low.
- Remember that whatever role you have (i.e. working with the child or their parents/carers or as a member of the public) be clear that it is not acceptable to do nothing when a child may be in need of help.

These cornerstones of good practice provide an excellent basis on which to build competence and confidence in safeguarding and child protection work. They can also usefully be accommodated within clinical supervision to help to ensure that the focus remains on the child and their lived experiences. The following sections add to this by first considering the related concept of authoritative practice and then the more practical, but equally important, aspects of information sharing and record keeping.

REFLECTION POINT

What are the issues that lead professionals to feel sympathy for parents? How might these issues impact the well-being of the child?

AUTHORITATIVE PRACTICE

Safeguarding and child protection practice is first and foremost dependent on the establishment of a compassionate and trusting relationship with families (Munro 2011). However, there is also a need to ensure that, where necessary, parents and carers are appropriately challenged about their provision of 'safe and effective care' to their children. Authoritative practice is a concept that has been widely promoted in the wake of the high-profile death of Peter Connelly (Haringey Local Safeguarding Children Board 2009). This is an important principle for practice, whereby practitioners are encouraged to demonstrate 'curiosity and respectful uncertainty' about potentially concerning presentations or stated progress and ensure that their focus remains on the child and their daily lived experiences. As Tuck (2013) notes, authoritative practice is particularly significant in addressing the drift or lack of progress, often caused by disguised or partial compliance that is seen in some complex safeguarding and child protection cases. It may also be important to be able to triangulate information about the child and family's needs and strengths with other colleagues, and perhaps other agencies.

SHARING INFORMATION

Children and young people's nurses, and other health care professionals may feel anxious about sharing information, particularly with those from outside of the immediate circle of carers or from other agencies, such as children's social care services. However, the reality of safeguarding and child protection practice is that emergent concerns may triangulate with other pieces of information that are already known and that together suggest a picture of a child who may be at risk of or suffering from harm. Sharing information can also help to identify sources of strength and support and ensure timely help for a family. Information-sharing guidance is available to help practitioners share information appropriately, securely and within the limits posed by legislation (i.e. Data Protection Act 1998) and their professional code (e.g. Nursing and Midwifery Council 2015) while promoting the importance of being open and seeking consent to share, unless it would place the child at greater risk (HM Government 2015b). A failure to share information in a timely manner is an important message from reviews of cases where children have suffered serious harm, including death from maltreatment.

RECORD KEEPING

As with inadequacies in information sharing, poor record keeping is also a feature of learning from serious cases. Good records not only provide a clear, factual and contemporaneous account of care, but also provide an opportunity to justify professional actions, including decisions to share or not share information. Importantly they also provide an opportunity to record the views and wishes of the child. The professional code outlines expected standards and provides guidance on the use of electronic as well as paper records, including data storage (Nursing and Midwifery Council 2015).

REFLECTION POINT

How can you document a decision to take no further action?

RECOGNITION AND RESPONSE

Referring a child who may be at risk of or suffering from child maltreatment to the lead statutory agencies (social care or the police) is known to be a source of much anxiety to health care professionals, not least because of their concerns about their relationship with families (Gilbert et al. 2008). But, as noted earlier, it is the breadth of exposure to the range of normality within childhood and family life, together with an understanding of child health and development, that place children and young people's nurses (and other child health practitioners) in a good position to recognize and respond to concerns. What is important is to do so in a timely and proportionate way.

EARLY HELP

The use of the term *early help* is gaining prominence within safeguarding and child protection practice, not least as a term that reflects collaboration and partnership with families, rather than the 'doing to' suggested by the notion of early intervention (Munro 2011). According to statutory guidance, a framework of early help services can ensure that families receive the right help, at the right time, and prevent additional needs (over and above universal provision) from becoming more acute, requiring children's social care involvement and the potential for compulsory intervention in family life, i.e. child protection proceedings (HM Government 2015a).

Local authorities (in England) are currently replacing the Common Assessment Framework (CAF) with an Early Help Assessment (EHA) which similarly helps frontline practitioners from a range of agencies to work with families to identify needs and strengths within the domains of 'child development', 'parents and carers' and 'family and environment' and to provide services accordingly. EHA is undertaken with parental (and where appropriate the child's) consent. As part of the assessment agreement will be sought to share information within and across agency boundaries to ensure that the right services are provided in a timely manner. Where several people are working with a family a meeting, often referred to as a 'Team around the Child' (TAC) or 'Team around the Family' (TAF), will occur. The child and family, and any 'significant others' will normally be invited to the meeting.

The EHA aims to prevent the delays and frustration caused by a lack of integrated working that previously may have resulted in children, young people and their families having to be re-assessed, being confused by fragmented or overlapping services or falling through gaps in 'the system'. The development of multi-agency safeguarding hubs (often known as MASHs), where services are co-located, is also leading to improved opportunities to coordinate early help provision and a timely response to need. MASHs may refer children and families of concern for early help rather than requiring a statutory response from children's social care. However, for a minority of children and young people the presenting concerns (which may include a lack of parental consent for an EHA or signs of a lack of compliance with early help planning) are such that a referral to children's social care (and in an emergency the police) will be necessary. Children and young people's nurses can seek help in making such a referral from their manager or local safeguarding children leads.

RECOGNITION OF CHILD MALTREATMENT

As we have stated, children and young people's nurses are well placed to recognize and respond to cases of possible child maltreatment. Not all concerns about the welfare and safety of children can be responded to within the early help provision outlined above; there will be cases that need to be referred to lead statutory agencies as needing further inquiries as to the possibility of significant harm. The following section considers some of the indicators of different types of child maltreatment that practitioners may come across in the course of their practice. However, given the constraints of chapter space and the availability of a number of excellent resources, the descriptions are deliberately brief. The NICE guidance (National Collaborating Centre for Women's and Children's Health 2009) is recommended as an essential resource to aid decision making in whether you should be considering, suspecting or indeed excluding the likelihood of child maltreatment. The emotive nature of the work, the likely absence of a clear history, and above all, the fact that child health practitioners would normally expect and accept parental explanations of their child's presentation with an injury or illness make this an area of practice where it is essential to seek supervision and support from a manager or safeguarding lead (e.g. the named nurse). Referral can be made on the basis of children being at risk of or suffering significant harm; the main purpose of child protection proceedings is to put in place a statutory plan for the child's safety.

PHYSICAL ABUSE

According to statutory guidance, physical abuse involves 'hitting, shaking, throwing, poisoning, burning, scalding, drowning, suffocating or otherwise causing physical harm to a child' (HM Government 2015a: 92). Bruising is of particular significance, and therefore an understanding of patterns of accidental versus non-accidental (sometimes called intentional) injuries is helpful in identifying this form of abuse.

CASE STUDY

Ronald, aged 14 weeks, has been brought to the emergency department by his parents. His father explains that he has been 'off his feeds' and sleepier than usual. Your first thought is that Ronald has a mild viral infection. However, when he is undressed to be weighed and examined you notice a small bruise on his upper arm. Mother thinks that he may have rolled onto a small toy.

REFLECTION POINTS

- At what age do children roll from front to back or back to front?
- Why is an understanding of development important for assessment for possible child maltreatment?
- What is the significance of bruising in a not independently mobile child?

Fabricated or induced illness (FII) is also classified as physical abuse, and the response to any concerns of FII should be undertaken within the framework provided by statutory guidance. More details on FII are provided in supplementary guidance (HM Government 2008). A further form of abuse which has long since been recognized as maltreatment (and is illegal in the UK) is female genital mutilation (FGM). Children and young people's nurses should have an awareness of the need to recognize and respond to girls at risk of FGM. Again readers are referred to national guidance on FGM (Department of Health 2015), as well as the excellent resource provided by Royal College of Midwives et al. (2013).

EMOTIONAL ABUSE

Identification of emotional abuse can be challenging, not least because it relates to a 'context' rather than an incident. There are links to neglect, and also to the presence of domestic violence and abuse (in seeing or hearing the ill treatment of another). According to Davies and Ward (2012) emotional abuse can be the most damaging form of abuse because it directly impacts a child's need to be loved and nurtured.

SEXUAL ABUSE

Child sexual abuse (CSA) reflects both contact and non-contact sexual activity involving a child, whether or not they are aware of what is happening (HM Government 2015a). The number of children subject to child protection proceedings because of CSA per se remains disproportionately low at the current time. Child sexual exploitation (CSE) is a form of CSA that, at the time of writing, has a high profile in the media as a result of criminal trials in several major towns and cities. CSE victims are not necessarily responded to through statutory child protection channels, not least because many of the victims will be adults before they come forward. CSE is a form of maltreatment that is widespread, i.e. not just confined to certain areas of the country, rural and urban. It is initially difficult to recognize, is pernicious in its effects and has raised some very important debates about the way in which services have viewed and responded to the victims, who have essentially been seen as 'bad' children, rather than children who bad things have happened to. The use of the term *child prostitution* is now (quite rightly) scorned. Jütte et al. (2015) have noted the increase in the number of calls to help lines regarding CSE in the wake of the increased publicity. Readers are advised to familiarize themselves with the supplementary guidance (HM Government 2009) as well as more recently published practice guidelines from the Department for Education (2012).

NEGLECT

Neglect is the most common reason for children and young people to be subject to child protection proceedings. Like emotional abuse, neglect is contextual. The definition found in the statutory guidance includes failing to ensure access to medical care and treatment, an issue which led to a call to reframe missed appointments for children and young people as 'was not brought' (WNB) rather than 'did not attend' (DNA) (Powell and Appleton 2012). Research undertaken with children who have suffered neglect has highlighted the impact as making them feel 'depressed, unloved and invisible' (Action for Children 2014), and the association with suicide and self-harm has been noted.

CHILD DEATH AND SERIOUS CASE REVIEWS

The final part of this chapter considers the importance of learning from child deaths; two processes are described. The first, the serious case review (SCR), is detailed in Chapter 4 of the statutory guidance (HM Government 2015a), which considers all forms of 'learning and improvement' reviews in safeguarding and child protection, with SCR being undertaken when a child dies or is seriously injured as a result of child maltreatment (or the case is otherwise of public interest). The second process, child death review (Chapter 5 of the statutory guidance), applies in the case of all deaths of children. This is essentially a public health function that fits under the broader safeguarding umbrella, albeit cases can be referred to Local Safeguarding Children Board (LSCB) serious cases committees for consideration of an SCR if the review process finds concerns that are indicative of child maltreatment.

REFLECTION POINT

Visit your local LSCB website to access a local SCR. What are the recommendations and how do they impact your practice? Note: If there are no local reviews you can find a published review via the NSPCC repository for SCRs.

BOX 2.1: Victoria Climbié

Victoria Adjo Climbié was born on the Ivory Coast on 2 November 1991. She was said to be a lovable and intelligent child who, in 1998, was taken by a great aunt to France, and then to England, to ensure that she had access to a good education and better opportunities for the future. What followed was an almost unbelievable sequence of escalating violence and maltreatment that led to her death on 25 February 2000, at 8 years of age. Her postmortem was undertaken by a home office pathologist, who described this as the 'worst case [of child abuse] he had ever dealt with … or heard of.' He found a total of 128 separate injuries on her body (Laming 2003: 1). Victoria had been beaten with implements such as shoes, football boots, a coat hanger, a wooden cooking spoon and a bicycle chain. She was also said to have spent long periods of time tied up in a bin-bag, covered in urine and faeces and made to eat left-over food off a piece of plastic 'like a dog'. When Victoria was admitted to hospital in a moribund condition she was found to be bruised, deformed, hypothermic and malnourished. Kouao (the great aunt) and Manning (a boyfriend of the aunt) are both serving life sentences for her murder.

The report of Lord Laming's subsequent inquiry into the death of Victoria Climbié makes for distressing reading, both in terms of the details of the appalling maltreatment she suffered and because it highlights the missed opportunities that a variety of agencies had to intervene. Laming described the extent of failures in the child protection system as 'lamentable' (Laming 2003: 3). Victoria was seen at a general practice and admitted to two different hospitals: the first time because of concerns about various cuts and marks on her face and hands, and the second time following a scald to her face. The second admission was for nearly 2 weeks. In addition to the contact with statutory agencies (including health, children's social care and housing), she was seen from time to time by distant relatives and also members of the church. For a brief period of time Victoria was also cared for by a childminder; however, she did not attend school. It is fair to report that the possibilities of child maltreatment were raised by individual health professionals during both hospital admissions. However, as the inquiry into her death noted:

> The concerns that medical and nursing staff at the hospital told me [Laming] that they felt about Victoria never, in my view, crystallised into anything resembling a clear, well-thought-through picture of what they suspected had happened to her and that would have helped social services in determining how best to deal with her case.

Laming 2003: 274

A number of children and young people's nurses were called to give evidence to the inquiry panel. Here they reported observing (although not documenting) indicators of physical abuse. These included lesions that they later considered to be indicative of intentional harm, such as burns, belt marks and bites. As worrying were their reports of witnessing Victoria's demeanour in the presence of Kouao and Manning. This was described as a 'master and servant' relationship. The inquiry made a number of recommendations for health services, including addressing the need for good record keeping, the reconciliation of differences of opinion, proper planning for discharge and arrangements for follow-up. A particularly challenging finding was the lack of opportunity for Victoria to communicate what was happening to her, and in reading the report it is clear that 'adult-centric' needs (e.g. for housing) took priority over the needs and wishes of this tragic child and that misconstruction of cultural issues prevailed.

The case of Victoria Climbié has been instrumental in changing policy and practice in safeguarding children that continues to this day. The Victoria Climbié Foundation UK, which campaigned to support these changes, has opened a school in Victoria's memory in her home village of Abobo. Details of their website are given at the end of this chapter.

Public inquiries into child deaths were at the forefront of the development of SCRs, with the Maria Colwell Inquiry (Department of Health and Social Security 1974) being of note.

Today SCRs are normally published in full, via LSCB websites, but the cases are not necessarily high profile, and details of the child, family and involved professionals are generally anonymized. However, the case of Victoria Climbié was considered to be of such importance that it was subject to a major public inquiry, chaired by Lord Laming (2003). The case has particular resonance for learning for child health and paediatric practitioners, but it also had, and continues to have, an impact on national and local child protection policies and procedures. Box 2.1 provides details.

SERIOUS CASE REVIEWS

SCRs are not an investigation into why a child died or was seriously injured, or who was responsible – these are processes that will be dealt with by the criminal or coroner courts. The primary purpose of an SCR is to consider how agencies have worked together to safeguard a child (or children) and whether or not there is learning for improving practice. The focus should be on the viewpoint and actions of those caring for the child and family at the time, rather than with the benefit of hindsight (Munro 2011; HM Government 2015a). SCRs are also not part of any disciplinary inquiry; i.e. this is not about apportioning 'blame' (although if an individual's practice is found to be wanting, then this will be dealt with by their agency's internal processes). Current guidance is supportive of a range of models that provide a proportionate review, although there remains an expectation that the process will be led independently. A systems approach to reviews is gaining favour, with the more traditional individual management reviews that may contribute to an overview report no longer mandated. The new methodologies generally provide an opportunity for greater practitioner involvement in the learning (Fish et al. 2008). Families and children (including child victims in some cases) should be invited to make a contribution. A common theme arising from SCRs is that of parental mental health problems, substance misuse or domestic violence, often in the context of poverty, deprivation and social isolation. While not all children who are subject to an SCR are known to children's social care, it is extremely unusual for health services (for both the child and adults in the family) not to have had contact, and thus their contribution is crucial.

Children and young people's nursing professionals may be asked to make a contribution to SCRs. If this is the case, they should be appropriately supported by safeguarding children leads (usually the named professional) during the process. This includes being given a full explanation of the process, the need to 'secure records' at the point of the likelihood of a case going to an SCR, and receiving feedback on their contribution and the learning from the case. There is an expectation that recommendations are made and that these will be translated into action plans, which will be closely monitored and scrutinized in terms of improvements for practice (e.g. through audit). Although the aims of the SCR process are to prevent future tragedies and seek improvements in practice, there is an ever-present danger that the focus on SCR and 'what went wrong' can detract from learning lessons from the vast majority of safeguarding cases where daily improvements are being made to the lives, and the life chances, of some of our most vulnerable children, young people and their families, often in very challenging circumstances.

CHILD DEATH REVIEW

The *Working Together* (HM Government 2015a) guidance also requires LSCBs to set up processes to review all childhood deaths, both expected and unexpected, that occur in each local authority area in England. Perhaps unsurprisingly, child death has been found to be linked with marked social inequalities (Wolfe et al. 2014). Sidebotham et al. (2008), who outlined the work of so-called 'early starter' panels prior to the child death review being mandatory, found that the learning has a very real potential to improve child health and prevent child deaths in the future. Child death review involves a multi-agency 'rapid response' to all unexpected deaths, and the setting up of local child death overview panels (CDOPs) to review all childhood deaths and determine whether there are any 'modifiable factors' that may have prevented the death (while seeking to ensure local learning has taken place, including how bereaved families are being supported).

Children and young people's nurses need to be familiar with the aims and objectives of child death review processes, as it is highly likely that they will both be in a position to make a notification to a local CDOP coordinator and be approached to contribute case information to inform the CDOP's work. The Lullaby Trust (2013) has produced a helpful leaflet for parents and carers that explains the purposes of a child death review; this should be available in all child health settings – and may also help children's practitioners understand why, although a rare occurrence, the death of a child is of sentinel importance. Learning from a child death review may reflect the need for improvements in local service provision, but it may also reflect the requirements for national policy developments to improve child health.

KEY POINTS

- One child dies as a result of child maltreatment each week in England and Wales.
- Serious case reviews consider lessons to be learned about the ways in which agencies and organizations work together to safeguard and promote the welfare of children.
- Child death review processes reflect the broader definitions of safeguarding and provide an additional opportunity to improve the ascertainment of child deaths from maltreatment.
- Modifiable factors in a child death review include actions that could be taken through national or local initiatives to reduce the risk of future child deaths.

CONCLUSION

This chapter began by setting out how the United Nations Convention on the Rights of the Child 1989 has influenced and supported the development of legislation, policy and guidance that keeps the focus firmly on children's best interests and their right to be safe and protected. It has provided definitions of key terms, including what is meant by *safeguarding*, *child protection*, *child maltreatment* and *significant harm*; it is anticipated that this has provided clarity in terms of the frequent, somewhat confusing, conflation of these key concepts. The challenges of measuring the prevalence of maltreatment have also been discussed. The principles for practice, including those promulgated by Laming (2009), have been highlighted with particular reference to promoting an understanding of the role of 'authoritative practice' in keeping children and young people safe.

An overview of the provision of assessment-based early help that can promote children's well-being and safety and diminish the risk of significant harm followed. A description of the key categories of child maltreatment, including CSE, was then provided; this section was somewhat brief in recognition of the availability of supplementary guidance (including the NICE guidelines) and references have been given accordingly. The case of Victoria Climbié was outlined as providing seminal learning that has cast long shadows forward in changing policy for children and improving practice. The chapter closed with an overview of the purpose of SCR and the statutory child death review process. The ultimate aim of this chapter has been to inform and improve practice to benefit the children, young people and families in our care. In doing so, it fits within the other chapters of this text, which together provide both a critical appraisal of policy and practice and an opportunity to influence and improve service provision into the future.

SOURCES OF HELP/ADVICE

British Association for the Study and Prevention of Child Abuse and Neglect: http://www.baspcan.org.uk/
Children are Unbeatable! http://www.childrenareunbeatable.org.uk/
National Association for People Abused in Childhood (NAPAC): http://napac.org.uk/
National Society for the Prevention of Cruelty to Children (NSPCC): http://www.nspcc.org.uk
Victoria Climbié Foundation UK: http://vcf-uk.org/

REFERENCES

Action for Children (2014) *The scandal that never breaks.* Watford: Action for Children.
All Wales Child Protection Procedures Review Group (2008) *All Wales child protection procedures.* Available at http://www.awcpp.org.uk/wp-content/uploads/2014/03/All-Wales-Child-Protection-Procedures (accessed 5 December 2015).
Archard D (2004) *Children: rights and childhood.* London: Routledge.
Brandon M, Bailey S, Belderson P, Larsson B (2014) The role of neglect in child fatality and serious injury. *Child Abuse Review* 23: 235–245.
Butchart A, Harvey AP, Furniss T (2006) *Preventing child maltreatment: a guide to taking action and generating evidence.* Geneva: WHO and ISPCAN.
Children Act 1989. London: HMSO.
Children's Society (2014) *The good childhood report 2014.* London: Children's Society.
Corby B, Shemmings D, Wilkins D (2012) *Child abuse: an evidence base for confident practice base.* 4th ed. Maidenhead: Open University Press.
Cowley S, Frost M (2006) *The principles of health visiting: opening the door to public health.* London: CPHVA and UKSC.
Davies C, Ward H (2012) *Safeguarding children across services: messages from research.* London: Jessica Kingsley.
Department for Education (2012) *What to do if you suspect a child is being sexually exploited: a step by step guide for frontline practitioners.* London: DfE.
Department of Health (2015) *Female genital mutilation risk and safeguarding; guidance for professionals.* London: DH.

Department of Health, Department for Children, Schools and Families (2009a) *Healthy Child Programme: Pregnancy and the first five years*. London: DH.

Department of Health, Department for Children, Schools and Families (2009b) *Healthy Child Programme from 5–19 years old*. London: DH.

Department of Health and Social Security (1974) *Report of the Committee of Inquiry into the care and supervision provided in relation to Maria Colwell*. London: HMSO.

Fish S, Munro E, Bairstow S (2008) *Learning together to safeguard children: developing a multi-agency systems approach for case reviews* London: Social Care Institute for Excellence.

Gilbert R, Kemp A, Thoburn J, Sidebotham P, Radford L, Glaser D, MacMillan HL (2008) Recognising and responding to child maltreatment. *The Lancet*. Available at http://dx.doi.org/10.1016/S0140-6736(08)61707-9 (accessed 23 May 2015).

Gray D, Watt P (2013) *Giving victims a voice: joint report into sexual allegations made against Jimmy Savile*. London: Metropolitan Police Service/NSPCC.

Haringey Local Safeguarding Children Board (2009) *Serious case review: child 'A'*. London: DfE.

HM Government (2008) *Safeguarding children in whom illness is fabricated or induced. Supplementary guidance to working together to safeguard children*. London: DCSF.

HM Government (2009) *Safeguarding children and young people from sexual exploitation*. London: DCSF.

HM Government (2015a) *Working together to safeguard children: a guide to inter-agency working to safeguard and promote the welfare of children*. London: DfE.

HM Government (2015b) *Information sharing: advice for practitioners providing safeguarding services to children, young people, parents and carers*. London: DfE.

Hogg S (2014) *All babies count: the Dad Project*. London: NSPCC.

Jütte S, Bentley H, Tallis D, Mayes J, Jetha N, O'Hagan O, Brookes H, McConnell N (2015) *How safe are our children? The most comprehensive overview of child protection in the UK*. London: NSPCC.

Kennedy I (2010) *Getting it right for children and young people: overcoming cultural barriers in the NHS so as to meet their needs*. Available at https://www.gov.uk/government/uploads/system/uploads/attachment_data/file/216282/dh_119446.pdf.

Laming, Lord (2003) *The Victoria Climbié inquiry: report of an inquiry by Lord Laming*. Cm 5730. London: Stationery Office.

Laming, Lord (2009) *The protection of children in England: a progress report*. London: Stationery Office.

Lampard K (2014) *Independent oversight of NHS and Department of Health investigations into matters relating to Jimmy Savile*. London: DH.

Lullaby Trust (2013) *Child death review: a guide for parents and carers*. London: Lullaby Trust.

Munro E (2011) *The Munro Review of Child Protection final report: a child-centred system*. London: Stationery Office.

National Collaborating Centre for Women's and Children's Health (2009) *When to suspect child maltreatment*. London: RCOG Press.

Nursing and Midwifery Council (2015) *The code: professional standards of practice and behaviour for nurses and midwives*. London: NMC.

Office of the Children's Commissioner/Young Minds (2007) *Pushed into the shadows: young people's experiences of adult mental health facilities*. London: Office of the Children's Commissioner.

Office of the First Minister and Deputy First Minister Northern Ireland (2009) *Safeguarding children: a cross-departmental statement on the protection of children and young people*. Belfast: Children and Young People's Unit.

Powell C (2007) *Safeguarding children and young people: a guide for nurses and midwives*. Maidenhead: Open University Press.

Powell C (2016) *Safeguarding and child protection for nurses, midwives and health visitors: a practical guide*. 2nd ed. Maidenhead: Open University Press.

Powell C, Appleton J (2012) Children and young people's missed health care appointments: reconceptualising 'did not attend' to 'was not brought' – a review of the evidence for practice. *Journal of Research in Nursing* 17(2): 181–192.

Royal College of Midwives, Royal College of Nursing, Royal College of Obstetricians and Gynaecologists, Equality Now, UNITE (2013) *Tackling FGM in the UK: intercollegiate recommendations for identifying, recording, and reporting*. London: Royal College of Midwives.

Royal College of Paediatrics and Child Health (2014) *Safeguarding children and young people: roles and competences for health care staff*. Intercollegiate guidance. 3rd ed. London: RCPCH.

Scottish Government (2014) *National guidance for child protection in Scotland*. Edinburgh: Scottish Government.

Sidebotham P, Atkins B, Hutton J (2012) Changes in rates of violent child deaths in England and Wales between 1974 and 2008: an analysis of national mortality data. *Archives of Disease in Childhood* 97(3): 193–199.

Sidebotham P, Fox J, Horwath J, Powell C, Perwez S (2008) *Preventing childhood deaths: a study of 'Early starter' child death overview panels in England*. London: DCSF.

Tuck V (2013) Resistant parents and child protection: knowledge base, pointers for practice and implications for policy. *Child Abuse Review* 22: 5–19.

United Nations (1989) United Nation's Convention on the Rights of the Child. Available at http://www.unicef.org.uk/UNICEFs-Work/UN-Convention/ (accessed 30 August 2015).

Welsh Assembly Government (2007) *Safeguarding children: working together under the Children Act 2004*. Cardiff: WAG.

Wolfe I, Macfarlane A, Donkin A, Marmot M, Viner R (2014) *Why children die: death in infants, children, and young people in the UK*. London: RCPCH and National Children's Bureau.

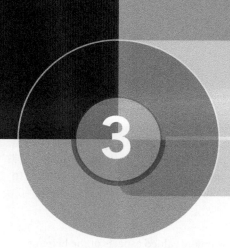

The use of restraint in children and young people's nursing

SALLY HORE

OVERVIEW

This chapter discusses fundamental issues surrounding the use of restraint on children and young people for clinical procedures and examines some of the complex moral, legal and ethical principles associated with this aspect of clinical practice. This is an issue that affects all those working with children and young people across a range of clinical settings. Appropriate guidance, policies and practical alternatives which the nurse should consider are reviewed. The lack of research into the use of restraint is also highlighted and the consequences discussed. The conclusion is that there is a need for parity and development of national policy and guidelines across the spectrum of healthcare services for the use of physical restraint (United Nations 1989). The case for this and the training and education of all those involved is put forward, as is the need for further research in this area of practice, especially from the child's perspective.

DEFINING RESTRAINT

The use and interpretation of what constitutes 'restraint' with patients/clients differs according to the type or remit of the clinical area. It is therefore pertinent to first analyze several definitions of *restraint* and consider these definitions as to their appropriateness for use within children and young people's nursing. In children and young people's nursing, healthcare professionals refer to the use of restraint specifically for facilitation of both diagnostic and therapeutic procedures. The restraint of children within healthcare settings for painful or painless procedures may be required to prevent significant and greater harm to the children themselves, practitioners or others (Royal College of Nursing [RCN] 2010).

The *Oxford Concise English Dictionary* (2015) defines *restraint* as

a measure or condition that keeps someone or something under control: Deprivation or restriction of personal liberty or freedom of movement: 'he remained aggressive and required physical restraint'.

This definition gives the reader the image of the maintenance of some sort of predetermined normality, yet also implies some use of force to suppress what might happen if the object were not restrained, i.e. a loss of control. The definition goes some way to recognizing that there may be a 'need' to restrain, with 'he remained aggressive' suggesting a possible rationale for its use. This has some relevance in the use of restraint in a clinical setting, where there has to be a morally acceptable rationale and the purpose for use deemed 'necessary' in order to achieve some justifiable goal or purpose. The literature, however, intimates the complexity of defining and justifying the moral principles underpinning these actions, especially in the realm of paediatric care, where often children are deemed to lack the ability to be able to consent and are therefore reliant on the advocacy of both those with parental responsibility and healthcare professionals to act in 'their best interests' (Hull and Clarke 2010; Page and McDonnell 2015; Bray et al. 2015).

Wright (1999, p. 462) suggests that

physical restraint implies the violation of other socially and professionally valued aspects of the helping relationship, such as the promotion of the client's dignity, autonomy and self determination, even if it is to preserve life and prevent suffering after other means of stopping the dangerous behaviour have failed.

This definition identifies the difficult dichotomy of roles for caring staff which exist in many care settings, including care of the elderly. The fundamental principles of biomedical ethics, beneficence, non-maleficence, justice and respect for autonomy (Beauchamp and Childress 2012), reflected in the professional code of conduct (Nursing and Midwifery Council 2015), which nursing staff herald as pivotal within healthcare practice, are in essence violated in many instances where restraint is employed. The rationale for such actions is usually supported by the premise that the member of staff is acting in accordance with prescribed medical care and the overarching professional and moral responsibility which suggests a nurse has a duty of care and must 'act in the best interests of people at all times' (Nursing and Midwifery Council 2015, p. 5).

Healy's (1997, p. 8) definition of restraint may also be considered pertinent within a nursing context:

Restraint occurs whenever a client has his or her movement physically restricted by the use of intentional force by a member of staff. Restraint can be partial; restricting and preventing a particular movement; or total; as in the case of immobilisation.

Within the literature reviewed the terms *restraint* and *holding still* may be used to describe the necessary restraint of a child or young person. The Department of Health (1995) and the Royal College of Nursing (1999) in the past have tried to provide some clarity on the differentiation between these two terms. *Physical restraint* is defined in terms of a minimum force necessary to overpower a child/young person with a guiding rationale of preventing the child/young person from harming themselves or others or from causing serious damage to property. In contrast, *holding still* is identified as using necessary force to ensure the safety of a child/young person throughout a clinical procedure. This may not require the 'overpowering' of the child in totality, but merely the restraint of only part of the child/young person's body. In 1999 the Royal College of Nursing went on to suggest that essentially the difference is related to the degree of force the nurse uses, as well as the intention of the nurse, which could be regarded as very subjective and difficult to externally verify and justify if necessary.

The term *restraint* within paediatric nursing and healthcare is increasingly being replaced by the term *restrictive physical intervention*, which the Royal College of Nursing (2010) suggests encompasses a range of approaches. These can include direct physical contact between persons where reasonable force is positively applied against resistance for the intended purpose to either restrict movement or mobility or to disengage from harmful behaviour displayed by an individual (Welsh Assembly Government 2005). The Royal College of Nursing (2010) cautions, however, that restrictive physical intervention should only be used to prevent serious harm.

More recently in an attempt to demystify and describe the ambiguous concept, Kangasniemi et al. (2014) undertook a qualitative study on the phenomenon of restraint in paediatric somatic care and suggest it is useful to consider *restraint* as referring to an action where a child has been held with the aim of promoting treatment or care; it is based on the principle of consent from the parent and aims to ensure the safety of the child and controlled care. They describe restraint as the positive application of force with the intention of overpowering the child, thus preventing the child from hurting themselves or others; in conclusion the actions necessary have been applied without the child's consent. This is compared to the term *therapeutic holding*, which the literature confers involves a different degree of force and differing intentions (Folkes 2005) which may not involve overpowering the child. However, *clinical holding* appears less ambiguous and is deemed the act of positioning the child so that a medical procedure can be carried out in a safe and controlled manner and necessitates consent of both the parent and child wherever possible (RCN 2010; Lambrenos and McArthur 2003).

Therefore for restraint to be justified in a paediatric nursing context the nurse would have to use restraint for the purpose of holding a child still against their will, with clearly identifiable intentions, which would be supported by the minimal use of force required for the intervention to be both successfully and safely performed. However, as recognized by Wright's (1999) definition, there are issues of violation of the 'helping relationship' and biomedical ethical principles which conflict with a nurse's professional identity and their ability to respect the child or young person's right to autonomy and self-determination. The act of restraint could therefore prove emotionally difficult for the nurse involved, even when the above criteria, the purpose and intention of the restraint, are clearly defined.

The use of restraint is further complicated in paediatric nursing where the concept of acting in the patient's best interests becomes a devolved responsibility. The majority of children have an altered view of what may be in their 'best interests', according to their age and cognitive development. A child and young person's cognitive stage has a huge impact on their ability to understand, assent to and participate in their care, which often involves many medical and nursing procedures and can cause distress, discomfort and even pain. These procedures are often deemed essential for the accurate diagnosis and treatment of both acute and chronic conditions. As the case study below demonstrates, in emergency situations children and young people's nursing staff may need to use clinical holding to ensure the safety of a child or young person during a necessary procedure.

CASE STUDY

Jade is an 18-month-old girl who is admitted to hospital with suspected urinary tract infection. On assessment she is noted to be pale, lethargic and appears generally very unwell with tachycardia, tachypnea and pyrexia. The advanced nurse practitioner recognizes Jade needs immediate intravenous access, bloods and cannulation to prevent further deterioration. She will then commence intravenous fluids and antibiotics. Topical anaesthetic creams, such as Ametop, would normally be applied prior to cannulation or venepuncture of a child, to help minimize the pain experienced during the procedure. These creams take between 20 and 60 minutes to produce an effective topical anaesthetic response. Owing to a lack of time and the seriousness of the child's condition the paediatric nurse present during the admission procedure restrains Jade by holding her arm firmly, with the child sitting upright in her mother's lap. The hospital play leader 'blows bubbles' in Jades direct line of vision to distract her. This allows the nurse practitioner to safely and successfully perform the intravenous cannulation. Jade would undoubtedly struggle during the experience as a result of the increased pain and her inability to cognitively understand the necessity of the procedure and thus cooperate by keeping still. However, in this situation it is seen as 'in the best interests of the child' to immediately treat such a serious suspected infection; therefore the use of clinical holding is deemed necessary and justified, but is managed in conjunction with the involvement and consent of the parent and use of the hospital play leader. The use of distraction in the form of blowing bubbles to help Jade cope with the experience can minimize the potentially damaging psychological effects of both the increased pain and experience of being held.

Many clinical interventions use only partial restraint for older children, whose cognitive development and understanding would enable some appreciation of the purpose of the intervention. The older child would generally be encouraged to collaborate with the nursing staff, allowing assent and where possible consent to be gained and therefore minimal restraint to be used. However, as already identified in the above case study, the degree of cooperation and compliance is drastically reduced in children under the age of 5 years who may require total immobilization to allow the safety of the child during clinical interventions. This is usually undertaken in conjunction with the informed consent and compliance of parents or primary care giver, who may be required to assist the nursing staff in actively restraining the child.

The term *restraint* will be used throughout this chapter and is intended to encompass the practices of what is also described in the literature as 'restrictive physical intervention', 'holding still', 'immobilizing' and 'clinical holding'.

PRINCIPLES FOR PRACTICE

- The use, interpretation and definition of *restraint* within paediatric nursing vary. Other terms for restraint may include *restrictive physical intervention*, *holding still*, *immobilizing* and *clinical holding*.
- The physical restraint of children and young people may be justified in clinical practice, but on a case-by-case basis.
- The use of restraint by children and young people's nurses must involve clearly identified intentions supported by the use of minimal force.

LEGAL, ETHICAL AND MORAL ISSUES

The legality of restraining children and young people has to be viewed in light of any pertinent legislation which seeks to promote children's rights within society. Issues surrounding the perceived use of power to overcome a child who chooses not to comply with treatment, such as the child in the case study where sutures were removed without sedation or anaesthesia, are raised by Charles-Edwards (2003), who illustrates how both a child and the parent can be overawed in the power-coercive environment of a hospital. She suggests that individual practitioners should examine the ethical principles followed by a workplace in determining when restraint can be justified.

There are obvious consequences to the restraining of older children without their prior consent. The dangers of harming not only the child but also the staff involved are real and even accentuated owing to the size of the child. There are also ethical implications for restraining children for the purpose of undertaking procedures, without the child's consent, which is described as a last-resort practice in a child of this age (Jeffery 2002).

Gaining a child's consent for the restraint and procedure has been identified as the ideal (Collins 1999; Department of Health 2003; Lambrenos and McArthur 2003; RCN 2010). This can possibly be achieved with older children who could be defined as 'Gillick competent' in the UK and therefore able to understand and rationalize the need for treatment. However, it can be argued that the majority of children who require restraining for a clinical procedure are cognitively unable to adequately comprehend the need for treatment. This is supported by Robinson and Collier (1997), whose study identified the age of less than 6.7 years as those most likely to require restraint.

SUMMARY OF GILLICK COMPETENCE, UK

In UK law, a person's 18th birthday draws the line between childhood and adulthood, so that in healthcare matters an 18-year-old enjoys as much autonomy as any other adult. To a more limited extent 16- and 17-year-olds can also take medical decisions independently of their parents. The right of younger children to provide independent consent is proportionate to their competence, but a child's age alone is clearly an unreliable predictor of his or her competence to make decisions as set out in Chapter 1.

A judgement in the High Court in 1983 (Wheeler 2006) laid down criteria for establishing whether a child, irrespective of age, had the capacity to provide valid consent to treatment in specified circumstances. Two years later these criteria were approved in the House of Lords and became widely acknowledged as the 'Gillick test', after the name of a mother who had challenged health service guidance that would have allowed her daughters aged under 16 to receive confidential contraceptive advice without her knowledge. For many years the criteria that have been referred to as the test for Gillick competence have provided clinicians with an objective test of competence. This identifies children aged under 16 who have the legal capacity to consent to medical examination and treatment, providing they can demonstrate sufficient maturity and intelligence to understand and appraise the nature and implications of the proposed treatment, including the risks and alternative courses of action (Wheeler 2006).

The issue of consent could be partially addressed if nurses were obliged to formally assess and document their rationale for restraining a child, with collaboration from the parents (Bland 2002; Jeffery 2002; RCN 2003). This could be structured to show a deliberated assessment of the child's age and understanding, the rationale for use of specified and agreed techniques as well as details of alternatives which could be considered appropriate and shown as being tried before resorting to restraint, which should only be considered as a last resort (Lambrenos and McArthur 2003; RCN 2010). Examples of these have been developed by Lambrenos and McArthur (2003) and Folkes (2005), both of which take the form of a clinical flow chart to aid the decision-making process, coupled with supporting documentation for recording, explaining and gaining consent for the process. However, Lambrenos and McArthur (2003) acknowledge that the increasing legal knowledge gained through implementation of teaching sessions accompanying the implementation of the new policy has 'heightened' some practitioners' concerns regarding their vulnerability to litigation.

The use of restraint by adults to overpower children and young people in any context is an emotive subject which raises complex moral, legal, ethical and practical issues. Clear guidance is required to help protect the rights and safety of the child, the practitioner involved in restraining the child or young person, as well as the parent who is often asked to assist. Current guidance within the UK is limited to locally based guidance, with many institutions developing their own frameworks to help define best practice (Hart 2004). This has heralded a call for the UK government to undertake a comprehensive review of the practice of restraint by all institutions involved, to ensure compliance with the United Nations (UN) Convention on the Rights of the Child (Committee on the Rights of the Child 2002) set out below. The latest report by this committee specifies a request for a review of all uses of restraint of children (Hart and Howell 2004). This has implications for the health service, which has been identified as one such area which needs to review current procedures and guidance, and has special relevance for all areas involved in the regular care and subsequent restraint of children and young people.

The UN Convention on the Rights of the Child (United Nations 1989), although not a 'law', has been ratified by the UK, which is committed to its implementation.

THE UN CONVENTION ON THE RIGHTS OF THE CHILD (1989) STATES:

Article 12

1. Parties shall assure to the child who is capable of forming his or her own views the right to express those views freely in all matters affecting the child, the views of the child being given due weight in accordance with the age and maturity of the child.

Article 19

1. Parties shall take all appropriate legislative, administrative, social and educational measures to protect the child from all forms of physical or mental violence, injury or abuse, neglect or negligent treatment, maltreatment or exploitation, including sexual abuse, while in the care of parent(s), legal guardian(s) or any other person who has the care of the child.

2. Such protective measures should, as appropriate, include effective procedures for the establishment of social programmes to provide necessary support for the child and for those who have the care of the child, as well as for other forms of prevention and for identification, reporting, referral, investigation, treatment and follow-up of instances of child maltreatment described heretofore, and, as appropriate, for judicial involvement.

The Human Rights Act (1998) and criminal law also seek to protect the rights of children and young people from abuse and excessive unjustifiable physical force to restrict them, their liberty and their autonomy. Again clear guidance on permissible forms of restraint is urgently needed by practitioners to help them clarify their role in restraining children and young people for clinical procedures, ensuring that minimal force is utilized. The Royal College of Nursing (2010) suggests practitioners seek guidance on the legal implications of any locally produced restraint policies. There is some evidence of the Education Act 1996 (Department for Education and Employment 1996) and mental health and mental handicap recommendations being used for guidance in formulation of teaching sessions on restraint (Valler-Jones and Shinnick 2005) owing to the lack of specific guidance for children and young people's nursing at present.

In the UK, the nurses' professional code of conduct (Nursing and Midwifery Council 2015) also provides guidance on a nurse's role within his or her professional capacity. It identifies a practitioner as personally accountable for ensuring that the nurse promotes and protects the interests and dignity of patients and clients. The code also reminds the professional to deliver safe and competent care, and to respect patients' and clients' autonomy. While guidance on restraining children appropriately for clinical procedures remains inadequate, nurses might be considered at risk of breaching their own code of conduct (Nursing and Midwifery Council 2015).

The code of conduct (Nursing and Midwifery Council 2015) also reinforces the nurse's role in obtaining clear documented consent for treatment from the patient or a person with parental responsibility. Good record keeping is identified as helping to protect patients and clients by providing an accurate account of treatment and care planning and delivery (Nursing and Midwifery Council 2009). With the current lack of documentation regarding the assessment, management and evaluation of restraint techniques used, nurses cannot prove that they comply with their professional and legal duty of care. The Nursing and Midwifery Council (2009) states that accurate documentation provides evidence that a nurse has honoured his or her duty of care, and that he or she has taken all reasonable steps to care for a patient and not compromise the patient's safety in any way. The Nursing and Midwifery Council (2009) reminds nurses to use their professional judgement to decide what is relevant and what to record. With the difficulties that arise from ensuring consent from children, young people and their parents, and the physical contact nature of restraining children and young people against their will, it would seem logical that this should be considered a vital area to clearly document within children and young people's nursing.

The physical restraint of children and young people for clinical procedures by nursing staff remains common practice within healthcare settings (Bland 2002; Folkes 2005; Pearch 2005). The child's ability to comprehend the need for the procedure, and thus his or her compliance, is directly linked to the child's age and developmental stage, as set out in Table 3.1, which is based on Piaget's cognitive developmental stages.

Younger children, as exemplified in the above case study, are unable to understand the rationale for procedures such as venepuncture; their non-compliance is exhibited by behaviours associated with the primal responses to fear – fight and flight – making any procedure difficult to perform without the use of clinical holding. It is common practice for parents, nurses, doctors and other multidisciplinary team members to engage in the forceful restraint of the uncooperative child to ensure the completion of a multitude of clinical procedures, e.g. taking the child's temperature, blood and X-rays. Nurses identify a need to hold the child to reduce the risk of additional injury from medical equipment being used to perform the task (Collins 1999). It can be argued that the moral rationale for holding the child still is 'in the best interests of the child' depending on the urgency underpinning the necessity of such clinical investigation (Robinson and Collier 1997; Collins 1999), with care being exercised to ensure that the child suffers minimal physical and psychological harm as a result.

However, it may be argued that in situations where the child does not require urgent therapeutic intervention an overreliance on the primary use of restraint becomes questionable. The taking of blood for non-urgent investigations, for example, may mean the use of excessive restraint which can be seen as unjustified. Bray et al. (2015) conducted a systematic review of the current evidence in relation to restraint in clinical paediatric care and concluded that healthcare professionals, although aware of ethical issues in relation to restraint, may choose to ignore them, arguing that frequency and repetitive exposure render the health professional immune to the actual short-term distress and ignorant of the longer-term psychological effects associated with restraint. They go on to argue that at present holding a child or young person against their wishes to complete a procedure is currently not framed as an ethical or moral issue, and that health professionals' individual ethical competence and moral agency (their ability to engage in ethically appropriate actions to respect patients' rights) (Poikkeus et al. 2014) have become eroded by institutionally unquestioned practice (Bray et al. 2015).

Table 3.1 Cognitive development and main characteristics as described by Piaget

Age of child in years	Piaget's stage of cognitive development	Main characteristics as described by Piaget
0–2	Sensorimotor	Simple reflexes, first habits, circular reactions, novelty and curiosity, internalization of schemes, object permanence
2–7	Preoperational	Magical thinking predominates, acquisition of motor skills, egocentrism; child cannot conserve or use logical thinking
7–12	Concrete operational	Child begins to think logically but only with practical aids; child is very concrete in his or her thinking, begins to conceive, no longer egocentric
12+	Formal operational	Development of abstract reasoning; children develop abstract thought, can easily conserve and think logically

Source: Bee, H., Boyd, D., *The Developing Child*, 13th ed., Pearson Education, Harrow, 2012.

There is a suggestion that when using the best interests principle, this needs to be firmly centred around the child's best interests considering both short- and long-term physical and psychological effects of restraint and the consideration of all available alternatives (Bray et al. 2015). In some circumstances the children and young people's nurse should consider and explore the use of alternative techniques such as distraction, and when necessary the appropriate use of sedation to undertake the procedure (Scottish Intercollegiate Guidelines Network [SIGN] 2004), thus minimizing the use of restraint at all times.

PRINCIPLES FOR PRACTICE

- The compliance of children and young people in clinical procedures is related to their stage of cognitive development.
- Although the use of restraint may be justified 'for the greater good of the child', care must be exercised to ensure that the child or young person does not suffer harm.
- When appropriate, the nurse must consider the use of suitable alternatives to restraint to minimize the need for inappropriate levels of restraint in all non-urgent procedures.

USE OF RESTRAINT ACROSS THE CLINICAL SPECTRUM

The use of restraint in other areas of nursing is well documented. The fields of both adult psychiatry and care of the older person describe the difficulties associated with the use of restraint in a practical care context, acknowledging both the physical problems associated with restraint (Molassiotis 1995; Bell 1997a) and the potential psychological effects on the patient (Gallinagh et al. 2001). Patients were identified as feeling a sense of entrapment, and they described a loss of autonomy and felt controlled by the nursing staff who used restraint habitually on the ward. These detrimental effects on the psychosocial well-being of the patients are further compounded by physical problems identified by Molassiotis (1995), which include contractures of major joints of locomotion, oedema of lower extremities, pressure sores, changes to bone demineralization and electrolyte loss. Although these studies relate to adult patients, the consequences of restraint may be equally applicable to children and young people.

The issue of restraint clearly extends beyond the UK and has international implications. Cleary (2001) acknowledges the commonplace use of restraint in healthcare facilities in the US, highlighting concerns over the lack of research supporting the efficacy of physical restraints in maintaining the safety of patients. Cleary (2001) suggests that the increasing development of legislation to protect patients' rights has been promoted as concern for the use of restraint among the elderly population is raised; in the context of this chapter, this is also relevant to children and young people. These changing trends are recognized and supported by other authors (Stilwell 1991; Tinetti et al. 1992; Mason et al. 1995). Cleary (2001) also identifies the role of individual members of the multidisciplinary team in considering the ethical and legal implications of using any prescribed restraint in practice.

There are clearly parallels to be drawn from the use of restraints in elderly care and in paediatrics. Although at differing ends of a chronological spectrum, the loss of autonomy which exists within elderly patients with dementia often results in regression, a lack of mental capacity and inappropriate behaviour that cannot be reasoned with. This lack of understanding, abnormal actions and limited mental capacity can cause an adult to display types of cognitive characteristics similar to those of a young child whose ability to comprehend context is limited to their own particular perception of the world. Both of these age groups become disempowered and lack the status and political leverage of the majority of the adult population. The public perception of the appropriateness of overpowering and controlling their behaviour through restraint appears more socially acceptable than if nurses choose, for example, to restrain an adult without any deficit in understanding, who is deemed to have full mental capacity. This would be regarded as a serious assault, as opposed to a necessary restraint.

In their more recent publication to enhance guidance to healthcare professionals on the appropriate and ethical use of restraint in elderly care, the Royal College of Nursing (2008) describes other variations of restraint. These can be broadly differentiated into four different categories: mechanical restraint, technological surveillance, chemical restraint and psychological restraint. Mechanical restraint involves the use of everyday equipment such as bed rails or mittens in ITU, but also involves controls on freedom of movement – such as baffle locks and keypads to prevent harm. Technological surveillance is often used to alert staff that a person is trying to leave or to monitor movements, for example door alarms, electronic tagging and video monitoring. Chemical restraint involves the appropriate use of both prescribed and over-the-counter medication. Psychological restraint by constantly reinforcing what a person is not allowed to do can involve depriving individuals of equipment or possessions necessary to do what they want to do. The Royal College of Nursing (2008) maintains that restraint may be necessary to prevent harm, and there should be an awareness of the ethical, legal, practical and professional issues surrounding the individual patient's needs, which can help prevent the malicious, abusive or inappropriate use of any form of restraint. The key is, however, to strike the right balance between independence, autonomy and ensuring safety, while acknowledging potential benefits and harm associated with any form of restraint.

The Mental Capacity Act 2005 sets out a legal definition for a person who lacks capacity and stipulates the responsibility of the healthcare provider to uphold the five principles which it stipulates protect capacity. The Mental Capacity Act (2005) clearly sets out three conditions which must be satisfied when considering an act which may be planned that would constitute restraint of a patient or client who lacks capacity:

1. The client lacks capacity in relation to the matter in question.
2. The nurse reasonably believes that it is necessary to do the act in order to prevent harm to the client.
3. The act is a proportionate response to (a) the likelihood of the client suffering harm and (b) the seriousness of that harm.

The Royal College of Nursing warns that if a nurse restrains any client or patient without a sound professional and legal basis they could be open to legal prosecution for negligence or physical or psychological harm, in civil law. In criminal law the restraint of another person without consent could be deemed a criminal activity. The need for professional guidance, education, reasonable force, clear intention and documentation is paramount (RCN 2008).

There is, however, a growing body of evidence that suggests that there are successful alternatives available, which could be used in clinical practice to reduce the need for physical restraint in elderly care (Molassiotis 1995; Bell 1997a; Stephens et al. 1999; RCN 2008). It has been suggested that alternative techniques could easily be incorporated into clinical areas through improved environmental design, person-centred care, adequate staff training and education to reduce the need for any form of restraint wherever possible (Robbins 1986; Stilwell 1991; Stephens et al. 1999; RCN 2008).

The call for the use of alternatives to restraint is echoed in paediatric care. This suggests that the nursing profession as a whole is beginning to question the routine use of restraint throughout practice and engaging in the process of identifying and questioning current standards, promoted by the quest for more ethically and morally acceptable, evidence-based, person-centred practice.

PRINCIPLES FOR PRACTICE

- There are clear parallels between the use of restraint in the elderly and that in children and young people.
- Detrimental effects on the physical and psychological well-being of the elderly caused by the use of physical restraint may be applied equally to its use on children/young people.
- The case for alternatives to physical restraint in the elderly is echoed in children and young people's nursing practice with regard to children and young people.

RESTRAINT OF CHILDREN AND YOUNG PEOPLE ACROSS A RANGE OF SETTINGS

The literature has highlighted methods for the safe restraint of children and young people, and their appropriate use, in several areas of society which deal with children and young people, such as education, residential care, dentistry and radiography.

The developing interest in physical restraint has also been fuelled by already documented historical investigations into serious restraint-related injuries sustained by children at Aycliffe Children's Centre by the Department of Health (1993a). Such reviews accelerated the call for a revision of techniques used by staff to restrain children (Department of Health 1993b), prohibiting control and restraint techniques which originated in the prison service (Epps et al. 1999). In the government's response to coroners' recommendations following the inquests of Gareth Myatt and Adam Rickwood, restraint was identified as a contributing factor to both boys' deaths in secure units in England (Ministry of Justice 2008, p. 3). It states:

Gareth Myatt, aged 15, died in hospital on 19 April 2004, following a restraint incident at Rainsbrook secure training centre. Gareth's death revealed a number of shortcomings in relation to Physical Control in Care (PCC), the approved method of restraint in secure training centres, and wider safeguarding issues were highlighted at the inquest into his death. Several months afterwards, on 9 August 2004, Adam Rickwood, aged 14, committed suicide at Hassockfield secure training centre. The jury at the inquest into Adam's death found that a restraint incident some hours before Adam's death had not contributed to it and that staff at Hassockfield had behaved appropriately throughout the time he was at the centre – but it was clearly a distressing incident for Adam. A number of safeguarding issues arose from the inquest and the coroner made a number of recommendations.

The Department for Education and Employment has sought to clarify the use of restraint as a means for controlling children within an education environment. The Education Act 1996 (Department for Education and Employment 1996) prohibits the use of 'corporal punishment' at any local education authority, independent, special or grant-maintained school. Circular 10/98, produced by the Department for Education and Employment (1998), seeks to address Section 550A of the Education Act 1996 and discusses the issue of using 'reasonable force' to prevent pupils committing a crime, causing injury or damage or causing disruption, stating that such powers have already existed under common law but have been misunderstood.

The concept of reasonable force has been determined through a court of law and can be described as an objective test determined by the jury (Police National Legal Database 2004). A jury is asked to determine whether the amount of force used, under given circumstances, can be justified by the defendant, as detailed in Box 3.1. However, civil rights lawyers interpret 'reasonable' as meaning 'minimal' and, under the Human Rights Act 1998, have disputed the interpretation of 'reasonable'.

The degree of force used to restrain a child or young person for clinical procedures is also of concern to professions allied to medicine. In radiographic examinations children and young people are required to undergo diagnostic tests which require immobilization, often against the will of the child (Hardy and Armitage 2002). There are concerns raised about the legal and moral implications for restraining children and young people within this field, acknowledging that the majority of radiographers lack any formal paediatric education and training, thus increasing the reliance on parents and other healthcare staff, namely nurses, to ensure adequate restraint of a child for radiographic imaging.

The same holds true for other professions. A quantitative questionnaire survey of 179 dental practitioners conducted by Newton et al. (2004) indicated that 39% felt that physical restraint was an acceptable practice for very young patients, with an even greater number acknowledging its appropriateness in handicapped children (62%). The results showed the decline in use of a previously more common practice – hand over mouth – which is broadly defined as a practitioner placing his or her hand over a patient's mouth while behavioural expectations are calmly explained to the child, and ensuring

---

BOX 3.1: Section 3(1) of the Criminal Law Act 1967, United Kingdom

A person may use such force as is reasonable in the circumstances in the prevention of a crime, or in effecting or assisting in the lawful arrest of offenders or suspected offenders or of persons unlawfully at large.

A jury must decide whether a defendant honestly believed that the circumstances were such as required him to use force to defend himself from an attack or threatened attack; the jury has then to decide whether the force used was reasonable in the circumstances.

Note that this is basically an 'objective test' determined by the jury. The jury does not have to consider whether the defendant thought his/her actions were reasonable in the circumstances. They just have to consider what *they* believe was reasonable.

the airway remains patent. This decline is linked to increased education of practitioners, concerns over the legal status of the technique and increasing parental concerns. Interestingly, 51% of these dental practitioners felt that long-term psychological problems might occur, such as fear of further treatment, which has direct relevance to restraint in paediatric nursing and the potential long-term impact of such practices as described in the case study below. More recently, the latest guidance from the British Society of Paediatric Dentistry (Nunn et al. 2008), *Consent and the Use of Physical Intervention in the Dental Care of Children*, is far more explicit, addressing issues around consent as well as the use and justification for physical intervention (restraint) in dental care of children. The general principles governing the use of physical intervention in this latest guidance include child factors, which are described as the actual necessity to accomplish the procedure, the notion of minimal use, full preparation of child and parent as well as consideration of legal frameworks which may be pertinent.

CASE STUDY

An 8-year-old girl attends a local paediatric admissions unit for removal of sutures following complex abdominal surgery performed in another district general hospital. The sutures were due to be removed 10 days postoperatively. However, the child attends the unit on day 15 postoperatively and her parents explain that she is very frightened about having the sutures removed owing to a previous 'bad experience' when she was caused considerable pain during suture removal after the last operation. The parents apologize, but explain that it has taken them 15 days to persuade their daughter to attend the hospital. They are now worried about the implications of trying to remove the sutures as the skin has already started to embed around them, making any attempts at removal very difficult. Local anaesthetic and systemic pain relief appears ineffective. The anaesthetic medical team are reluctant to give a general anaesthetic to allow for suture removal, stating that it is medically too risky to give a second general anaesthetic to this particular child for such a minor procedure. They suggest holding the child down to enable suture removal. The child complains of extreme pain during the procedure and reacts in a physically and verbally aggressive manner to the restraint, resulting in five clinical staff being required to hold her still to enable safe suture removal. This action can be seen as compounding the fear and anxiety in a child who already suffers with procedural anxiety related to prior experience. The child will need further surgery and this experience will undoubtedly psychologically significantly affect the child and could lead to profound long-term effects.

REFLECTION POINTS

- What are your feelings and emotions after reading the above case study?
- What other measures could staff have considered and employed to minimize the pain and distress experienced by the 8-year-old girl having embedded sutures removed from her abdomen?
- What may be the long-term consequences of this experience for the girl, her family and staff?

USE OF RESTRAINT IN PSYCHIATRIC SETTINGS

There is a plethora of research into the restraint of children which exists within a psychiatric context (Bell 1997b; Allen 2002; Kenny 2004). However, the purpose behind some of the restraints used within this field is identified as a therapeutic treatment. Child psychotherapists use forceful restraint to help children express emotions through confrontation, as a treatment for conditions such as autism, schizophrenia and attachment disorders (Mercer 2002).

Other aspects of society, such as education, have also begun to grapple with some of the legal and moral dilemmas of restraining children (Hamilton 1997; Fletcher-Campbell et al. 2003; Gold 2004; Hart 2004). With the advent of the Education Act 1996 (Department for Education and Employment 1996), which prohibits the use of corporal punishment within schools, teachers have sought clarity on the issue of using reasonable force in restraining pupils to prevent them committing crimes or causing disruption, injury or damage. There is much confusion and ambiguity surrounding how much force can be considered reasonable while restraining pupils. It is essential to define the concept of reasonable force, which has become the accepted theoretical moral ruler by which each case is measured and considered in light of an increasingly litigious society (Hantikainen and Kappeli 2000; Jeffery 2002; Charles-Edwards 2003; RCN 2010). As the following case study shows, restraint may be ruled unlawful and has consequences for the individual patient/client, professionals involved and their organization.

The inquest into the death of 25-year-old Godfrey Moyo, while on remand at HMP Belmarsh, concluded in July 2009 with the jury deciding that the medical cause of his death was (1) positional asphyxia with left ventricular failure following restraint and (2) epilepsy. The jury's verdict reflects the shocking evidence of what happened on 3 January 2005. In their damning narrative verdict the jury found:

On 3 January 2005 at approximately 2.50 am at Belmarsh prison Mr Godfrey Moyo suffered an epileptic fit in his cell. Prison officers were alerted and together with a nurse were dispatched to the cell. Upon regaining consciousness, Mr Moyo experienced post-ictal behavioural disturbance and attacked a cellmate. Prison officers entered the cell to bring Mr Moyo under control. A vigorous struggle ensued between Mr Moyo and five prison officers in which three officers sustained injuries. Prison officers brought Mr Moyo to the floor on the landing outside the cell. Full control was achieved immediately. Mr Moyo was then restrained in the face down prone position for approximately 30 minutes.

During this time Mr Moyo suffered at least two further fits, followed by periods of unconsciousness in which his breathing was restricted as a result of his position.

Mr Moyo began to suffer from the effects of positional asphyxia. The first nurse on the scene failed to adequately monitor Mr Moyo's condition during the restraint, which contributed to his death by neglect.

The prison officers also failed to recognize the signs of distress being shown by Mr Moyo during the restraint, as highlighted by their control and restraint training. At no time during the restraint by any persons present was an attempt made to move Mr Moyo off his front as per the control and restraint guidelines or place him in the recovery position during periods of unconsciousness.

REFLECTION POINT

Consider how the death of Mr Moyo could have been averted and the nurse's role in this situation as the client's advocate.

Other deaths caused by physical restraint have also been reported in the US, as set out below.

CASE STUDY

Angelika (Angie) Arndt suffocated while in a control hold at the Rice Lake Day Treatment Center, Wisconsin, in May 2006. The case went to trial and was reported in the local newspaper, *The Chronotype*, on 14 May 2009 (Coalition Against Institutionalized Child Abuse 2009).

Angelika was born in Milwaukee. She was subjected to severe physical and sexual abuse while living with her biological parents, stated the complaint. She was diagnosed with a variety of psychological disorders and developmental problems, including a short attention span. Her parents terminated their parental rights in 2004. She was placed with foster parents Donna and Daniel Pavlik in January 2005 and immediately became a part of their family. Angelika was placed in the Rice Lake Day Treatment Center for academic assistance on 24 April 2006.

From that day until 25 May 2006, Angelika was placed in the control hold at least a dozen times lasting from a minimum of 17 minutes up to a maximum of 98 minutes. She was placed in the control holds for such behavior as putting her hands down the front of her pants, putting her arms and head inside her shirt, not sitting properly, talking to others and gargling her drink.

Angelika was a client of the center, which provided intensive intervention and preventative mental health services for youths. The defendant, 29-year-old Bradley Ridout, with other staff members had placed Angelika in a control hold as a disciplinary measure at the clinic on 25 May 2006. She was forced to lie face down on the floor and was restrained by at least three staff members, including Ridout lying across the 67-pound girl's back and shoulders. She suffocated from the pressure and could not be revived. During the last control hold, Angelika lost consciousness, stopped breathing, sustained a tear to the cornea and suffered blunt trauma to the head. She went into cardiac arrest, sustained internal bleeding and brain death.

The clinic pleaded no contest to a subsequent charge of homicide under the patient abuse statute. It was fined $100,000. As part of the plea agreement, the Rice Lake Clinic closed its doors. Ridout pleaded no contest to misdemeanour negligent patient abuse. He was placed on 1 year of probation with 60 days in jail.

KEY POINTS

- Physical restraint is used on children and young people in a psychiatric setting as part of therapy, educational settings and the penal system.
- Deaths caused by physical restraint have been recorded in the UK and US.

USE OF RESTRAINT IN PSYCHOTHERAPY

Within the psychotherapy field restraint can be used for a different purpose. Mercer (2002) reviews four main techniques used within child psychotherapy, whose long-term goal is to 'create family warmth and affection', but the action is described as 'uncomfortable physical restraint and intrusive emotional confrontations that verge on violence' (Mercer 2002, p. 304).

The assumption behind these therapies is that they treat emotional problems by releasing accumulated negative emotions that would otherwise inhibit positive emotion and affection for others (Mercer 2002). The four techniques include Z-process therapy, Welch method attachment therapy, Colorado-style attachment therapy and Federici's therapeutic holding. In essence, the child is physically restrained by usually more than one adult and encouraged to express their emotions. They are then verbally and physically overpowered until the child becomes calm. These treatments were claimed to be successful for autism, schizophrenia, attachment and attention disorders (Mercer 2002). The potential for harming the child and the inappropriate use of the techniques as punishment are highlighted; there are, however, descriptions of extensive forceful restraint, coupled with emotional challenge, which exist far beyond the scope of the types of restraint used for clinical interventions within nursing, and so they are not clearly comparable. The author's description of 10-year-old Candace Newmaker's death as a result of such psychotherapy restraint techniques does, again, bring the question of reasonable force to the forefront of restraint of children. Such cases, covered extensively by the media, have helped highlight the issue to a wider audience.

CASE STUDY

Candace Newmaker died on 18 April 2000 in Evergreen, Colorado. She was the victim of child abuse as a young child and was 5 years old when she was removed from her parents. She was adopted by Jeane Newmaker 2 years later; however, there were concerns about her behaviour and attitude at home. She was eventually enrolled in a 2-week intensive session of 'attachment therapy' involving a 70-minute 'rebirthing' session during which she was wrapped in a flannel sheet to simulate a womb and told to extract herself from the sheet, while four adults used their hands, feet and large pillows to push against her to prevent her from freeing herself. The experience of rebirthing was supposed to help Candace 'attach' to her adoptive mother.

The session was videotaped and Candace repeatedly tells the adults involved that she is having difficulty breathing. She even states on the tapes that she thinks that she is dying.

Candace Newmaker died as a result of being asphyxiated during the restraint.

Mercer's (2002) conclusions regarding the appropriateness of such restraint techniques within child psychotherapy are supported by Sourander et al. (2002). This study examines the use of restraints, holding, seclusion and timeout within child and adolescent psychiatric inpatient units in Finland from the perspective of the consultant psychiatrist responsible for the child/young person's care. About 40% of the sample (n = 504) had experienced some form of restraint procedure during an inpatient stay, with 'aggressive acts' being the rationale for instigating the restraint of the child or young person. This study again raises concern surrounding the lack of 'research-based understanding' of the impact of restraining children and young people.

KEY POINTS

- There are legal implications for the use of physical restraint in practice.
- Research and real-life case studies identify worrying practices such as the use of hand over mouth and questionable psychotherapeutic techniques.

Hart and Howell (2004, p. 4) undertook a comprehensive review of the topic for a report commissioned by the National Children's Bureau. The report states:

The use of direct physical contact in order to overpower a child raises complex legal, ethical and practical issues. There are times when such intervention is necessary in order to protect the child or others from harm but clear guidance is essential in order to safeguard both the child concerned and the practitioner exercising the restraint. It is debatable whether such clarity currently exists in the UK.

Hart and Howell (2004) call for more research into the implications of restraint on children and the safety and effectiveness of techniques, most of which are derived from adult control and restrain policies originating from prisons and which can be considered an inappropriate basis that fails to acknowledge the different physical and psychological status of children and young people. The authors also highlight the need for research into the actual incidence of restraint within a variety of contexts, including healthcare, and the effectiveness of their use.

The concerns about the lack of research are compounded by Epps et al. (1999), who also suggest that most childcare organizations are left to develop techniques and procedures with little external support or guidance. They blame the deficit in research for the lack of systematic practice development. The lack of clear policy and practical guidelines appears to be an issue across many childcare facilities and is not therefore regarded as uniquely a deficit in children and young people's nursing. These findings compound Hart and Howell's (2004) conclusion that at present there is a lack of guidance surrounding the issue of restraining children across many institutions.

KEY POINTS

- The use of physical restraint in children has been questioned by the National Children's Bureau, UK.
- A lack of research into the use of physical restraint has been identified.

NEED FOR GUIDELINES ON RESTRAINT TO INFORM PRACTICE

Within paediatric nursing there appears to be little research analyzing the issue of restraining children and young people for clinical procedures. Some authors suggest this could be due to the difficult nature of the topic, questioning whether restraining children/young people was tantamount to identifying poor practice within children and young people's nursing (Robinson and Collier 1997; Folkes 2005; Homer and Bass 2010). There has been a request for greater critical reflexivity surrounding this uncontested and almost invisible aspect of common paediatric nursing practice (Bray et al. 2015), with a need for urgent investigation into the exploration of the child and young people's perception and experiences. Bray et al. (2015) also call for a critical exploration of how children's best interests are balanced against their need for increasing autonomy and developing agency.

There remains at present very little practical guidance for children and young people's nurses in restraint techniques from a policy perspective. The Royal College of Nursing has published several documents which help inform and guide nurses in practice. *Restraining, Holding Still and Containing Children and Young People* (RCN 2003) and *Restraint Revisited: Rights, Risks and Responsibility* (RCN 2004) have a moral and ethical remit; however, they fail to give any direct advice in the practical management and correct procedures for restraining children or young people. This leaves nurses questioning the basis from which commonly used techniques have been developed (Valler-Jones and Shinnick 2005).

There is a clear acknowledgement of the lack of local and national policies regarding suitable techniques for use by nursing staff. This could be attributed to the continued lack of clarity currently available from relevant professional bodies, such as the Royal College of Nursing (2010). The latest guidance highlights the principles of good practice but also recognizes a need for local organizations to develop local policies which give guidance to health professionals regarding restraint which are pertinent to the clinical area and the specific client group. It concludes that while the guidance on good practice should help guide local policy, it should also form the basis for educational programmes and practical training as necessary. It can be suggested that, as yet, no one has assumed responsibility for directing this practical aspect of professional practice within the UK, with both national and local institutions seeking guidance from each other. The literature surrounding the development of local policies in the US regarding restraint suggests that without clear national guidance a lack of parity can occur nationally. This can create problems for both staff and patients as experiences and expectations differ from area to area (Selekman and Snyder 1995). The current guidance, however, fails to give advice on correct techniques and methods suitable for use in clinical settings.

There are several examples in the children and young people's nursing literature that discuss the introduction of local policies to guide practice on restraint within specific clinical areas. Most reflect the Royal College of Nursing (2010) principles of good practice and highlight the need for adequate staff training.

The introduction of a clinical holding policy within a teaching hospital in England (Lambrenos and McArthur 2003) and the use of clinical benchmarking in defining best practice concerning restraint in health authorities in northwest England (Bland 2002) are both good examples of local organizations taking the initiative in developing their own guidance to help define and guide best practice when restraining children for clinical procedures, as described in Table 3.2. Guidance is also readily available from other NHS Trusts, such as Portsmouth, Newcastle upon Tyne and East and North Hertfordshire, indicating a growth in local policies.

REFLECTION POINTS

- What guidelines or clinical protocols are used in your clinical area in relation to the physical restraint of children and young people?
- Have the training needs of yourself and your professional colleagues have been met in relation to appropriate techniques for restraining children and young people and the use of alternatives such as distraction?

The development of a clinical protocol to help guide best practice is discussed by Bland (2002) in the use of 'clinical benchmarking' as a process to develop an action plan to initiate best practice in restraining children for procedures. The process is similar to the research paradigm action research in its cyclical, re-evaluative approach to clinical development. His work defines six core factors that are used to consider the most appropriate management of restraint within a clinical area (Bland 2002), as set out in Box 3.2.

A scoring system of statements identified along a continuum from A to E allows a practitioner to clearly isolate best practice (A on the scale), and then in comparison highlight where the particular unit's practice lies. For example, under training, best practice is defined as 'mandatory' on restraint management for all staff, whereas poor practice highlights that there would be no evidence of training or education surrounding

Table 3.2 Summary of key attributes associated with best practice in restraining children for clinical procedures

Lambrenos and McArthur (2003)	Bland (2002)
Flow chart to assist decision making on clinical holding used in each procedure for each individual child	Development of an evidence-based clinical benchmark as a tool to be used to identify best practice in procedural restraint
Narrative document developed defining terms, responsibilities, training needs and need for audit	Promotes equal partnership with the child and family; ensures the rights of the child are maintained
Consent form and information document are completed prior to the procedure	Assessment to minimize risk to the child and clear documentation of the processes involved to reduce potential for litigation
Professional training package developed specifically designed for the purpose of clinical procedural holding	Implementation of a formalized education and training package
Developmental needs of the child are highlighted as well as alternative approaches to consider	Physical and psychological developmental needs assessed and alternative techniques considered where possible

---

BOX 3.2: Six core factors in relation to physical restraint

1. Equal partnership with child and family
2. Methods of restraint
3. Alternatives to restraint
4. Training and education
5. Assessment and documentation
6. The rights of the child

Source: Bland, M., *Professional Nurse*, 17(12), 712–5, 2002.

the topic (Bland 2002). Staff training, education and implementation would need to be supported, both financially and practically, to ensure success of this type of local intervention. This type of local policy development can help ensure practice is evidence based.

REFLECTION POINTS

- Whose responsibility is it to ensure all healthcare professionals have training and education in restraint?
- What may be the consequences of a lack of training and education?

KEY POINTS

- There is a lack of national policy or guidelines in relation to physical restraint in the US and UK.
- Although the guidelines outlined so far may inform practice, there is a need for national policies and guidelines applicable to all areas where physical restraint is used.

IMPACT OF RESTRAINT: UNDERSTANDING PARENTS' EXPERIENCES

There is growing evidence of the effects of parental involvement in restraint which the literature suggests can have both short- and long-term consequences. Longitudinal research by McGrath et al. (2002) suggests parental involvement in restraint can have a negative longer-term effect on the parent–child relationship. There is evidence of parents of children with long-term conditions arguing 'whose turn it is' this time to hold their child for a procedure with neither wishing to be the one who has to restrain (Swallow et al. 2011). Some suggest the parents feel as though after the event they have 'let their child down' or acted as accomplices in some crime, and experience feelings of disempowerment, guilt, regret and even anger (Lundqvist and Nilstun 2007; Alexander et al. 2010; Brenner 2013; Bray et al. 2015).

In previous research 98% of nurses questioned felt that the parent's presence was beneficial to the child during a procedure (Robinson and Collier 1997), yet extreme emotional responses by the parents would probably only upset the child further. This is a difficult professional decision when deliberating at the time of the event: whether a parent should stay with the child and be involved in the restraint or merely be present while the nurse holds the child.

Such an ad hoc approach to the preparation of the parents and child could be minimized if staff were encouraged to formally assess and document the patient's individual needs prior to the restraint for any necessary procedures (Lambrenos and McArthur 2003; RCN 2010). This would automatically require discussion between parents, the child/young person and the nursing staff on how best to approach the patient.

The need for documentation and assessment has been highlighted by several authors (Bland 2002; Jeffery 2002; Lambrenos and McArthur 2003; RCN 2010). When children and young people are deemed unable to reliably give consent for the use of the restraint, the parents should at least have an opportunity to discuss and agree on the types of restraint to be used and the degree of force appropriate. This would serve only to improve the communication between parents and the nursing staff concerned. If the nurse involved is obliged to discuss and gain prior consent for the restraint from the parents, this at least should serve as a period of time for psychological preparation of the parents, forewarning them what to expect (Lundqvist and Nilstun 2007).

Ideally, the staffing levels on the children and young people's ward need to reflect sufficient personnel to help support parents through these difficult experiences rather than rely on them to physically help with the restraint of their own child. There is an acknowledged need for parents to remain with their children wherever possible during clinical procedures to ensure their child has emotional support. Parents become essentially compromised, both emotionally and physically, when giving hands-on help to restrain their child (Lundqvist and Nilstun 2007). Without proper risk assessment and documentation of this role for parents, there appear to be considerable risks for all concerned.

There is a clearly identified need for children and young people's nurses to gain the consent of the parents and, if possible, the child to ensure the ethos of collaborative family-centred care. Many of the procedures and restraints that are undertaken could be considered intimately invasive, and respecting the need for consent for such events is essential in defining best practice for children and young people's nursing, as highlighted in Table 3.2. There could also be benefits from staff training in the risk and potential of any litigation through improvements in child safety (Bland 2002; RCN 2010). This might also address the astounding lack of awareness of the legal responsibility of the children and young people's nurse when restraining a child (Robinson and Collier 1997).

PRINCIPLES FOR PRACTICE

- All staff involved in clinical procedures must carefully assess whether the use of physical restraint is necessary and consider all other approaches.
- Parents must be involved in any discussion and be supported by staff.
- If physical restraint is used, consent must be sought from parents.

IMPACT OF RESTRAINT: UNDERSTANDING NURSES' EXPERIENCES

Prolonged exposure to events such as traumatic restraints of children can alter the nurse's perception (Benner and Wrubel 1989). This confirms and supports Sabo (2006), who likened the health professional's response to repetitive traumatic events to post-traumatic stress disorder and describes this behaviour as 'compassion fatigue'. Student nurses and parents are often well placed to describe the potential impact of traumatic restraint experiences as they have yet to be overexposed to such emotionally difficult situations and often perceive the experience differently from a more experienced nurse.

As noted by Benner and Wrubel (1989, p. 60):

Stress management approaches that deal only with the altering emotional states by dampening, controlling or distracting may be helpful in the short term to interrupt a stressful response set, but in the long run, such strategies foster an alienated stance towards emotion.

Perhaps this explains why a student's response can appear so emotionally raw to more experienced staff who, over time, can become more emotionally detached. Maybe this is why more experienced practitioners have been slow to question their actions during such episodes of restraint, after prolonged exposure has dampened their response to such situations as part of a developing coping strategy. Again such apathy toward the issue of restraining children and young people could be part of the reason why policy and guidance has been so slow to evolve surrounding the topic.

Nurses have been described as feeling 'uncomfortable' in their role when actively restraining children (Lambrenos and McArthur 2003; Coyne and Scott 2014). This feeling is echoed by student nurses (Valler-Jones and Shinnick 2005) and supported by the experiences of practitioners in other fields of nursing (Bonner et al. 2002). Again this could be attributed to the violation of other socially and professionally valued aspects of the 'helping relationship', as suggested by Wright (1999), and the basis of the code of conduct (Nursing and Midwifery Council 2015), beneficence and non-maleficence. This is often coupled with concerns over the dichotomy of their relationship with children they provide care for, which is developed through a gradual formation of mutual trust, only to have that fragile bond shattered through the need to restrain a child for a painful clinical procedure (Bricher 1999).

Nurses can experience feelings of guilt that are difficult to explain without further in-depth research focusing on why nurses feel guilty when restraining children. This could be partly attributed to what Bricher (1999) refers to as the perceived loss of trust within the nurse–patient relationship which has been carefully formed while caring for a child or young person. The nurse then has to abuse that trust by causing the child pain or distress during a necessary procedure (Darby and Caldwell 2011; Coyne and Scott 2014).

The feeling of guilt could also be linked to the interpersonal conflict with our professional and personal self-images, or as Wright (1999) terms as a result of the 'violation' of other socially and professionally valued aspects of the helping relationship. To cause intentional harm to a child in any other context could be construed as physical abuse; this behaviour also conflicts with any inherent nurturing instinct the nurse may have which encourages him or her to protect the child (Darby and Caldwell 2011; Coyne and Scott 2014).

This moral sense of wrongdoing is reflected in the literature by both paediatric authors (Lambrenos and McArthur 2003) and authors writing about other fields of nursing (Bonner et al. 2002). It was also one of the issues raised through informal discussions with child branch nursing students by Valler-Jones and Shinnick (2005). Nurses involved in the restraint of children for clinical procedures can feel they need to have a moral 'rationale' for their actions. They describe the moral dilemma of restraining the child to enable clinical procedures as a need to 'be cruel to be kind'. This kind of rationale is supported by Robinson and Collier (1997), who found that the majority of nurses used restraint as a means to protect the child from accidental injury and out of necessity for the procedure to be undertaken safely. However, this rationale can still be seen as causing moral and professional dilemmas for the individual nurse (Darby and Caldwell 2011; Coyne and Scott 2014).

Robinson and Collier's (1997) study also highlights the ambiguity of the nurse's understanding regarding legal and professional responsibilities. Only 12% of their sample ($n = 153$) identified the nurse as legally responsible when restraining a child for a clinical procedure, and 52% of the study sample stated that they 'didn't know' who was responsible. Such confusion in the legal and ethical aspects of restraint can be clearly attributed to a lack of formal training and national or local guidance surrounding the issue.

USE OF ALTERNATIVES TO PHYSICAL RESTRAINT

The use of chemical restraint in paediatrics involves various types of medication and even consideration of sedation if necessary to prevent both excessive use of restraint and psychological harm. The Scottish Intercollegiate Guidelines Network (SIGN) (2004) has published the national guidance *Safe Sedation of Children Undergoing Diagnostic and Therapeutic Procedures*. SIGN (2004) recommends combining both pharmacological and non-pharmacological methods and using an individualized approach, which recognizes that the child's needs may vary considerably and an approach based purely on the age of the child should be avoided. Individual assessment can allow a more holistic approach, considering the child's age, physical size, cognitive ability, maturity, past experience and coping strategies.

SIGN (2004) clearly identifies that sedation is not without risk; however, the guidance provides detailed evidence to support all levels of sedation from anxiolysis through to general anaesthesia. The guidance also describes the benefits and risks of both pharmaceutical agents and parental presence and the necessary training, safety checks and equipment which must be in place in any area considering the use of sedation for enabling diagnostic and therapeutic interventions involving children.

Cummings (2015) also concludes that there is a need to use 'experts' when undertaking procedures on children. In her ethnographic study of restraint for painful procedures in an emergency department in the US she observed that children were restrained for up to 40 minutes on occasions, depending on the procedure or severity of the injury. She also observed that in some cases up to three adults could be involved. One of the findings recommends the use of expert practitioners, described as having technical expertise when dealing with children, which enabled procedures to be undertaken swiftly.

Young (2000) also studied the use of sedation for clinical procedures and compared the effectiveness of two pharmacological sedatives, ketamine and midazolam, in minimizing the need for restraint of 644 children during interventions such as suturing, stapling, Steri-Strips and gluing of minor wounds in the emergency department. The results show that ketamine was more effective, with children requiring less restraint and reporting an overall better behavioural experience throughout the whole procedure (Young 2000). There is, however, an acknowledgement that some children and young people will be unsuitable for sedation and will continue to be restrained for procedures.

When practitioners are unable to use sedation or other alternative techniques and restraint is deemed necessary to ensure the safety of the child or young person during a procedure, it is vitally important that nurses have clear guidance available to help ensure best practice (Darby and Caldwell 2011). A clinical tool is necessary to help guide practitioners in the safe and appropriate choice of techniques and to ensure consent is properly gained from the parents and documented prior to the procedure. The effect of the experience on the parents must be recognized and their needs also taken into consideration at all stages of the procedure.

PRINCIPLES FOR PRACTICE

- There would seem to be a need for national and even international guidance in relation to the use of physical restraint.
- Research shows that the use of physical restraint on the child can cause more distress than the actual clinical procedure.
- To minimize distress clinical staff could consider the use of sedation in children.

Table 3.3 Alternative techniques and their application in practice

Technique	Example
Play/distraction techniques	Use of bubbles, noisy toys, TV, conversation, cuddly toys, mimicry, role play
Guided imagery	Use of pictures, images, sounds, smells
Relaxation techniques	Use of deep breathing, progressive muscular relaxation, relaxation imagery and meditation
Pharmacological management	Use of sedatives/hypnotics

The use of restraint of younger patients for necessary clinical procedures has been described as problematic. When patient-restraining techniques are used without proper pharmacological support this potentially makes the procedures more difficult to perform. The use of alternative techniques, for example distraction by a nurse or play therapist, can prove valuable, but it also has to be viewed as only part of any solution to avoid or minimize use of physical restraint (Table 3.3).

The provision of play services in hospitals where children are cared for is recognized as a Department of Health requirement (Department of Health 2003). Play specialists have the appropriate skills and knowledge to engage children of all ages with the use of appropriate techniques to understand even complex clinical interventions, minimizing the child's fear and engaging the child through the medium of play to increase cooperation. The simple use of blowing bubbles around the clinical setting while children are undergoing venepuncture, combined with the adequate use of a topical anaesthetic gel or cream, can provide enough distraction to be able to perform the necessary investigation without the child really being aware of the procedure. This minimizes the use of restraint and allows the experience to be less traumatic for both the child and the parent.

REFLECTION POINTS

- Are any of the alternative techniques to restraint listed above used in your clinical area?
- If not, why not?
- What may be some of the barriers to using these techniques in clinical practice?

As previously discussed in this chapter children and young people's nurses need adequate training, preparation and support within clinical areas to enable confidence in utilizing the above techniques. Other multidisciplinary members could also be trained to use these techniques within clinical areas such as medical staff, play staff and other therapists. With correct training and support parents could also be taught how to use these alternative techniques both at home and within the clinical environment.

KEY POINTS

- Training and education in the use of physical restraint and alternatives is urgently required in practice.
- Training and education will improve the hospitalization experience for children and their parents.

EDUCATION AND TRAINING OF PROFESSIONALS INVOLVED IN RESTRAINT

The need for further training was highlighted in the literature by several authors (Bland 2002; Lambrenos and McArthur 2003; Willock et al. 2004; Darby and Caldwell 2011; Coyne and Scott 2014), whose findings all suggest a lack of knowledge of perceived alternatives to restraint by qualified nursing staff currently working with children. This is highlighted as contributing to the high reliance on the use of restraint within children and young people's nursing at present in the UK. Most of the authors highlight a need for staff training which needs to be evidence based and developed from national guidelines (Collier and Pattison 1997; Robinson and Collier 1997; Collins 1999; Jeffery 2002; Valler-Jones and Shinnick 2005). Even the policy put forward by the Royal College of Nursing (2003), *Restraining, Holding Still and Containing Children and Young People*, highlights the need for adequate staff training and refers practitioners to their designated workplace risk managers and named executive directors to implement the provision of locally based training programmes, of which, to date, none are specifically designed (Lambrenos and McArthur 2003; Folkes 2005; Pearch 2005; Valler-Jones and Shinnick 2005).

There is a suggestion that practitioners use the guidance from the Royal College of Nursing (2010) when restraining a child, but this causes confusion for practitioners when the guidance fails to be the prescriptive clinically detailed advice they urgently need in practice. Valler-Jones and Shinnick (2005) conclude that with the current lack of guidance it is pertinent to question what guidelines practitioners are currently working to. And who has designated the current techniques used as safe and acceptable? Does current policy and practice breach the UN Convention (Hart and Howell 2004)?

Within the field of nurse education pre-registration nursing students are currently taught manual handling and receive violence and aggression training, but the issue of restraining children and young people is not directly addressed within the indicative content of most UK child nursing programmes. Page and McDonnell (2015) suggest there is a theory–practice gap. Intimating clear variation in training and preparation of student nurses on restraining children, their research describes evidence of students feeling poorly prepared and therefore experiencing emotional trauma when involved in restraint in practice.

What training exists at present has been classed as 'lacking in quality' (Robinson and Collier 1997) and lacking clear application to the specific situation of clinical restraint for procedures (Lambrenos and McArthur 2003). With 90.8% of their study group identifying a clear need for guidance, Robinson and Collier (1997) are supported in raising this as an important issue for the profession. The issue of 'credibility of trainers' again raises concern (Lambrenos and McArthur 2003; Valler-Jones and Shinnick 2005) with some evidence in the literature of individual areas developing their own training programmes (e.g. Valler-Jones and Shinnick 2005) to meet the specific needs for pre-registration child branch nurses. Again, although this is admirable, the lack of clear guidance nationally will lead to differing standards and educational preparation which may disadvantage other students. The training needs of current practitioners must also be recognized, as they serve as mentors to the students during clinical practice.

The evidence suggests that clear guidance and training will not only benefit staff and students but ultimately improve the hospitalization experience for the child and family (Collier and Pattison 1997; Robinson and Collier 1997; Collins 1999; Page and McDonnell 2015). However, limited research and ambiguous guidance on the practical application of restraint remain problematic and result in a lack of clear evidence-based practice from which to develop teaching models and programmes (Kangasniemi et al. 2014; Page and McDonnell 2015). This experience could be further improved if the educational training programmes, once developed, also sought to raise nurses' awareness of moral, ethical and legal considerations as well as possible alternatives, such as distraction techniques and guided imagery (Willock et al. 2004), which many nurses feel unable to use because of limited training in their use and application (Bland 2002; Lambrenos and McArthur 2003). Another reason for limited use of alternatives is a lack of resources, with staff suggesting high workload, low staffing levels and tradition all responsible for nurses to use restraint rather than spend time with the child using explanations and play therapies to adequately prepare a child for an intervention (Collins 1999; Sparks et al. 2007; Kangasniemi et al. 2014). Collins (1999) argues that parents might be taught to use distraction prior to admission, under certain circumstances, which would be assessed as ideal practice under Bland's (2002) clinical benchmark criteria, supporting the nursing ethos of collaborative 'family-centred care'.

CONCLUSION

This chapter has discussed some of the fundamental issues surrounding the use of restraint of children for clinical procedures. The complex moral, legal and ethical components which are weaved throughout the topic have been critically analyzed and their implications explored. A clear lack of research into the issues pertinent to the use of restraint in paediatric nursing has been highlighted and the consequences discussed.

There remains a need for clear national policy as well as national guidelines from which educational and training programmes for nurses in pre- and post-registration could be developed. The current situation of locally developed guidance could prove problematic in the future, when a lack of national parity could create confusion for practitioners, parents and patients, as has occurred in the US (Selekman and Snyder 1995).

Educational and training programmes on the safe restraint of children and young people in all settings could potentially benefit students and professionals as well as families. The current situation of poorly informed practitioners which lack adequate preparation within this field of practice cannot persist.

Training and education in the use of alternative techniques could be expanded to include other multidisciplinary members and parents.

Above all, parents need to be supported in their role as emotional aids to their children, and not coerced into participation involving emotionally and physically alien roles as collaborators to their child's distress during restraint for a procedure. A need for assessment and documentation of the types and situations within which restraint could be used can also be deemed essential from both a practitioner's and the patient's/family's perspective. This would also help to clarify the necessary informed consent prior to the actual experience occurring.

Lastly, it is questionable whether the current use of restraint in children and young people's nursing as described and explored within this chapter complies with current guidance from the UN Convention on the Rights of the Child (United Nations 1989), the Human Rights Act (1998) and criminal law. With calls for the government to undertake a comprehensive review of the practice of restraint by all institutions involved (Committee on the Rights of the Child 2002), children and young people's nursing must identify the urgency of this issue. Practitioners are best placed to instigate change within this area, by highlighting current practice and their concerns to those responsible and ensuring local policies and training within their areas (RCN 2010).

It is clear that restraint is used on children and young people across a range of settings and that children and young people's nurses as well as other health and social care practitioners need to be aware of all the issues surrounding this. There remains a need for further research and clear practical guidance.

SUMMARY OF PRINCIPLES FOR PRACTICE

- Children and young people's nurses must avoid using restraint wherever possible.
- Children and young people's nurses must advocate other means that do not involve restraint and view actual restraint as the last resort.
- Children and young people's nurses must ensure that any method of restraint does not cause the child or young person actual harm.
- Children and young people's nurses must consider the moral, ethical and legal issues involved, and there is a need for training and education in restraint.

REFERENCES

Alexander E, Murphy C, Crowe S (2010) What parents think about physical restraint of their child to facilitate induction of anesthesia. *Paediatric Anaesthesia* **20**: 1056–8.

Allen B (2002) *Ethical approaches to physical interventions: responding to challenging behaviour in people with intellectual disabilities*. Kidderminster: British Institute of Learning Disabilities, p. 239.

Beauchamp T, Childress J (2012) *Principles of biomedical ethics*. 7th ed. Oxford: Oxford University Press.

Bee H, Boyd D (2012) *The developing child*. 13th ed. Harrow: Pearson Education.

Bell J (1997a) The use of restraint in the care of elderly patients. *British Journal of Nursing* **6**: 504–8.

Bell L (1997b) The physical restraint of young people. *Child and Family Social Work* **2**: 37–47.

Benner P, Wrubel J (1989) *The primacy of caring: stress and coping in health and illness*. Reading, MA: Addison-Wesley.

Bland M (2002) Procedural restraint in children's nursing: using clinical benchmarks. *Professional Nurse* **17**(12): 712–5.

Bonner G, Lowe T, Rawcliffe D, Wellman N (2002) Trauma for all: a pilot study of the subjective experience of physical restraint for mental health inpatients and staff in the UK. *Journal of Psychiatric and Mental Health Nursing* **9**: 465–73.

Bray L, Snodin J, Carter B (2015) Holding and restraining children for clinical procedures within an acute care setting: an ethical consideration of the evidence. *Nursing Inquiry* **22**(2): 157–67.

Brenner M (2013) A need to protect: parent's experiences of the practice of restricting a child for a clinical procedure in hospital. *Issues in Comprehensive Pediatric Nursing* **36**: 1–2, 5–16.

Bricher G (1999) Paediatric nurses, children and the development of trust. *Journal of Clinical Nursing* **8**: 451–8.

Charles-Edwards I (2003) Power and control over children and young people. *Paediatric Nursing* **15**(6): 37–42.

Cleary KK (2001) The use of restraint in health care: background, regulations, ethical implications and legal considerations. *Acute Care Perspectives* **10**(4): 11–4.

Coalition Against Institutionalized Child Abuse (2009) Available at http://lizditz.typepad.com/i_speak_of_dreams/2007/01/coalition_again.html.

Collier J, Pattison H (1997) Attitudes to children's pain: exploding the 'pain myth'. *Paediatric Nursing* **9**(10): 15–8.

Collins P (1999) Restraining children for painful procedures. *Paediatric Nursing* **11**(3): 14–6.

Committee on the Rights of the Child (2002) *Consideration of reports submitted by states parties under Article 44 of the convention. Concluding observations of the Committee on the Rights of the Child: United Kingdom of Great Britain and Northern Ireland*. Geneva: United Nations.

Coyne I, Scott P (2014) Alternatives to restraining children for clinical procedures. *Nursing Children and Young People* **26**(2): 22–7.

Cummings JAF (2015) Pediatric procedural pain; how far have we come? An ethnographic account. *Pain Management Nursing* **16**(3): 233–41.

Darby C, Cardwell P (2011) Restraint in the care of children. *Emergency Nurse* **19**(7): 14–7.

Department for Education and Employment (1996) *Education Act, Section 548*. Available at http://www.legislation.hmso.gov.uk/acts/acts1996/96056-cn.htm.

Department for Education and Employment (1998) *Section 550A of the Education Act 1996: the use of force to control or restrain pupils*. Circular 10/98. London: DfEE.

Department of Health (1993a) *A place apart: an investigation into the handling and outcomes of serious injuries to children and other matters at Aycliffe Centre for Children, County Durham*. London: Social Services Inspectorate, DH.

Department of Health (1993b) *Guidance on permissible forms of control in children's residential care*. London: DH.

Department of Health (1995) *Support force for children's residential care. Good care matters: ways of enhancing good practice in residential child care*. London: DH.

Department of Health (2003) *Getting the right start: national service framework for children 'standards for hospital services'*. London: DH.

Epps K, Moore C, Hollin C (1999) Prevention and management of violence in a secure youth centre. *Nursing and Residential Care* **1**(5): 261–7.

Fletcher-Campbell F, Springall E, Brown E (2003) *Evaluation of circular 10/98 on the use of force to control or restrain pupils*. London: National Foundation for Educational Research, Department of Education and Skills.

Folkes K (2005) Is restraint a form of abuse? *Paediatric Nursing* **17**(6): 41–4.

Gallinagh R, Nevin R, McAleese L, Campbell L (2001) Perceptions of older people who have experienced physical restraint. *British Journal of Nursing* **10**(13): 852–9.

Gold K (2004) Dark shadows. *TES Extra: Special Needs* June: 6–7.

Hamilton C (1997) Physical restraint of children: a new sanction for schools. *Childright* **138**: 14–6.

Hantikainen V, Kappeli S (2000) Using restraint with nursing home residents: a qualitative study of nursing staff perceptions and decision making. *Journal of Advanced Nursing* **32**(5): 1196–205.

Hardy M, Armitage G (2002) The child's right to consent to x-ray and imaging investigations: issues of restraint and immobilisation from a multi-disciplinary perspective. *Journal of Child Health Care* **6**(2): 107–19.

Hart D (2004) Forcing the issue. *Community Care* **1519**: 38–40.

Hart D, Howell S (2004) *Report on the use of physical intervention across children's services*. London: National Children's Bureau. Available at http://www.ncb.org.uk/resources/res.

Healy A (1997) The prevention and management of violence. In Hayden C (ed.) *Physical restraint in children's residential care*. Report no. 37. Portsmouth: Social Services Research and Information Unit, University of Portsmouth.

Homer J, Bass S (2010) Physically restraining children for induction of general anaesthesia: survey of consultant pediatric anaesthetists. *Pediatric Anesthesia* **20**: 638–46.

Hull K, Clarke D (2010) Restraining children for clinical procedures: a review of the issues. *British Journal of Nursing* **19**(6): 346–50.

Human Rights Act (1998) London: Stationery Office.

Jeffery K (2002) Therapeutic restraint of children: it must always be justified. *Paediatric Nursing* **14**(9): 20–2.

Kangasniemi M, Papinaho O, Korhonen A (2014) Nurses' perceptions of the use of restraint in pediatric somatic care. *Nursing Ethics* **21**(5): 608–20.

Kenny C (2004) Can mental health nursing ever give up the option of restraint? *Community Care* **1553**: 14–5.

Lambrenos K, McArthur E (2003) Introducing a clinical holding policy. *Paediatric Nursing* **15**(4): 30–3.

Lundqvist A, Nilstun T (2007) Human dignity in paediatrics: the effects of health care. *Nursing Ethics* **14**(2): 215–28.

Mason R, O'Conner M, Kemble S (1995) Untying the elderly: response to quality of life issues. *Geriatric Nursing* **16**: 68–72.

McGrath P, Forrester S, Fox-Young S, Huff N (2002) Holding the child down for treatment in paedaitric haematology: the ethical, legal and practice implications. *Journal of Law and Medicine* **10**: 84–96.

Mental Capacity Act (2005) London: Stationery Office.

Mercer J (2002) Child psychotherapy involving physical restraint: techniques used in the four approaches. *Child and Adolescent Social Work Journal* **19**(4): 303–14.

Ministry of Justice (2008) *The government's response to coroners' recommendations following the inquests of Gareth Myatt and Adam Rickwood.* Available at https://www.gov.uk/government/uploads/system/uploads/attachment_data/file/362700/response-inquest-myatt-rickwood.pdf.

Molassiotis A (1995) Use of physical restraints 2: alternatives. *British Journal of Nursing* **4**(4): 201–2, 219–20.

Newton JT, Patel H, Shah S, Sturmey P (2004) Attitudes towards the use of hand over mouth (HOM) and physical restraint amongst paediatric specialist practitioners in the UK. *International Journal of Paediatric Dentistry* **14**: 111–7.

Nunn J, Foster M, Master S, Greening S (2008) *Consent and the use of physical intervention in the dental care of children.* London: British Society of Paediatric Dentistry.

Nursing and Midwifery Council (2009) *Guidelines for records and record keeping.* London: NMC.

Nursing and Midwifery Council (2015) *Code of professional conduct.* London: NMC.

Oxford concise English dictionary. 9th ed. (2015) Oxford: Oxford University Press.

Page A, McDonnell A (2015) Holding children and young people: identifying a theory-practice gap. *British Journal of Nursing* **24**(8): 447–51.

Pearch J (2005) Restraining children for clinical procedures. *Paediatric Nursing* **17**(9): 36–8.

Poikkeus T, Leino-Kilpi H, Katajisto J (2014) Supporting ethical competence of nurses during recruitment and performance reviews – the role of the nurse leader. *Journal of Nursing Management* **22**(6): 792–802.

Police National Legal Database (2004) Available at https://www.pdms.com/track-record/case-studies/police-national-legal-database/

Robbins LJ (1986) Restraining the elderly patient. *Clinical Geriatric Medicine* **2**(3): 5919.

Robinson S, Collier J (1997) Holding children still for procedures. *Paediatric Nursing* **9**(4): 12–4.

Royal College of Nursing (1999) *Restraining, holding still and containing children: guidance for good practice.* London: RCN.

Royal College of Nursing (2003) *Restraining, holding still and containing children and young people. Guidance for nursing staff.* Available at www.rcn.org.uk.

Royal College of Nursing (2004) *Restraint revisited: rights, risks and responsibility. Guidance for nursing staff.* Available at www.rcn.org.uk.

Royal College of Nursing (2008) *Let's talk about restraint: Rights, risks and responsibilities.* London: Author.

Royal College of Nursing (2010) *Restrictive physical intervention and therapeutic holding for children and young people: guidance for nursing staff.* London: RCN.

Sabo B (2006) Compassion fatigue and nursing work: can we accurately capture the consequences of caring work? *International Journal of Nursing Practice* **12**(3): 138–42.

Scottish Intercollegiate Guidelines Network (2004) *Safe sedation of children undergoing diagnostic and therapeutic procedures. A national clinical guideline.* Edinburgh: Scottish Intercollegiate Guidelines Network.

Selekman J, Snyder B (1995) Nursing perceptions of using physical restraints on hospitalized children. *Pediatric Nursing* **21**(5): 460–4.

Sourander A, Ellila H, Valimaki M, Piha J (2002) Use of holding, restraints, seclusion and time out in child and adolescent psychiatric in-patient treatment. *European Child & Adolescent Psychiatry* **11**: 162–7.

Stephens B, Barkey M, Hall H (1999) Techniques to comfort children during stressful procedures. *Accident and Emergency Nursing* **7**(4): 226–36.

Stilwell E (1991) Nurses education related to the use of restraint. *Journal of Gerontology Nursing* **17**(2): 236.

Sparks L, Setlik J, Luhman J (2007) Parental holding and positioning to decrease IV distress in young children: a randomized controlled trial *Journal of Pediatric Nursing* **22**(6): 440–7.

Swallow V, Lambert H Santacroce S, MacFadyen A (2011) Fathers and mothers developing skills in managing children's long-term medical conditions: how do their qualitative accounts compare? *Health and Development* **37**: 512–23.

Tinetti ME, Wen-Liang Lui, Ginter SF (1992) Mechanical restraint use and fall related injuries among residents of skilled nursing facilities. *Annals of Internal Medicine* **116**(5): 369–76.

United Nations (1989) Convention on the Rights of the Child. Adopted under General Assembly Resolution 44/25. Geneva: UN.

Valler-Jones T, Shinnick A (2005) Holding children still for invasive procedures: preparing student nurses. *Paediatric Nursing* **17**(5): 20–2.

Welsh Assembly Government (2005) Framework for restrictive physical intervention: policy and practice. Available at www.wales.gov.uk (accessed on 3 November 2015).

Wheeler R (2006) Gillick or Fraser? A plea for consistency over competence in children. *British Medical Journal* **332**: 807.

Willock J, Richardson J, Brazier A, Powell C, Mitchell E (2004) Peripheral venepuncture in infants and children. *Nursing Standard* **18**(27): 43–50.

Wright S (1999) Physical restraint in the management of violence and aggression in in-patient settings: a review of issues. *Journal of Mental Health* **8**(5): 459–72.

Young S (2000) Comparing the use of ketamine and midazolam in emergency settings. *Paediatric Nursing* **12**(2): 18–21.

PART

2

FAMILY-CENTRED CARE
IN PRACTICE
Being Inclusive

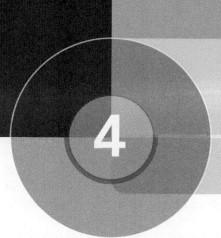

Being family centred: Inclusive practice with mothers, fathers and others

4

SUE HIGHAM

OVERVIEW

In this chapter the evidence relating to the current practice of family-centred care is examined within the context of social change relating to families, and in particular the increasing involvement of both fathers and grandparents in children's lives. Fathers' and grandparents' experiences when a child is ill are explored. The challenges to children and young people's nurses seeking to practice truly family-centred care are identified.

INTRODUCTION

Family-centred care is central to children and young people's nursing across the world, yet it has been described as an ideal rather than a reality in practice. Crawford (2012) has highlighted the tension for children and young people's nurses inherent in espousing family-centred care while also practicing evidence-based care, given the lack of evidence to support the efficacy of family-centred care. Furthermore, as a concept, family-centred care has its origins in the development of understanding the relationships between mothers and children in the early decades of the twentieth century (Shields 2011). Yet social change in more recent decades has led to greater diversity in the family structure and the roles that family members fulfil are becoming more diverse in the twenty-first century. Thus the practice of family-centred care has become more complex, presenting challenges to children and young people's nurses, and revealed in this chapter through a critical appraisal of the evidence of the reality of current practice of child- and family-centred care in relation to different family members.

MEANING AND ORIGINS OF FAMILY-CENTRED CARE

Family-centred care is widely held as the cornerstone of children's nursing practice, within the UK and across the world (Shields 2011), yet it is argued that it is a consistently ill-defined concept (Darbyshire 1994; Hutchfield 1999; Franck and Callery 2004; Shields 2011).

Progress in the care of children in hospital also dates from the 1950s, stemming from a growing understanding of the psychological trauma caused in part by mother–child separation in hospital (Jolley 2007), and heavily influenced by the social norm of the traditional nuclear family.

A key conceptual advance was the development of the partnership model by Casey during the late 1980s. The partnership model is based on the belief that 'the care of children, well or sick, is best carried out by their families, with varying degrees of assistance from members of a suitably qualified healthcare team whenever necessary' (Casey 1988, p. 9).

The concept of family-centred care has further developed since Casey's work, with Smith et al. (2002, p. 22) offering the definition of family-centred care as 'the professional support of the child and family through a process of involvement, participation and partnership underpinned by empowerment and negotiation'.

Recently, a new terminology – *child- and family-centred care* – has begun to emerge in policy (e.g. in the National Service Framework for Children and Young People [Department of Health 2004]) and literature in the UK (Smith and Coleman 2010), reflecting the influence of both increasing regard for children's rights and consumerism on healthcare policy. Child- and family-centred care therefore incorporates the notion that children are active participants with their parents and nurses in negotiation and decision making in healthcare (Coleman 2010).

A weakness in the nursing research on families in hospital is that, despite the centrality of the concepts of parent and family to children's nursing, by and large the terms *parent* and *family* have been uncontested and undefined, with the exception of Darbyshire (1994) and Callery (1995). The gender balance of participants in research on families' healthcare experiences also merits consideration. In a meta-analysis of research in paediatric palliative care, MacDonald et al. (2010) found mothers constituted 75% of the overall sample of parents, so unless gender balance is sought, research on parental perspectives does not fully reflect fathers' and mothers' needs and experiences.

CHANGING FAMILIES

WHAT IS A FAMILY?

Family is a central concept for nurses working with babies, children and young people. Whether they practice child- and family-centred care, family-centred care or family systems nursing, family is central. *Family* is also a term used every day in personal life, and therefore it is easy to assume that the meaning of *family* is obvious. While in terms of practice, Shields (2011) is right to argue that family comprises whatever the particular family perceives it to be, given its centrality to children and young people's nursing practice, there is a need for children and young people's nurses to have a theoretical understanding of the concept.

The philosopher Archard (2003, p. 69) defines family as 'essentially a stable multigenerational association of adults and children serving the principal function of rearing its youthful members'. Arguably, this is the meaning with which 'family' is most usually used. Yet, thinking about this further, a group of adult siblings and their partners may regard themselves as a family, as might a couple without children. Nonetheless, the social unit of adults and children has persisted across history and throughout vastly different societies and cultures (Archard 2003). Within that continuity, however, there is also considerable variation and change in family form across time and cultures.

SOCIAL CHANGE INFLUENCING FAMILY COMPOSITION

The key changes to family life affecting children in Britain include the following:

- The 2001 census revealed 65% of children live with both their natural parents, 11% in a stepfamily and 23% in a lone-parent family (Office for National Statistics 2004).
- The proportion of families comprising children and cohabiting opposite-sex parents increased to almost 30% by 2014 (Office for National Statistics 2015).
- There has been an increase in the number of stepfamilies (Ferri and Smith 1998), from both marriage and cohabitation breakdown, so that one child in eight will experience living in a stepfamily by the age of 16 (Ferri and Smith 1998).
- 10% of families with dependent children are stepfamilies (Cabinet Office and Department for Children, Schools and Families 2008).
- A small but increasing number of families comprise children and same-sex parents (Office for National Statistics 2015).
- There has been increased participation in paid work by mothers and a rapid increase in the number of families in which both parents work full time (Cheal 2002).

Social change therefore means that there is now considerable variation in relationships within the structure of an outwardly traditional nuclear family, although the extent to which such change varies across different ethnic groups is unclear (Mann 2009). The parents may be cohabiting, one or more of the children may be adopted, one adult may be a stepparent and some children may be the couple's biological children while others are stepchildren. Thus some young people may experience multiple changes in family structure as they grow up. After divorce, many children manage life in two families, maintaining good relationships with both parents and both wider family networks (Morton et al. 2006). Family structure is further complicated by reproductive technologies such as egg, sperm and embryo donation, which may create outwardly traditional nuclear families in which there may be a range of genetic relationships between parents and birth children.

Mac an Ghaill and Haywood (2007) argue that family is now understood as a negotiated relationship rather than an institution defined by blood and marriage ties, although its function is unchanged. Changes in family form over the last 50 years mean that membership of a family today can be much more fluid and diverse, with groups of individuals defining themselves as a family according to their own criteria. One size of family-centred care clearly does not fit all families; children's nurses need to treat each family as an individual unit and make no assumptions about roles and responsibilities.

DIVERSITY OF FAMILIES

The term *nuclear family* has traditionally been used to refer to a heterosexual married couple and their dependent biological children (Muncie and Sapsford 1997), in which the adults adopt breadwinner/homemaker roles along traditional gender lines (Cheal 2002). This type of family has often been portrayed as an ideal and is a powerful social norm. Yet Hobson and Morgan (2002) claim that, in fact, this was the majority family type in western Europe and the US for only a short time during the 1950s and 1960s.

The most common pattern of family life in modern Britain is of families who are technically nuclear but also have extensive contact with a kin group (i.e. people to whom they are directly or indirectly related by descent) who live nearby (Muncie and Sapsford 1997). Such kinship groups have the potential to provide practical and emotional support during stressful times, such as a child's admission to hospital.

'Extended family' is a phrase normally used to refer to biologically related family members of three generations living together, usually grandparents, parents and children, but sometimes including others such as uncles and aunts (Dallos and Sapsford 1997). While this type of family may be traditionally associated with some minority ethnic groups, it occurs across society. Within the extended family, the child has recourse to close relationships with adults beyond his parents, and the closest child–adult relationship may not be child–parent. Responsibilities for childcare and decision making may be shared between parents and grandparents, or parents may defer to grandparents in relation to child-rearing practices and decisions. With increasing longevity, an increasing number of four-generation families is being seen (Cheal 2002), which may mean that parents have responsibility for caring for their own grandparents as well as their children. Extended families may therefore be either a source of support for the parents of a sick child or an additional responsibility.

Lone-parent families, i.e. one parent living in a household with his or her dependent children, have always been a feature of British society, currently numbering 2 million, with 91% of lone parents rearing children being mothers (Office for National Statistics 2015). Lone-parent families are more likely to experience poverty (Department for Education and Skills 2007) which has a negative impact on children's health. Over half of lone parents had their children in marriage or a long term relationship, the average of lone parents is 38%, and 21% are from black or minority ethnic communities (Gingerbread 2016). In order to practice truly family-centred care, nurses would need to know the nature of the child's usual relationship with the non-resident parent and encompass consideration of that parent's needs into the plan of care.

A small but increasing number of families comprise same-sex couples and their dependent children, and may be biological, step, adoptive or in vitro in origin. There is some evidence that same-sex parents tend to balance work and home responsibilities more equally than heterosexual couples and involve more extended family networks of kin and friends in their parenting (Scottish Government 2009). Fairtlough (2008) concluded from a literature review concerning children and young people's experiences that, although they experienced homophobia, they were predominantly positive about their parenting experiences. Yet in a Swedish study, lesbian parents were embarrassed by the assumptions of heterosexuality made by maternity healthcare professionals, who the parents also thought were embarrassed by their clients' sexuality (Röndahl et al. 2009).

Some children and young people, including unaccompanied sanctuary-seeking children, live apart from their families, in the care of a local authority. In England there are approximately 60,000 children in care at any one time, of whom approximately 70% live with foster carers and 11% in children's homes (Department of Health and Department for Children, Schools and Families 2009). The local authority acts as a corporate parent for such children, and each child or young person has a personal health plan (Department of Health and Department for Children, Schools and Families 2009). Some children and young people have continued contact with family members and others do not. Nurses need to understand an individual child or young person's circumstances and identify who has parental responsibility, and consider what information should be shared, how and with whom. As parents routinely take such active roles in the care of their children in hospital, children's nurses need to pay heed to the risk that some of the needs of unaccompanied looked after children may go unmet, and how they might compensate for the absence of parental care for some looked after children.

There are 51,000 young carers in the UK, with an average age of 12 years. While being a young carer does not necessarily have a negative impact on a young person, there is evidence that excessive care demands may have a negative impact on a young person's physical, emotional, social and educational well-being (Children's Society and Princess Royal's Trust for Carers undated). Stigma and fear of the consequences of disclosure may make the young carer reluctant to reveal their circumstances. When young carers are themselves in need of healthcare, nurses need to be aware that there may not be someone able to fulfil the normal parental role for that young person and also that alternative caring arrangements may need to be made for the person for whom the child normally provides care.

Some parents may face particular challenges in participating in care in the way that nurses may expect and may need additional support in order to participate in care. These may include, for example, those with learning difficulties, parents with enduring mental health problems, parents with impaired mobility, parents who misuse substances, recent migrants and families who do not speak English.

REFLECTION POINTS

- To what extent do the forms and paperwork where you work demonstrate assumptions about family structure and relationships?
- Do the questions you ask when admitting a child or meeting a family for the first time convey an assumption that every child has one mother and one father?
- How do you adapt your negotiation of care to accommodate some parents' needs for extra support?

CHANGING ROLES WITHIN FAMILIES

Children's nurses frequently use the term *parents* rather than specifically talking of mothers and fathers. Again, parenting is an everyday concept, but it is worth taking time to explore what the concept really means; for example, is parenting the same as mothering or fathering?

PARENTING

Parents exert a profound influence on their children's development and health (Ramchandani and McConaghie 2005). In addition to genetic health, dietary habits, lifestyle and attitudes are acquired within the family; aspects of behaviour and emotional health are dependent on relationships with parents. Hence, 'good parenting' is seen as vital for children's well-being and achievement, as defined in *Every Child Matters* (Department for Education and Skills 2003). In the Common Assessment Framework, dimensions of parenting are identified as the capacity to provide basic care safety and protection; emotional warmth and stability; and guidance, boundaries and stimulation (Department for Children, Schools and Families 2009).

Much of the research on parenting has been derived from attributes of the maternal role; i.e. it has been conducted through a matrifocal lens, meaning that aspects of mothering have been regarded as the norms against which fathers' parenting is measured, resulting in what Golden (2007) has termed a 'deficit model' for fathering. Golden (2007) therefore argues that a masculine concept of caregiving needs to be developed.

MOTHERS

Children's nurses will be aware that the Platt Report (which began the changes that led to the development of family-centred care) on the care of children in hospital (Central Health Services Council 1959) was heavily influenced by the work of child psychiatrist John Bowlby. In 1950, Bowlby was commissioned by the World Health Organization to write a report on the effects of maternal deprivation on infant and child mental health. He says of mothers: 'What is believed essential for mental health is that an infant and young child should experience a warm, intimate and continuous relationship with his mother' (Bowlby 1965, p. 13); and of fathers: 'In the young child's eyes father plays second fiddle' and 'his value as the economic and emotional support of the mother will be assumed' (Bowlby 1965, p. 15).

Although Bowlby modified his ideas in later years, and his attachment theory has been refined to encompass a primary attachment to the father and include multiple attachments (Featherstone 2009), his understanding of the mother–child relationship was highly influential at the time.

A focus on the child's relationship with his or her mother continued in psychological and social science research for many years and is reflected in the early literature on parents in hospital. Here, the interest in parental presence has been firmly on mothers being the resident parent and performing what were described as mothering tasks, such as providing comfort, entertainment and meeting hygiene and nutritional needs (Craig and McKay 1958; Brain and Maclay 1968). However, these brief descriptive papers do show an awareness of the impact of a child's hospitalization on other family members (Moncrieff and Walton 1952; Craig and McKay 1958). Meadow (1964) reported an investigation into whether *mothers* wanted to stay with their child, reporting that only 44% did, with many citing their husband's needs as a reason why they could not. Brain and Maclay (1968) found only 20% of *mothers* agreed to take part in their clinical trial in which mothers accompanied children admitted for tonsillectomy.

By the 1980s researchers were using the term *parent*, rather than *mother*, although in reality their participants were almost entirely mothers (e.g. Webb et al. 1985; Sainsbury et al. 1986). This usage has continued in much of the later research until very recently.

FATHERS

Fatherhood, like motherhood, is both a biological and socially defined phenomenon. Across cultures, societies and times, the father role is seen as encompassing procreation, provision and protection (McNeill 2007). This would suggest that models of parenting derived from mothering are not appropriate for fathering. In his overview of fatherhood research, Lamb (2000) has argued that the defining aspect of fathering has shifted over decades from the provision of moral guidance through breadwinning, sex-role modelling and marital support to nurturance and the emergence of 'new fatherhood' in the 1970s. There has been growing academic interest in fatherhood and in relationships between fathers and children since that time. Early fatherhood research focused on father absence (Krampe 2009), whereas, more recently, researchers have explored the effects of fathers' personal characteristics, employment and behaviour on child development (Equal Opportunities Commission 2007). Earlier father research focused on early childhood, although more recently evidence suggests that father input during adolescence is associated with positive outcomes for young people (Videon 2005; Utting 2007).

INVOLVED FATHERHOOD

The notion of 'involved fathering' has become widespread within children's services including health, social care and education. Flouri (2005) has identified involved fathering to entail being there for children, providing for physical needs and providing psychological support and moral guidance. Father involvement is claimed to be good for children and to lead to higher self-esteem, better friendships, more empathy, better life satisfaction, higher educational achievement, decreased risk of criminality and decreased risk of substance abuse (Layard and Dunn 2008). Videon (2005) also found involved fatherhood to have a positive influence on young people's well-being.

While *involved fatherhood* as a term derives from the academic or policy sphere, there is evidence that it is reflected in the values and aspirations of wider society. For example, new fathers viewed a good father as present in the home, involved with their children and sensitive to their needs (Henwood and Proctor 2003). A clear expectation that fathers should be 'involved' in the family was evident in research carried out by Warin et al. (1999), although the reality of involvement was tempered by a reluctance of both sexes to surrender traditional roles.

Social structures have an influence on individual decisions: better paid fathers have more freedom in balancing the provider role with other aspects of fathering than those who have to work long hours to provide sufficient income for their family (Marsiglio and Cohan 2000). A substantial number of men in couple relationships are the main carers for their children all or some of the time (Fatherhood Institute 2011). These factors will also influence an individual father's ability to be present and involved in the care of his sick child.

Fathers' own beliefs and commitment are also important factors determining the level of involvement with children (Gaunt 2008), and these are influenced by age, race, views of gender, socioeconomic circumstances and relationships (Marsiglio and Cohan 2000). Williams (2009) also argues that white working class men and African-Caribbean fathers, who may have different understandings of masculinity and fathering, have been overlooked in fatherhood research. Within a child–adult relationship, fathering practices change as the child and father age, develop and experience different circumstances (Palkovitz and Palm 2009). Children's own perspectives on their experiences of being fathered are also underresearched.

A further factor influencing the extent of fathers' involvement is maternal gatekeeping. This is the concept that mothers regulate fathers' involvement through their own supportive or resistant behaviour (Allen and Hawkins 1999). Such gatekeeping may not be conscious or intentional (Gaunt 2008), and is in turn influenced by the mother's own beliefs and attitudes particularly in relation to gender role and beliefs about fathers (Cannon et al. 2008). Although the concept of maternal gatekeeping is controversial, there is some evidence to support it. Ellison et al. (2009) found that more mothers than fathers viewed childcare as primarily the mother's responsibility, and Henwood and Proctor's (2003) found some new fathers felt they were less involved in decision making than they wanted to be or that they had to ask mothers' permission to be involved in baby care. Zvara et al. (2013) found that the influence of maternal gatekeeping and beliefs about gender roles extended to fathers' involvement in children's healthcare. This highlights the point that involved fathering requires mothers to 'move over' to make space for them.

Family change means more men live apart from their children and more men are living with children to whom they are not biological fathers. An individual child may have a biological father, separated from his mother but involved in the child's life, and an unrelated male who assumes the father's role in his life. Burgess (2008) asserts that child and family services commonly fail to identify important males in children's lives and their relationships with the child, particularly when the father is living in another household. Nurses may feel awkward asking such intrusive questions, yet failing to do so can leave a child at risk or exclude a father who has a right to information about his child.

Ferri and Smith (1998) found that stepfathers were more involved in childcare than biological fathers, and Pickford (1999) found no difference between married and cohabiting fathers in their involvement or commitment to their children. Burghes et al. (1997) use the term *social fathers* to encompass all the variations of the non-biological father–child relationship. Using such a term reminds nurses not to make assumptions about relationships based on biology alone and conveys acknowledgement that a male adult may have a significant relationship and play an important role in a child's life while having no biological or legal status.

In reality therefore family status and structure may make little difference in the stability, commitment to each other and relationships within the family. Ahmann (2006, p. 88) urges healthcare professionals to be open-minded and inclusive in their approach in relation to the father role in families, arguing that 'the person or persons who see themselves in the paternal role, whether or not they are biologically related to the child, are the persons most likely to be involved participants in the child's care'.

REALITY OF CONTEMPORARY FATHERS' ROLES IN FAMILIES

It is recognized by the United Nations that the perceptions of the role of women and men in families have changed; men are no longer just economic providers to families (United Nations Department of Economic and Social Affairs 2011). In the UK, strongly gendered attitudes toward family roles were revealed by Ferri and Smith (1996) in their analysis of data from the National Child Development Study; however, a study on fathers' needs and expectations at home and work for the Equal Opportunities Commission found widespread acceptance of traditional roles alongside a wide diversity of fathers' roles within families, with couples making pragmatic decisions relating to childcare and work based on earning capacity (Hatter et al. 2002).

A national study for the Equality and Human Rights Commission (Ellison et al. 2009) revealed:

- 47% of fathers thought the father's role is to provide for the family
- 23% of fathers thought that childcare is the primary responsibility of mothers
- 62% of fathers thought that fathers in general should spend more time caring for their children
- 58% believed that it is possible for partners to share responsibilities around work and care equally
- Fathers of children with disabilities were less likely to work full-time and twice as likely to say they had primary responsibility for caring for their child

This research therefore demonstrates that while attitudes are changing toward a co-parenting model, couples' actual decisions reflect a more traditional division of responsibilities. Although there have been changes in male and female work patterns, Dex (2003) argues that the 1.5 earner household (i.e. a father who works full-time and a mother who works part-time) has become the norm, with the greatest change being the increase in the number of mothers of children under 5 in paid work, 40% of mothers with young children work part-time and 17% work full-time (Cabinet Office and Department for Children, Schools and Families 2008). In one study, fathers in dual-full-time-earner households were found to be more likely to share childcare and domestic work and, in some families, shift parenting occurred where fathers were responsible for childcare while mothers worked and vice versa (Ferri and Smith 1996). However, many fathers in the Equal Opportunities Commission study described work as a welcome escape from family life (Hatter et al. 2002), and, in another study, 75% of mothers stated that they had primary responsibility for childcare in day-to-day life (Ellison et al. 2009).

So while evidence is contradictory on specific aspects of work and parenting, trends toward more shared responsibility for earning and childcare are evident. For many parents, the day-to-day reality of bringing up children involves complex decision making. Ellison et al. (2009) concluded that parenting was widely seen as a team effort and that practicalities, rather than beliefs and values, drove decision making regarding roles and responsibilities – the person who is available at the time does what needs to be done. Therefore parents of both sexes may experience tension between paid work, family responsibilities and the care of the child in hospital.

CASE STUDY

Jay, aged 5, is on a children's ward with appendicitis. His mother and father both work: Sahira, his mother, is a head teacher of a primary school and his father, Ramesh, is a website designer. They have no other family members in the country. They agree that Jay should have someone with him at all times, but both are also continuing to work during Jay's stay in hospital. They manage this by doing shifts. Ramesh stays with Jay during the day, arriving at 0730, leaving at 1800 and working at home late into the night. Ramesh also tries to work when he can on the ward during the day. Sahira comes to the ward after work at 1730, receiving a brief 'handover' from Ramesh. Sahira, in turn, goes straight to work from the hospital at 0800, after handing over to Ramesh.

Jay develops postoperative complications and has a prolonged stay in hospital. After 5 days, nurses have found the parents to be increasingly critical of care and irritable with each other and the staff. Sahira tells a staff nurse that she feels left out and is dependent on secondhand information because she cannot be on the ward for the surgeon's ward round. Jay seems settled and happy, although some nurses think he is 'clingy' for his age.

REFLECTION POINTS

- How would you practice family-centred care with a dual-earner two-parent family who both continue to work?
- What would your personal reaction be to two working parents who both wanted to continue working while their child is ill?
- In your workplace, how easy would it be for a parent who works 0900 to 1700 to speak to a senior practitioner or make a clinic appointment outside of the parent's own working hours?
- How do your answers relate to partnership and collaboration with parents or carers?

PRINCIPLES FOR PRACTICE

- Fathers' involvement in the care of their children in hospital will be influenced by the broader context of their normal family lives, including working patterns, their usual levels of involvement with their children and other commitments.
- Nurses need to be aware of how their own values and beliefs in relation to fathers influence their own practice.
- Maternal gatekeeping behaviour may occur in everyday life and in relation to the child's hospitalization.
- Families make decisions on a pragmatic basis rather than from their beliefs and values.

GRANDPARENTS

Of course, grandparents have always been a part of family life, although Whitworth (2005) has argued that grandparents have been overlooked in social and economic policies. Arguably this applies to children's healthcare too; there is very little discussion of grandparents in the children's nursing or literature on family-centred care.

As people live longer, it is increasingly the case that the grandparent–grandchild relationship may last 30 years or more. Fifty percent of older Americans can expect to become great grandparents (Stelle et al. 2010).

There is a trend toward greater grandparental involvement with their grandchildren than in the past (Griggs et al. 2009), and grandparents are becoming increasingly important in family life across Europe (Glaser et al. 2010). Grandparents are the largest source of informal childcare in the UK (Smethers 2015), and across Europe they provide childcare which enables parents to work (Glaser et al. 2010). Griggs et al. (2009) found from a national survey in England and Wales that a high level of involvement with grandparents was reported for most grandchildren, with a positive association between grandparental involvement and child well-being. Some grandparents who provide care also benefit from an enhanced sense of purpose, even if the childcare itself may be demanding and exhausting (Statham 2011). With half of grandparents aged under 65 years in the UK, this means that grandparents may be juggling the demands of work and childcare in a way similar to that of parents (Smethers 2015).

An increasing number of grandparents are also taking on parental or near-parental roles with their grandchildren, when parents are unable to fulfil that role (Ravindran and Rempel 2011); however, this has been shown to have a negative impact on the health of grandparents (Smethers 2015).

PRINCIPLES FOR PRACTICE

- The prevalence of the concept of involved fathering and changing parental responsibilities within families means that fathers are more likely to be present with their child in hospital than in earlier decades. Even if they are not present in hospital or normally resident with the child, their child's hospitalization has an impact on fathers.
- In order to support fathers, nurses need to understand their experiences and needs, yet the British literature on parents' involvement in their children's care in hospital reveals little of them.
- Without evidence from research, nurses have to depend on their personal knowledge and experience. The discussion in this chapter thus far has demonstrated that nurses need to be aware of their own assumptions and expectations in relation to fathers' roles, and guard against imposing these on families in practice.
- Grandparents may be directly involved in providing childcare and can be an important resource for the child and the parents.

FAMILY MEMBERS' EXPERIENCES OF CHILDREN'S ILLNESS AND HEALTHCARE

DOES ONE SIZE FIT ALL?

The 'family' in family-centred care is often taken to mean 'parents', and 'parents' equals mothers, underpinned by the assumption of a nuclear family structure. The appropriateness of family-centred care for minority ethnic families, among whom there may be more varied patterns of responsibility for childcare, has been questioned (Ochieng 2003). If parent equals mother reflects children's nursing thinking, it could lead to the exclusion from care of individuals who are significant for the child, for example a social father, a grandparent or an older sibling.

CASE STUDY

A toddler is brought to the accident and emergency department with significant scalds. He is accompanied by eight adults of different ages, none of whom appear to speak English. The adults are all distressed, shouting at each other. It is not possible to establish who, if anyone, is the child's parent. Staff assess and treat the child amid considerable noise and confusion; it is apparent that the child will need to go to the paediatric intensive care unit (PICU).

When the interpreter arrives, the relationship to the child of each adult is established. Both parents are present and insist that the child's 19-year-old aunt accompany the child to PICU as she normally cares for the child along with others in the family while the parents work. Staff try to persuade the family that it should be a parent who stays.

REFLECTION POINTS

- What is the purpose of having a resident adult with a child?
- Who do you think should stay with the child in the case study above?
- What are the implications for nurses if the person staying with the child is not the parent?

Childhood illness and contact with medical services is stressful for families. It tests parental resilience (Ramchandani and McConaghie 2005) and may exacerbate existing difficulties in family functioning (Johnson et al. 2005). As there is evidence that adjustment following illness is frequently related to family functioning (Johnson et al. 2005), supporting mothers, fathers and other family members promoting effective family functioning can promote children's recovery. Children's nurses are in a position to support parents in exploring and accessing practical and emotional support from other family members and friends. Children's nurses may also need to be flexible in who is resident with a child, given the diversity of family structures and roles in the twenty-first century.

In the remainder of this chapter, current research in relation to fathers' and grandparents' experience during children's healthcare is explored in order to provide an evidence base for inclusive practice with families.

WHAT IS KNOWN ABOUT FATHERS' EXPERIENCES AND NEEDS WHEN THEIR CHILD IS ILL?

The needs and experiences of fathers of children in acute care have been largely overlooked by researchers. However, some of the research examining parents' experiences in this area has touched on fathers' experiences, although samples in these studies are predominantly mothers. Darbyshire's (1994) investigation of the experiences of parents who were resident in hospital with their child included 24 mothers and 4 fathers, reflecting the ratio of resident parents at the time. He suggests that fathers were marginalized by organizational policies which constructed 'parents' to mean mothers (e.g. the facility for resident parents was called the 'mothers unit'), and there is a suggestion that fathers were largely ignored by nurses (Darbyshire 1994). Callery (1995) also explored parental experiences, interviewing the member of the family most involved in the child's care, predominantly mothers but including a minority of fathers and a grandparent. He found that some fathers were involved in care but they were relegated to a secondary role, as substitutes for the real carers (that is mothers) or an optional extra. Coyne (2003) found fathers acted as supporters to mothers – by relieving them at the child's bedside and sharing duties at home.

FATHERS IN ACUTE SETTINGS

Although, initially, it was mothers who accompanied their children in hospital, the term *parents* has been commonly used since the 1980s, while research was actually being conducted with mothers. As society has changed, more fathers are likely to be present in hospital, and it has been assumed that what we know from research with parents (really mothers) is relevant to them. The oversight of fathers' needs appears to have resulted, at least in part, from a focus on understanding the perspectives of the parent who is resident in hospital, as in the past this has predominantly been mothers.

Nurses have been found to have clear but subconscious expectations of the roles that parents would play when in hospital with their child (Coyne 2007), which are often in accordance with stereotypical gender roles (Higham 2011). These expectations may lead both nurses and parents to presume that responsibilities for care will be shared in particular ways.

Board (2004) explored symptoms and sources of stress for fathers. Fathers reported symptoms including headaches, having unpleasant thoughts, being easily annoyed and worrying too much (Board 2004). Ninety percent of fathers identified 'seeing their child have needles' and 80% 'not knowing how to help' as stressful (Board 2004). Children's nurses can use this information to help prepare fathers for how they might feel and the practical ways they can help their child, as this might reduce the stress fathers experience.

Tourigny et al. (2004) video recorded mothers' and fathers' presence and actions in the first hour after their child's surgery, finding that, although mothers were present for longer, mothers and fathers demonstrated a similar range of helpful behaviours, though fathers showed them with less frequency (Tourigny et al. 2004). These findings suggest that mothers and fathers adopted similar roles in relation to their child in hospital.

Thompson et al. (2009) found higher agreement between fathers' preoperative predictions of their child's level of anxiety at anaesthetic induction and scores from a behaviour rating scale completed by researchers than mothers' predictions. At face value this would suggest that fathers were better able to predict their child's anxiety than mothers. However, rather than accept that finding, which perhaps does not fit with gender expectations, the researchers argue that mothers' predictions may have been based more on their child's internal state than behavioural state and that the children's anxiety cues were too subtle to be picked up by the assessment tool used, resulting in falsely low anxiety scores, so that in fact mothers' predictions were accurate (Thompson et al. 2009). This argument could be seen as attributing greater credibility to maternal knowledge of the child over paternal knowledge of the child.

'Being there' is a recurring theme in relation to the parents of children in hospital, yet Kars et al. (2008) found differences in the meaning of being there for mothers and fathers. Mothers focused on empathy, involvement and child and parent staying together, whereas, for fathers, being there had a more active meaning, seeing it as advocating and supporting their children in a more practical way, i.e. 'doing something' (Kars et al. 2008). This masculine conceptualization of being there is concordant with the widely recognized protector aspect of the father role and is also shown in Higham's study of fathers' roles with children in hospital (Higham 2011).

> **REFLECTION POINT**
>
> Nurses may interpret fathers' actions such as asking questions about treatment plans or questioning professionals' actions and decisions as their way of being there, as part of their role as a protector, not necessarily a criticism of care.

FATHERS IN NEONATAL UNITS

The birth of a sick or preterm infant is always a shock for parents, with long-term consequences for both parents. Fathers whose babies are admitted to neonatal units face particular challenges in addition to the shock and stress of the birth of a sick or preterm infant which they have to confront in the very visible context of the neonatal unit. If they are first-time fathers, their transition to fatherhood takes place in the public setting of the unit, as does their bonding with their baby. There may be physical barriers which prevent or inhibit them from holding their child. If they have other children, they will be concerned about how to tell them that their anticipated sibling will not be coming straight home or may not survive. In addition to concern for their infant, they will be concerned for the welfare of their partner post-delivery, who may have undergone a caesarean section or may be ill, and may be in a different hospital to the child. The father is frequently the parent who is able to be most present in the earliest hours of a child's stay in a neonatal unit. Children's nurses have a crucial role to play in supporting mothers, fathers and other family members at this challenging time.

Johnson (2008) has argued that engaging fathers in the care of their infants in neonatal intensive care is much more challenging than involving mothers. Identification of family care needs is part of nursing assessment and contributes to developmental care (Johnson 2008), yet just as in the acute setting, most studies of parents' experiences in neonatal units focus on mothers (Deeney et al. 2009). Arockiasamy et al. (2008) suggest that existing parental support mechanisms are based on healthcare providers' perceptions of what parents might need rather than having been developed with parental input. There is clearly a need to understand fathers' perspectives on their experiences and needs.

Fegran and Helseth (2009) argue that the neonatal intensive care unit is an environment in which two worlds meet. Parents are experiencing an ontological change, i.e. their way of being in the world is changing forever, whereas nurses are doing an ordinary day's work. While parents need privacy and individualized care, nurses need efficiency, visibility and access (Fegran and Helseth 2009). Approximately 40% of neonatal intensive care units in the UK allowed both parents to stay overnight whenever they chose (Greisen et al. 2009), suggesting that separation of mothers and fathers at this stressful time is common. Pöhlman (2009) found that the necessary precedence given to technological care of infants in neonatal intensive care left fathers feeling frustrated, afraid and alienated and that nurses were unaware of how fathers were feeling. Fathers have also reported feeling marginalized, more like a visitor than a parent (Poppy Steering Group 2009). Fathers wanted to be involved but felt there was little they could 'do' (Pöhlman 2003). Arockiasamy et al. (2008) found there was a universal sense of lack of control among fathers of extremely ill infants in neonatal intensive care. Fathers identified that relationships with the healthcare team; friends and family; and consistent information, including short, relevant written information, helped them regain a sense of control (Arockiasamy et al. 2008). A need for greater opportunity to discuss their own feelings was expressed by fathers in the Poppy study, an inquiry into parental views on neonatal services (Poppy Steering Group 2009). Fathers also reported taking on a protector role toward both their partner and child (Arockiasamy et al. 2008).

Sloan et al. (2008) found that fathers identified their partners and families as sources of emotional support. This research highlights the importance of parents' relationships with each other and with family members, and nurses need to consider how they can promote and support these. Information needs vary. Fathers in one study identified staff as sources of informational support, although less than half were satisfied with the information they received (Sloan et al. 2008). Some fathers actively sought information as a means of regaining some control, whereas others wanted limited information (Arockiasamy et al. 2008). Knowing how much and what sort of information to give – whether he needs a broad overview or specific details – is a further challenge. It is not surprising therefore that neonatal nurses experience interaction with parents as perhaps the most challenging part of their job (Fegran and Helseth 2009). In the UK, only 40% of neonatal intensive care units were found to permit completely open 24-hour parental visits, including during ward rounds (Greisen et al. 2009). While this policy may be predicated on the need to protect confidentiality, it may also exclude parents from important exchanges of information and decision making.

The formation of attachment bonds between parents and child is a crucial process during the neonatal period, which is disrupted if the child is born preterm or sick. In a natural setting, proximity, reciprocity and commitment are central characteristics of the attachment process (Goulet et al. 1998, cited by Fegran et al. 2008). Again, most of the literature on this topic is focused on mothers (Fegran et al. 2008). Fegran et al. (2008) argue that touch and visual contact are the most powerful tools by which parents communicate with their infants. Fathers in their study described how touching and holding their child, even if they were reluctant to do so initially, transformed their relationship with their child from an impersonal one to one of belonging and protection, having a positive effect on fathers' self-esteem and coping (Fegran et al. 2008).

FATHERS OF CHILDREN WITH CHRONIC ILLNESS

Father involvement in aspects of a child's chronic illness may positively influence marital, family and child psychological outcomes (Clarke et al. 2009), as well as the health of the ill child. As an example, paternal involvement in their children's asthma management had a moderating effect on their children's use of emergency care (Kuhn et al. 2014). Research with fathers of children with chronic illness has explored relationships with healthcare professionals and child health services, the social and emotional impacts of having a child with chronic illness, the coping strategies fathers use and fathers' role expectations.

Some fathers have seen health services as being oriented toward women (Clarke 2005; Ware and Raval 2007) and reported that they, as men, felt they had been treated differently from women to the extent of feeling ignored or abandoned by healthcare professionals (Ware and Raval 2007; Hayes and Savage 2008). Some men saw dealing with healthcare professionals as challenging (Chesler and Parry 2001; Clarke 2005; Waite-Jones and Madill 2008). Clarke (2005) identified outpatient appointment times within normal working hours as a barrier to fathers' greater involvement in medical care. In hospital, ward round times may mean that working fathers are unable to be present. This can mean that fathers have to depend on second-hand medical information from the child's mother, adding to stress and anxiety and potentially causing conflict between the parents (Chesler and Parry 2001).

The social effects on fathers of having a child with a chronic illness include social isolation, with family, friends and others seen as not understanding (Katz and Krulik 1999; Goble 2004; McNeill 2004; Waite-Jones and Madill 2008) or not as supportive as anticipated (Ware and Raval 2007). In some studies, fathers reported increased strain on the couple's relationship, but also increased closeness with their partner along with increased closeness to the ill child (McNeill 2004; Ware and Raval 2007) or to the other well children in the family (Goble 2004). Some fathers felt that having a chronically ill child had led to increased division of labour within the family along gendered lines (Goble 2004; Waite-Jones and Madill 2008) with consequent greater pressure on fathers to provide financially.

In terms of the emotional effects of childhood chronic illness on fathers, a sense of chronic sadness is evident, for example among fathers of children with diabetes (Sullivan-Bolyai et al. 2006) and of children with life-limiting illness (Ware and Raval 2007). Fathers have described multiple losses of a 'normal' family life, of an ideal healthy child, of their role as a protector and provider and of opportunities for shared family and father–child activities (Waite-Jones and Madill 2008). Fathers also faced anxiety arising from day-to-day uncertainty in relation to their child's condition (Cashin et al. 2008; Hayes and Savage 2008), and fears for the future (McNeill 2004; Sullivan-Bolyai et al. 2006).

Yet, fathers of children with chronic illness express reluctance to discuss or show their feelings with family members or professionals. This reluctance is identified by men as arising from a need to 'be strong' and support their partners (Chesler and Parry 2001; McNeill 2004; Sullivan-Bolyai et al. 2006; Ware and Raval 2007). In short, research with fathers reveals:

- A reluctance to burden partners with their feelings (McNeill 2004)
- A view that men generally do not and should not talk about or show their feelings (Ware and Raval 2007; Hayes and Savage 2008; Waite-Jones and Madill 2008)

- The attitude that it is better not to talk about issues in order to avoid painful emotions (Hayes and Savage 2008)

The range of coping strategies fathers of children identify include:

- Denial (Waite-Jones and Madill 2008)
- Distraction (McNeill 2004; Peck and Lillibridge 2005; Waite-Jones and Madill 2008)
- 'Time out' (McGrath and Chesler 2004)
- Focusing on the here and now (Peck and Lillibridge 2005; Hayes and Savage 2008)
- Taking positive action (McNeill 2004; Sullivan-Bolyai et al. 2006; Ware and Raval 2007)
- Maintaining a positive outlook (McNeill 2004)

Some fathers respond to their child's chronic illness by seeking information (Ware and Raval 2007; Cashin et al. 2008), whereas others avoid finding out more because such knowledge could increase stress and cause powerful emotions (Peck and Lillibridge 2005; Hayes and Savage 2008).

Many fathers of children with chronic illness are direct caregivers, for example providing routine childcare for the affected child, becoming the main carer for siblings when a mother's time was consumed by the needs of an ill child, becoming the main carer for the ill child (Clarke 2005; Bonner et al. 2007), performing medical aspects of care (Clarke 2005; Sullivan-Bolyai et al. 2006) and providing emotional support for all family members (Chesler and Parry 2001). Yet some fathers experience mothers as the 'experts' in the child's care (Pelchat et al. 2003; Pöhlman 2003), with the authority to include fathers or keep them on the periphery (Pöhlman 2003). Mothers have acknowledged not leaving room for fathers to participate in care and feeling that fathers were not able to adequately care for the ill disabled child (Pelchat et al. 2003). Thus there is more evidence to support the notion of maternal gatekeeping. Healthcare professionals may unwittingly perform gatekeeping of their own if they assume that 'mother knows best'.

The protector element of their paternal role can be challenged by their child's chronic illness, in relation to both the ill child and other family members (McGrath and Chesler 2004; McNeill 2004; Clarke 2005). One father in McGrath and Chesler's (2004) study spoke of how his role as a father was 'to fix things', and of the anger and frustration resulting from not being able to fix his son's cancer. In other research, fathers expressed the protector role through taking responsibility for keeping their child calm and minimizing stress during clinical procedures (Swallow et al. 2011), and in discussion of the need for advocacy for their ill child in healthcare situations (McNeill 2004; Clarke 2005). Such advocacy included asking awkward questions or monitoring the performance of hospital staff. Nurses who understand the protector role as a driver for aspects of paternal behaviour may be able to discuss this with fathers so that the potential for tension to arise between fathers and nurses is reduced.

There are some positive aspects of being a father of a child with a chronic illness. A sense of gradual adjustment, acceptance over time and personal growth is evident in some studies (e.g. Chesler and Parry 2001; McNeil 2004). Despite intra-family stresses and strain, mothers and fathers have reported stronger marriages and closer families (Chesler and Parry 2001). Fathers described opportunities to become more involved in family life that they would not have had if their child were healthy (Hayes and Savage 2008) and heightened relationships with their partner, the ill child (McNeill 2004; Ware and Raval 2007) or their healthy children (Goble 2004).

In the past, fathers of children with disability were evaluated by health professionals in terms of the support they gave to the mother (Pelchat et al. 2003), be that emotional, practical or financial, whereas health professionals need to recognize, value and support the father–child relationship in and of itself.

KEY POINTS

- Many healthcare professionals are largely unaware of fathers' needs.
- Fathers in acute care have been overlooked by researchers.
- Researchers are beginning to investigate the experiences and needs of fathers of sick or preterm neonates.
- Many fathers of chronically ill children are active givers of care who experience social and emotional consequences as a result of their child's condition.
- These consequences challenge the fulfilment of the father role.
- There is contradictory evidence in relation to fathers' information needs.

GRANDPARENTS

As discussed earlier, many grandparents contribute directly to the care of their grandchildren in addition to providing support for their own children's parenting. Therefore any illness of the grandchild has an impact on the grandparents and many grandparents might expect to be involved in the care of ill children. Yet, despite the espousal of family-centred care in children's nursing, Hall (2003) argues that grandparents, and particularly grandfathers, have been marginal in children's nursing research. This seems to be particularly the case in relation to acute care.

Wakefield et al. (2014) found that grandparents of children with cancer were seen as providing a 'safety net' for the whole family, although this was at a personal cost to the grandparents. Those of children with cancer were found to experience more psychological distress than a control group of grandparents, yet this distress was not disclosed to healthcare professionals and the authors suggested that without intervention, this distress could limit grandparents' capacity to support the whole family (Wakefield et al. 2014). Miller et al. (2012) found that the grandparents of children with disabilities put family needs ahead of their own wishes (for example by continuing to live near the family with the disabled child to provide support, rather than moving away in retirement).

'Double concern' – for both their own child and the grandchild – was identified among grandfathers of sick neonates in a study by Hall (2003). These men valued both information and presence with the child as support for their own coping. Yet in a UK-wide study, although sibling and grandparent visiting was permitted in many neonatal units, this was often conditional on being accompanied by parents (Greisen et al. 2009). Thus grandparents could be prevented by unit policy from staying with the neonate to enable parents to take a break and support one another, and inhibited from developing their own bond with their new grandchild.

CASE STUDY

Sixteen-year-old Becky has given birth at 27 weeks to Mia, who is admitted to a neonatal unit (NNU). Becky and Jake, Mia's father, live with Becky's parents, Phil and Jan. Becky is ill postnatally and is unable to visit the NNU. Jake seems overwhelmed with the situation. He visits the unit for short periods only and is yet to touch or hold Mia and does not speak to the staff. Phil and Jan are keen to be involved in Mia's care and frustrated that they cannot visit on their own. The staff are concerned about Jake's apparent lack of commitment to Mia. Jan tells a staff nurse that Jake feels like everyone is staring at and judging him. She asks staff to back off a bit and let her and Phil get Jake involved at his own pace.

REFLECTION POINTS

- How do you think nurses should react to Jan's request to 'back off a bit'?
- How might nurses support young fathers without making them feel under pressure or scrutiny?
- What contribution might Phil and Jan make to Mia's care?

KEY POINTS

- Many grandparents provide vital support to parents and sick children.
- Grandparents experience concern for both the sick child and their own child which healthcare professionals need to recognize.

CONCLUSIONS

Everyday practice of children's nurses involves working with families of all descriptions in which individual members undertake a wide range of roles. Roles and relationships within families cannot be assumed. Fathers are more involved in their children's lives than in previous generations and consequently are in contact with healthcare professionals more frequently. Fathering is both a role and a relationship, and the nurse needs to consider this child–father relationship independently of the child–mother and mother–father relationship, while respecting family functioning. Similarly, grandparents may have significant caring responsibilities for their grandchildren.

The use of the term *parents* rather than *mothers* in children's nursing literature has led nurses to apply understanding drawn from research with mothers to their work with fathers. This has been exacerbated by a tendency for researchers to examine the experiences of the parents of hospitalized children from the perspective of the resident parent only. Yet we know that the wider family is affected by the child's hospitalization and can support the parents. There is as yet very little research on the contributions that grandmothers, grandfathers and other family members make to the care of ill children.

In this chapter, some of the research evidence concerning fathers' and grandparents' experiences of their child's healthcare has been outlined. There is some evidence to support the notion that fathers' needs when their children are ill are different from those of mothers. Children's nurses need to be aware of this evidence and consider how they identify and meet fathers' needs, particularly given the evidence that some fathers feel the need to appear strong and may be reluctant to talk. Children's nurses need to learn to consider fathers in their own right and in relationship to the child, not just as support or a substitute for mothers. There is also a need for nurses to discuss with parents the extent of involvement of grandparents in the sick child's care.

There is also clearly a need for pre-registration and continuing professional development programmes to reflect the fact that parenting is in reality mothering and fathering and to prepare nurses to work effectively with mothers, fathers and other family members.

There is a need for further research with fathers, particularly in the acute setting, to improve understanding of their needs. Yet researchers undertaking such work face challenges, such as some men's reluctance to talk about their feelings. Approaches such as peer research may prove fruitful in the future.

In this chapter it has been argued that, even though fathers and grandparents play a vital role in caring for their child in sickness and in health, this has often been overlooked or disregarded by health and social professionals, including children and young people's nurses. Family-centred care, if it is to be implemented in its truest sense, must take value from and respect the contribution made by all members of the family.

REFERENCES

Ahmann E (2006) Supporting fathers' involvement in children's health care. *Pediatric Nursing* **32**: 88–90.

Allen SM, Hawkins AJ (1999) Maternal gatekeeping: mothers' beliefs and behaviors that inhibit greater father involvement in family work. *Journal of Marriage and the Family* **61**: 199–21.

Archard D (2003) *Children, family and the state.* Aldershot: Ashgate.

Arockiasamy V, Holsti L, Albersheim S (2008) Fathers' experiences in the neonatal intensive care unit: a search for control. *Pediatrics* **121**: e215–22.

Board R (2004) Father stress during a child's critical care hospitalization. *Journal of Pediatric Health Care* **18**: 244–9.

Bonner M, Hardy K, Willard V, Hutchinson K (2007) Brief report: psychosocial functioning of fathers as primary caregivers of pediatric oncology patients. *Journal of Pediatric Psychology* **32**: 851–6.

Bowlby J (1965) *Child care and the growth of love.* 2nd ed. Harmondsworth: Penguin.

Brain D, Maclay I (1968) Controlled study of mothers and children in hospital. *British Medical Journal* **1**: 278–80.

Burgess A (2008) *The costs and benefits of active fatherhood.* London: Fathers Direct. Available at www.fatherhoodinstitute.org/uploads/publications/247.pdf.

Burghes L, Clarke L, Cronin N (1997) *Fathers and fatherhood in Britain.* London: Family Policy Studies Centre.

Cabinet Office and Department for Children, Schools and Families (2008) *Families in Britain: an evidence paper.* London: DCSF. Available at http://www.cabinetoffice.gov.uk/media/111945/families_in_britain.pdf.

Callery P (1995) An investigation into the role of parents in hospital. PhD thesis, University of Liverpool, Liverpool.

Cannon E, Schoppe-Sullivan S, Mangelsdorf S, et al. (2008) Parent characteristics as antecedents of maternal gatekeeping and fathering behavior. *Family Process* **47**(4): 501–19.

Casey A (1988) A partnership with child and family. *Senior Nurse* **8**(4): 8–9.

Cashin G, Small S, Solberg S (2008) The lived experience of fathers who have children with asthma: a phenomenological study. *Journal of Pediatric Nursing* **23**(5): 372–84.

Central Health Services Council (1959) *The welfare of children in hospital.* Platt Report. London: Ministry of Health.

Cheal D (2002) *Sociology of family life.* Basingstoke: Palgrave Macmillan.

Chesler M, Parry C (2001) Gender roles and/or styles in crisis: an integrative analysis of the experiences of fathers of children with cancer. *Qualitative Health Research* **11**: 363–84.

Children's Society and Princess Royal's Trust for Carers (undated) *Making it work: good practice with young carers and their families.* London: Children's Society and Princess Royal's Trust for Carers. Available at www.youngcarer.com.

Clarke J (2005) Fathers' home health care work when a child has cancer: I'm her Dad; I have to do it. *Men and Masculinities* **7**(4): 385–404.

Clarke N, McCarthy M, Downie P, et al. (2009) Gender differences in the psychosocial experience of parents of children with cancer: a review of the literature. *Psycho-Oncology* **18**: 907–15.

Coleman V (2010) The evolving concept of child and family-centred healthcare. In Smith L, Coleman V (eds.) *Child and family centred-care: concept, theory and practice.* 2nd ed. Basingstoke: Palgrave, pp. 1–26.

Coyne I (2003) A grounded theory of disrupted lives. PhD thesis, King's College London, London.

Coyne I (2007) Disruption of parent participation: nurses' strategies to manage parents on children's wards. *Journal of Clinical Nursing* **17**: 3150–8.

Craig J, McKay E (1958) Working of a mother and baby unit. *British Medical Journal* **1**: 275–7.

Crawford D (2012) Evidence vs family centred care. *Nursing Children and Young People* **24**(10): 3.

Dallos R, Sapsford J (1997) Patterns of diversity and lived realities. In Muncie J, Wetherell M, Langan M, et al. (eds.) *Understanding the family.* 2nd ed. London: Sage, pp. 126–70.

Darbyshire P (1994) *Living with a sick child in hospital: the experiences of parents and nurses.* London: Chapman & Hall.

Deeney K, Lohan M, Parkes J, Spence D (2009) Experiences of fathers of babies in intensive care. *Paediatric Nursing* **21**: 45–7.

Department for Children, Schools and Families (2009) *Common Assessment Framework: practitioners' and managers' guides.* Nottingham: DCSF. Available at http://www.dcsf.gov.uk/everychildmatters/strategy/deliveringservices1/caf/cafframework/.

Department for Education and Skills (2003) *Every child matters.* London: DfES.

Department for Education and Skills (2007) *Every parent matters.* London: DfES.

Department of Health (2004) *The National Service Framework for children, young people and maternity services.* London: Department of Health.

Department of Health and Department for Children, Schools and Families (2009) *Healthy lives, brighter futures: the strategy for children and young people's health.* London: Department of Health.

Dex S (2003) *Families and work in the 21st century.* York: Joseph Rowntree Foundation. Available at http://www.jrf.org.uk/publications/families-and-work-twenty-first-century/.

Ellison G, Barker A, Kulasuriya T (2009) *Work and care: a study of modern parents.* Manchester: Equality and Human Rights Commission. Available at www.equalityhumanrights.com.

Equal Opportunities Commission (2007) *Fathers and the modern family.* Manchester: Equal Opportunities Commission.

Fairtlough A (2008) Growing up with a lesbian or gay parent: young people's perspectives. *Health and Social Care in the Community* **16**(5): 521–8.

Fatherhood Institute (2011) *Fathers, mothers, work and family.* Available at www.fatherhoodinstitute.org/2011/fi-research-summary-fathers-mothers-work-and-family/.

Featherstone B (2009) *Contemporary fathering: theory, policy and practice.* Bristol: Policy Press.

Fegran L, Helseth S (2009) The parent-nurse relationship in the neonatal intensive care unit context – closeness and emotional involvement. *Scandinavian Journal of Caring Sciences* **23**: 667–73.

Fegran L, Helseth S, Fagermoen M (2008) A comparison of mothers and fathers' experiences of the attachment process in a neonatal intensive care unit. *Journal of Clinical Nursing* **17**: 810–16.

Ferri E, Smith K (1996) *Parenting in the 1990s.* London: Joseph Rowntree Foundation. Available at www.jrf.org.uk/publications/parenting-1990s.

Ferri E, Smith K (1998) *Step-parenting in the 1990s.* York: Joseph Rowntree Foundation. Available at www.jrf.org.uk/sites/default/files/jrf/migrated/files/spr658.pdf.

Flouri E (2005) *Fathering and child outcomes.* Oxford: Wiley Blackwell.

Franck L, Callery P (2004) Re-thinking family-centred care across the continuum of healthcare. *Child: Care, Health and Development* **30**(3): 265–77.

Gaunt R (2008) Maternal gatekeeping: antecedents and consequences. *Journal of Family Issues* **29**(3): 373–95.

Gingerbread (2016) *Statistics: single parents today.* Available at www.gingerbread.org.uk/content/365/ statistics.

Glaser K, Montserrat E, Waginger U, Price D, Stuchberry R, Tinker A (2010) Grandparenting in Europe and the US. Available at http://www.gulbenkian.org.uk/files/13-12-10-FP5%20Grandparenting%20in%20 Europe%20Summary_Grandparents%20Plus.pdf.

Goble L (2004) The impact of a child's chronic illness on fathers. *Issues in Comprehensive Pediatric Nursing* **27**: 153–262.

Golden A (2007) Fathers' frames for childrearing: evidence toward a masculine concept of care-giving. *Journal of Family Communication* **7**(4): 265–85.

Goulet C, Bell L, Tribble D, Lang A (1998) A concept analysis of parent-infant attachment. *Journal of Advanced Nursing* **28**: 1071–81.

Greisen G, Mirante M, Haumont D (2009) Parent, siblings, grandparents in the neonatal intensive care unit: a survey of policies in eight European countries. *Acta Paediatrica* **98**: 1744–50.

Griggs J, Tan J-P, Buchanan A, et al. (2009) 'They've always been there for me': grandparental involvement and child well-being. *Children and Society* **24**: 200–14.

Hall E (2003) A double concern: Danish grandfathers' experiences when a small child is critically ill. *Intensive and Critical Care Nursing* **20**: 14–21.

Hatter W, Vinter L, Williams R (2002) *Dads on dads: needs and expectations at home and work.* Manchester: Equal Opportunities Commission.

Hayes C, Savage E (2008) Fathers' perspectives on the emotional impact of managing the care of their children with cystic fibrosis. *Journal of Pediatric Nursing* **23**(4): 250–6.

Henwood K, Proctor J (2003) The 'good father': reading men's accounts of paternal involvement during the transition to first-time fatherhood. *British Journal of Social Psychology* **42**(3): 337–55.

Higham S (2011) Protecting, providing and participating: fathers and their children's unplanned hospital admission. Unpublished PhD thesis, Swansea University, Swansea.

Hobson B, Morgan M (2002) Introduction. In Hobson B (ed.) *Making men into fathers: men, masculinities and the social politics of fatherhood.* Cambridge: Cambridge University Press, pp. 1–24.

Hutchfield K (1999) Family-centred care: a concept analysis. *Journal of Advanced Nursing* **29**(5): 1178–87.

Johnson A (2008) Engaging fathers in the NICU: taking down the barriers to the baby. *Journal of Perinatal and Neonatal Nursing* **22**(4): 302–6.

Johnson G, Kent G, Leather J (2005) Strengthening the parent-child relationship: a review of family interventions and their use in medical settings. *Child: Care, Health & Development* **31**(1): 25–32.

Jolley J (2007) Separation and psychological trauma: a paradox explained. *Paediatric Nursing* **19**(3): 22–5.

Kars M, Duinjnstree M, Pool A, et al. (2008) Being there: parenting the child with acute lymphoblastic leukaemia. *Journal of Clinical Nursing* **18**: 1553–62.

Katz S, Krulik T (1999) Fathers of children with chronic illness: do they differ from fathers of healthy children? *Journal of Family Nursing* **5**(3): 292–315.

Krampe E (2009) When is the father really there? A conceptual reformulation of father presence. *Journal of Family Issues* **30**(7): 875–97.

Kuhn V, Freitas C, France B Distelberg B (2014) Parents in fragile families: the influence of parental engagement in emergency care use in children with asthma. *Families, Systems and Health* **32**(4): 389–98.

Lamb M (2000) The history of research on father involvement: an overview. *Marriage and Family Review* **29**(2): 23–42.

Layard R, Dunn J (2008) *A good childhood: searching for values in a competitive age.* London: Children's Society/Penguin.

Mac an Ghaill M, Haywood C (2007) *Gender, culture and society: contemporary femininities and masculinities.* London: Palgrave Macmillan.

MacDonald M, Chilibeck G, Affleck W, Cadell S (2010) Gender imbalance pediatric palliative care research samples. *Palliative Medicine* **24**(4): 435–44.

Mann R (2009) *Evolving family structures, roles and relationships in light of ethnic and social change.* Available at www.citeseerx.ist.psu.edu/viewdoc/download;jsessionid=016FF194625A11F29FA169CBB8C82FF7? doi=10.1.1.366.832&rep=rep1&type=pdf.

Marsiglio W, Cohan M (2000) Conceptualizing father involvement and paternal influence. *Marriage and Family Review* **29**(2): 75–95.

McGrath P, Chesler M (2004) Fathers' perspectives on the treatment for pediatric hematology: extending the findings. *Issues in Comprehensive Pediatric Nursing* **27**: 39–61.

McNeill T (2004) Fathers' experience of parenting a child with juvenile rheumatoid arthritis. *Qualitative Health Research* **14**(4): 526–45.

McNeill T (2007) Fathers of children with a chronic health condition: beyond gender stereotypes. *Men and Masculinities* **9**: 409–24.

Meadow SR (1964) No thanks; I'd rather stay at home. *British Medical Journal* **2**: 813–4.

Miller E. Buys L, Woodbridge S (2012) Impact of disability on families: grandparents' perspectives. *Journal of Intellectual Disability Research* **56**(1): 102–10.

Moncrieff A, Walton A (1952) Visiting children in hospital. *British Medical Journal* **1**: 43–4.

Morton S, Jamieson L, Highet G (2006) *Cool with change: young people and family change*. Research Briefing 23. Edinburgh: Centre for Research on Families and Relationships. Available at https://www.era.lib.ed.ac.uk/bitstream/handle/184/2780/rb26.pdf?sequence=1&isAllowed=y.

Muncie J, Sapsford J (1997) The concept of the family. In Muncie J, Wetherell M, Langan M, et al. (eds.) *Issues in the study of the family*. 2nd ed. London: Sage, pp. 7–39.

Ochieng B (2003) Minority ethnic families and family-centred care. *Journal of Child Health Care* **7**(2): 123–32.

Office for National Statistics (2004) *Census 2001: national reports for England and Wales*. Part 2. London: ONS.

Office for National Statistics (2015) *Families and households*. Available at www.ons.gov.uk.

Palkovitz R, Palm G (2009) Transitions in fathering. *Fathering* **7**(1): 3–22.

Peck B, Lillibridge J (2005) Normalization behaviours of rural fathers living with chronically ill children: an Australian perspective. *Journal of Child Health Care* **9**: 31–45.

Pelchat D, Lefebre H, Perreault M (2003) Differences and similarities between mothers' and fathers' experiences of parenting a child with a disability. *Journal of Child Health Care* **7**(4): 231–47.

Pickford R (1999) *Fathers, marriage and the law*. London: Family Policy Studies Centre.

Pöhlman S (2003) When worlds collide: the meanings of work and fathering among fathers of premature infants. PhD thesis, St Louis University, St Louis, MO.

Pöhlman S (2009) Fathering premature infants and the technological imperative of the neonatal unit: an interpretive inquiry. *Advances in Nursing Science* **32**(3): e1.

Poppy Steering Group (2009) *Family-centred care in neonatal units. A summary of research results and recommendations from the Poppy project*. London: National Childbirth Trust

Ramchandani P, McConaghie H (2005) Mothers, fathers and their children's health. *Child: Care, Health and Development* **31**(1): 5–6.

Ravindran VP, Rempel GR (2011) Grandparents and siblings of children with congenital heart disease. *Journal of Advanced Nursing* **67**(1): 169–75.

Röndahl G, Bruhne E, Linde J (2009) Experiences of lesbian parents in the UK. *Midwifery Matters* **139**: Winter.

Sainsbury C, Gray O, Cleary J, et al. (1986) Care by parents of their children in hospital. *Archives of Diseases in Childhood* **61**: 612–5.

Scottish Government (2009) *The experiences of children with lesbian and gay parents – an initial scoping review of evidence*. Edinburgh: Scottish Government. Available at www.scotland.gov.uk/socialresearch.

Shields L (2011) *Family-centred care: effective care delivery or sacred cow?* Forum on public policy. Available at http://forumonpublicpolicy.com/vol2011.no1/archive2011.no.1/shields.pdf.

Sloan K, Rowe J, Jones L (2008) Stress and coping in fathers following the birth of a preterm infant. *Journal of Neonatal Nursing* **14**: 108–15.

Smethers S (2015) What are the issues affecting grandparents in Britain today? *Quality in Aging and Older Adults* **16**(1): 37–43.

Smith L, Coleman V (eds.) (2010) *Child and family centred-care: concept, theory and practice*. 2nd ed. Basingstoke: Palgrave.

Smith L, Coleman V, Bradshaw M (2002) Family-centred care: a practice continuum. In Smith L, Coleman V, Bradshaw M (eds.) *Family centred-care: concept, theory and practice*. Basingstoke: Palgrave, pp. 19–43.

Statham J (2011) Working paper 10: grandparents providing childcare. Available at www.cwrc.ac.uk/resources/documents/Grandparent_care_briefing_paper_Nov_11_WP_No_10.pdf.

Stelle C, Fruhau C, Orel N, Landry-Meyer L (2010) Grandparenting in the 21st century: issues in diversity in grandparent-grandchild relationships. *Journal of Gerontological Social Work* **53**(8): 682–701.

Sullivan-Bolyai S, Rosenburg R, Bayard M (2006) Fathers' reflections on parenting young children with type 1 diabetes. *Maternal-Child Nursing* **31**: 24–31.

Swallow V, Lambert H, Santocre S, Macfadyn A (2011) Fathers and mothers developing skills in managing children's long-term medical conditions: how do their qualitative accounts compare? *Child: Care, Health and Development* **37**(4): 512–22.

Thompson C, MacLaren J, Harris A, Kain Z (2009) Brief report: prediction of children's pre-operative anxiety by mothers and fathers. *Journal of Pediatric Psychology* **34**(7): 716–23.

Tourigny J, Ward V, Lepage T (2004) Fathers behaviour during their child's ambulatory surgery. *Issues in Comprehensive Pediatric Nursing* **27**: 69–81.

United Nations Department of Economic and Social Affairs (2011) *Growing importance of men in families.* Available at http://www.un.org/en/development/desa/news/social/men-in-families.html.

Utting D (2007) *Parenting and the different ways it can affect children's lives; research evidence.* York: Joseph Rowntree Foundation. Available at www.jrf.org.uk/publications.

Videon T (2005) Parent-child relations and children's psychological well-being: do dads matter? *Journal of Family Issues* **26**: 55–77.

Waite-Jones J, Madill A (2008) Concealed concern: fathers experiences of having a child with juvenile idiopathic arthritis. *Psychology and Health* **23**(5): 585–601.

Wakefield C, Drew D, Ellis S, Doolan E, McLoone J, Cohn R (2014) Grandparents of children with cancer: a controlled study of distress, support and barriers to care. *Psycho-Oncology* **23**: 855–61.

Ware J, Raval H (2007) A qualitative investigation of fathers' experiences of looking after a child with a life-limiting illness, in process and retrospect. *Clinical Child Psychology and Psychiatry* **12**(4): 549–65.

Warin J, Solomon Y, Lewis C, Langford W (1999) *Fathers, work and family life.* York: Joseph Rowntree Foundation. Available at www.jrf.org.uk/publications.

Webb N, Hull D, Madeley R (1985) Care by parents in hospital. *British Medical Journal* **291**: 176–7.

Whitworth D (2005) Grandparents are family too. *Community Care* 16–22 June: 20.

Williams R (2009) Masculinities and fathering. *Community, Work and Family* **12**(1): 57–73.

Zvara B, Schoppe-Sullivan S, Dush C (2013) Fathers' involvement in child health care: associations with pre-natal involvement, parents' beliefs and maternal gatekeeping. *Family Relations* **62**: 649–61.

Recognizing and supporting the needs of siblings

MARIA O'SHEA, MARY HUGHES, EILEEN SAVAGE AND
CLARE O'BRIEN

OVERVIEW

When fostering an ethos of family-centred care, nurses aspire to look after not only the child with the health concerns but also the family as a whole. While the primary focus is the sick child, the secondary focus is often the parents/carers, as these are the family members that health professionals have the most contact with. The needs of siblings of sick children are often overlooked or ignored. This situation is sometimes mirrored in the home environment as the sick child becomes the central family focus, leaving the well siblings feeling vulnerable and isolated. This chapter explores the needs of children who live with a child sibling with acute or chronic health care needs. It also explores the caring role of the well sibling for his or her brother or sister with a health issue or physical disability. The effect of bereavement on siblings is also examined and support groups for siblings are discussed.

INTRODUCTION

Most of the children that nurses and health professionals come in contact with in both acute and non-acute settings have siblings, i.e. brothers or sisters. The sibling relationship within a family unit is very important in terms of the emotional, social and behavioural development of both the child with the illness/disability and the sibling of the child being cared for. This sibling relationship, however, is often overlooked and sometimes ignored. This chapter begins by looking at the nature of sibling relationships and the concept of family-centred care (FCC). It challenges nurses to consider siblings as an important and integral component of the family unit. This chapter then closely examines the needs of healthy siblings when their brother or sister becomes ill or has a developmental disability. It highlights how the healthy sibling may often feel unnoticed or uncared for as parental attention and focus is on the child with the illness/disability. The effect of this situation on the well sibling in terms of role changes, taking on more responsibility and developing a protector role is also discussed.

This chapter concludes by examining the effects of the bereavement of a child on the remaining sibling(s). The death of a child brings about a multitude of emotions for families, communities and health care professionals. Both negative and positive effects are discussed. Support for bereaved siblings is also a focus of this section, highlighting the needs for age-appropriate support structures such as sibling support groups, as well as family supports, all of which are necessary to facilitate the grieving process.

REFLECTION POINTS

- Consider the impact of a child's illness/disability on his or her sibling(s).
- Have you ever considered siblings when planning, implementing and evaluating family-centred care?
- Have you contemplated the effects of a child's death on the remaining siblings?

THE NATURE OF SIBLING RELATIONSHIPS

Most children when growing up in their families live with at least one sibling, a brother or a sister. It is estimated that more than 80% of children in the Western world have at least one sibling (Howe and Recchia 2006). Sibling relationships are likely to be one of the longest-lasting relationships in one's life because they continue from childhood throughout adulthood. In summarizing the literature, Howe and Recchia (2006) identified three major characteristics of sibling relationships that commence in early childhood. They found that sibling relationships are (1) emotionally charged, (2) defined by intimacy and (3) have large individual differences in quality. It is through sibling relationships that young children learn to express positive and negative emotions in ways that are socially acceptable. According to Kramer (2014), sibling relationships in the early years provide a foundation for children to learn how to get on in the world. Through these relationships, children learn how to share joyous experiences; express opinions, desires and feelings; co-operate with one another; and address conflicts and rivalries (Kramer 2014). Because children spend large amounts of time with one another in family life, they come to know each other intimately which, as noted by Howe and Recchia (2006), translates into siblings being a source of emotional and instrumental support for one another. The quality of sibling relationships can vary considerably. For example, siblings of similar ages may have closer relationships than those with a wide age gap because of issues of power and control (Howe and Recchia 2006). However, an important factor influencing sibling relationships is differential parental treatment (Howe and Recchia 2006; Kramer 2014) and the family environment (Jenkins et al. 2012). For example, when a child perceives their parents' interactions with a sibling to be showing more attention or favouritism, sibling rivalry or conflict can arise. This situation may arise at any time including specific events in family life, such as the birth of a new baby or when one child becomes ill.

Sibling relationships can be positively or negatively affected in the event that a brother or sister becomes acutely ill, is hospitalized, is diagnosed with a chronic illness or has special needs. For example, in a study on parent–sibling communication in families of children with sickle cell disease (SCD), Graff et al. (2010) found that some parents described siblings to be loving, empathetic, close and affectionate toward the child with SCD. In contrast, other parents described sibling relationships to be characterized by jealousy, which they attributed to parental attention given to the child with SCD. Other siblings were described as experiencing anger and unhappiness because of the impact of SCD on the sick child and the family. Sibling relationships are therefore integral to family life in the event that a brother or sister becomes ill or has a disability. Just as a sick child has needs for emotional and social attention, so too does the sibling of that child. The needs of siblings of a sick child in a family are important and need to be addressed throughout the illness journey, the pathway to recovery, or in the sad event of the child dying, leaving the sibling bereaved.

KEY POINT

Sibling relationships can be affected positively or negatively when a child in the family becomes ill or has special needs.

REFLECTION POINTS

- Recall your relationships with your siblings as a child and provide examples of sharing, having fun, conflicts and rivalry.
- How did you and your siblings support one another during childhood and in what contexts?

WHOLE FAMILY PERSPECTIVES AND FAMILY-CENTRED CARE

The concept of FCC is not new to caring for children in the health services and has gained increasing interest as a model for practice in hospital settings since the 1950s. Prior to this, the care of children in hospital was largely exclusive of families, even parents, because of concerns about infection control and assumptions that sick children in hospital made faster recoveries without their mothers, and that the efficiency of a ward managed by nursing staff would be compromised by a 'cluttering up' effect if open visiting was allowed (Brandon et al. 2009). Restricted visiting for parents was the norm in children's wards prior to the 1950s.

For example, an audit of hospitals in the UK published in 1953 found that out of 1300 hospital units for children only 23% allowed daily visiting by parents and a further 12% actually prohibited visiting (Central Health Services Council 1953). Since then, practices have gradually changed, most notably influenced by the publication of the Platt Report following an inquiry commissioned by UK government, titled *The Welfare of Children in Hospital* (Ministry of Health 1959). In a paper commemorating the 50th anniversary of the Platt Report, Davies (2010) maps how the recommendations were achieved toward parents being accepted as central to the care of sick children and which she described as a move from 'exclusion to toleration' of parental participation.

Over time, thinking about involving families within the context of child health care services has shifted. Since the early 1990s, there has been more than a decade of research on the role of parents, particularly mothers, caring for the hospitalized child (e.g. Callery 1991; Shuttleworth 1997; Hughes 2007). There has been an increasing shift in research from the hospitalized child to understanding the needs of parents of children with long-term illnesses or disabilities (Kirk 2001; Tong et al. 2008; Wilkie and Barr 2008). However, most research on parents as the family members affected by a child's ill health or disability has been from mothers' perspectives. Until recent years, little was known about the role of fathers because they were seldom included in studies, a trend which has changed in recent years not just relating to hospitalized children (Higham and Davies 2013) but also for children with chronic illnesses (Hayes and Savage 2008; Swallow 2008) or disabilities (MacDonald and Hastings 2010). An area that has seen a marked growth of research since the early 2000s has been children's experiences of illness and their relationships with their parents and health care professionals in seeking active involvement in their care (Savage and Callery 2007; Lambert et al. 2008; Callery and Milnes 2012). A key driver for listening to the views of children in health care has been the United Nations Convention on the Rights of the Child (UNCRC) (United Nations 1989), which requires that children's views are heard and acted upon. Listening to the views of children and acting upon them is critical to developing child-friendly health care (Kilkelly and Savage 2013).

KEY POINT

The UNCRC applies to siblings of a sick or unwell child, which means that they have the right to have their views heard and acted upon.

So far, it can be seen that research on family roles when a child is ill has evolved from a principal focus on mothers to including the needs of fathers and of children in hospital or with a chronic health problem. What has emerged is a somewhat disparate clustering of research which at one level offers practitioners an understanding of how to implement child-friendly care and at another level offers them an understanding of how to implement care centred on parents, either mothers or fathers or both. While this research may be helpful to practitioners, it lacks a focus on the whole family, with siblings largely excluded from previous research. The trends that evolve from research are both interesting and useful to compare with trends in practice. In other words, how does the research emphasis on parental involvement in the care of an acutely or chronically ill child compare with current practices of involving the family? This question calls for reflection.

REFLECTION POINTS

- Recall a recent practice event when you were caring for a child and his or her family in a health care setting?
- What family members were involved and how?
- What family members were not involved and why?
- To what extent did the child's care take account of the needs of siblings?

In order to meet the needs of siblings, a whole family perspective is needed. While the needs of the unwell child remain central, the care must extend beyond the prevailing trend of just considering the parents as the child's family. This may be stating the obvious, and an outcome from the above reflection may be that the needs of families in caring for a child in health care are inclusive of the needs of siblings. If this is the case, then practice is closely aligned to or embedded in a culture of FCC.

FCC as a concept has emerged as the kernel to fostering a whole family perspective in child health care. The term *family-centred care* is no stranger to the field of child health and paediatrics and is espoused to be the cornerstone of children's nursing practice and health care, although difficult to implement (Shields 2010). Definitions of FCC offer some insights into its fundamental characteristics and what these mean for practice. Based on a concept analysis, Mikkelsen and Frederikson (2011, p. 1159) defined *family-centred care* as

the professional support of the child and the family through a process of involvement and participation, underpinned by empowerment and negotiation. FCC is characterized by a relationship between health care professionals and the family, in which both parts engage in sharing the responsibility for the child's health care.

Here the emphasis seems to be on the role of family as provider and carer, in which case the needs of individual family members may be overlooked. Words of caution from Lane and Mason (2014) are that the experiences and feelings of siblings need to be taken into consideration when a child member of the family becomes ill. Parents may be burdened by their own emotional upset in dealing with their child's illness, in which case the needs of siblings may not be recognized or prioritized. Furthermore, parents may be unsure of how best to address the emotional needs of siblings. According to Lane and Mason (2014), there is a need for professionals to support parents in ways that take account of sibling needs using a family-centred approach. However, the authors did not define what they meant by FCC and how this could be implemented to address the needs of siblings.

Shields et al. (2006, p. 1318) offers a different perspective drawing attention to families as recipients of care, with *family-centred care* defined as

a way of caring for children and their families within health services which ensures that care is planned around the whole family, not just the individual child/person, and in which all the family members are recognised as care recipients.

There remains a lack of clarity from the above definitions about who the 'family' is. Although Shields is explicit in her reference to the 'whole family', it cannot be assumed that this will translate into the needs of siblings being addressed in practice. Indeed, the literature on FCC is of little practical use to practitioners because there is a striking lack of attention to siblings and how best to work with them to address their needs within a framework committed to a whole family perspective. A lack of understanding about what is meant by FCC is considered one of the main barriers to implementing FCC in practice (Kuo et al. 2012). For example, in a study on nurses' and parents' perceptions of FCC (Stuart and Melling 2014), siblings were considered only in the context of tending to their needs at home by fathers. Gaps in research on the needs and role of siblings in FCC exist, making it difficult for practitioners to establish a whole family perspective inclusive of siblings.

REFLECTION POINTS

- What is your understanding of FCC in practice?
- To what extent does your understanding take account of the needs of siblings?
- What ideas do you have for making your practice a 'sibling friendly' model of FCC and what would need to change?

The above reflection points are intended to prompt you to critically examine your practice and the culture of your organization as a starting point to thinking about the inclusion of siblings in a 'whole family' perspective toward FCC. The third point of reflection is likely to be challenging especially if your model of FCC is largely centred around parents, a finding evident in practice based on what FCC means to nurses (Coyne et al. 2011). The nurses in Coyne et al.'s study valued FCC as a model of care, which was difficult to implement without organizational and managerial support. An interesting observation from the findings of this study is that the nurses' ideas about implementing FCC specific to siblings pointed to structural resource issues with reference to 'facilities for siblings such as crèches or minders in hospital to enable parents to spend time with the sick child and also have siblings nearby' (Coyne et al. 2011, p. 2567). What is interesting about this observation is that although the nurses were thinking about the siblings, their ideas imply meeting the needs of parents rather than the needs of siblings. If implemented as the only approach to addressing siblings' needs, siblings are likely to be left marginalized from the caring process. The negative impact of overlooking siblings when a child is ill is illustrated later in this chapter.

> **KEY POINT**
>
> Health care professionals need to support parents in helping them meet the needs of siblings as well as meeting the needs of the sick child.

NEEDS OF HEALTHY SIBLINGS

Having a sibling who is unwell is an additional element to the typical growing-up experience of living in a family for healthy siblings. The usual routine of life is altered as family functioning is changed due to the care needs of the unwell child. This can result in less time spent with parents and the unwell sibling, and result in higher levels of anxiety for the healthy sibling (O'Shea et al. 2012). This is because they often do not understand the reasons why their sibling requires such additional time and attention from parents and they feel left out. Communication is key to decreasing this level of anxiety among siblings, as it allows them to ask questions and develop an understanding of what is happening to their sibling, and their role in the family (Wilkins and Woodgate 2005). Having a child with a developmental disability or chronic illness alters the family function in terms of roles typically associated with parents and siblings. This is because of the caregiving demands of the unwell child, which can have a significant impact on the lives of healthy siblings (Dauz Williams et al. 2010; Graff et al. 2010; Wennick and Huus 2012). Significant amounts of parental attention are often focused on the needs of the unwell child, as they are unable to be met without assistance. Routines are followed to ensure that medications, therapies and treatments in addition to the child's fundamental care needs are met. This reduces the time available to parents for other activities, including those with other siblings. Families transform the way they function when one of the children are unwell, especially with a chronic illness such as asthma when medical intervention is required unexpectedly (Shaw and Oneal 2014). Knowledge and skills are developed to assist them in coping with alterations in the child's health resulting in a heightened level of functional awareness. Situational awareness is enhanced by the development of expertise in recognizing and responding to the unwell child's ques. There is often a change in the psychosocial function of healthy siblings because of the decrease in parental attention due to the needs of the unwell child in a family.

The developmental age of the healthy siblings is important in terms of level of understanding and cognition in adapting to changes in the family (Piaget and Inhelder 1969). Adolescents may seek out support from peers more than younger children, who have greater dependency on their parents and other adults to care for them (Erikson 1995). Siblings have been found to have needs in terms of how their lives have changed and managing intense feelings, and have unmet needs as a result of having an unwell sibling (Wilkins and Woodgate 2005; Norris et al. 2010). Differences have been found between proxy accounts of sibling experiences by parental perceptions and from the personal reports by healthy siblings themselves (Graff et al. 2010; Norris et al. 2010; Sleeman et al. 2010). This may be because siblings view the situation differently to their parents and contribute different information on the same event. This may also be due to a lack of understanding of the situation, or because they have developed coping strategies to allow them to make sense of the situation and reduce its gravity in their lives.

Studies have shown that the needs of the sibling at home are overlooked by the family and health care professionals, as the priority is the child who is unwell or has been injured (Wilkins and Woodgate 2005; Lehna 2010; Nabors et al. 2013). Parents have reported that healthy siblings engage in negative behaviours because they feel isolated from their parents, and are jealous of the attention the sick child receives (Williams et al. 2009). This fluctuation in emotions by healthy siblings can continue long after the acute treatment phase has elapsed and affect their psychosocial well-being (Buchbinder et al. 2011). Healthy siblings experience an overwhelming range of emotions including sadness, loneliness, rejection, fear, anxiety, anger, jealousy and guilt (Wilkins and Woodgate 2005). Healthy siblings have also reported that they feel resentment and anxiety associated with their sibling if they have a mental illness or display behaviours associated with autism when in public due to the reactions from strangers (Smith 2006).

O'Shea et al. (2012) found psychosocial, emotional or behavioural changes in healthy siblings following the diagnosis of cancer in a sibling. They found that siblings recognized the needs of their unwell sibling but they wanted attention from their parents also. This was difficult for children in one-parent families. This was noted particularly at the time of the diagnosis and the period of initial treatment. They were cared for by relatives at this time, which resulted in a disconnect in the family functioning, resulting in a lack of information, which increased their fears. The hospital visiting policies also did not help as they were not able to visit at certain times or if there was an outbreak of infection on the unit their sibling was resident in. The separation of the family affected sibling and parental bonding as the normal routine was disturbed for long periods of time. Age was found to affect how siblings reacted to illness. Toddlers wanted parents more, whereas older children wanted their sick sibling more or to be more involved and be able to ask questions. Not all emotional or behavioural changes were negative however; gains were found in family cohesiveness which may be a balancing factor. Findings indicated a failure by parents and nurses in meeting the needs of healthy siblings consistently on communication, in providing them with age-appropriate information about cancer, in supporting them to maintain their own interests and activities, and in allowing them chances to participate in the care of their sick sibling (O'Shea et al. 2012).

Bugel (2014) found that healthy siblings were experiencing crisis at a personal level as well as at a family systems level when their sibling experienced a traumatic injury. She studied the school-aged siblings of children who had a traumatic injury, in the recuperative period. Her findings indicate that healthy siblings experienced a change in their relationship with their sibling, realizing how much they loved their sibling and fighting with them less (Bugel 2014). There was an increase in the number of other adults caring for them as their parents were with the unwell sibling; grandparents in particular were very involved. Healthy siblings experienced changes in sleep and sleeping arrangements, even moving rooms so they were not alone at night. They slept in their sibling's bed for comfort or with a parent for comfort so they were not alone. Healthy siblings reported a change in daily routine as their parent was not there as before, and other family members now assisted them. They experience an increase in household chores and tasks, and they were proud of their contribution as it gave them a purpose which felt good. There was still sibling rivalry with jealousy apparent when the unwell sibling received gifts or attention. School and after-school activities were a constant in their lives and stayed the same, which was a mediating factor for their stress as it was normal activity for them.

Healthy siblings of children who have developmental disability were found to have negative responses to the family functioning in research by Dauz Williams et al. (2010). Manifestations included upset, anger resentment and frustration, which resulted in negative behaviours such as making unkind remarks, needing a lot of attention and withdrawing into self, regressing and whining or crying for attention and being rough with the child who had the disability. They also got lonely and sad and sometimes depressed as their sibling was not at their level, which caused them to feel embarrassed, and were envious of the attention the unwell sibling received. Parents felt the healthy sibling did this because they did not understand the reason for, or nature of, the disability, which left them physically or emotionally detached from their parents due to the attention the other child required (Dauz Williams et al. 2010).

However, healthy siblings have also been shown to have a positive response to the changes associated with having an unwell sibling (Williams et al. 2009; Buchbinder et al. 2011). Adaptive resilience is seen in many studies, not only maladjustment in healthy siblings. Sleeman et al. (2010) found a positive impact on behavioural, emotional and social adjustment of well siblings when a child in the family has type 1 diabetes. Their study showed better emotional and behavioural adjustment than their peers according to their parents (Sleeman et al. 2010). The duration of the sibling's illness was found to have an effect on healthy siblings' adjustment. This is because they had developed better coping skills and had adapted to the illness over time. It should also be noted that siblings in this study were all well controlled. Siblings in Sleeman et al.'s study were older than those in other studies discussed, which may explain the findings as they potentially had more developed cognitive ability and coping skills.

Siblings manifest a range of problems that could be helped by playing them out. Medical play was used in research by Nabors et al. (2013) to allow children to narrate their own stories and recall their experiences of having a sick sibling. Play activities indicated that they wanted the ill child to become well and typically had a positive outcome. They played at providing support to parents in demonstrating how they coped and giving a sense of control in the play situation. They played about missing their parent, and fear of the medical procedures. They played out about needing support and about being supportive to their unwell sibling. They also played out being 'left out' and discussed sensitive issues, such as their fears for their parents. They said they could not discuss these issues with their parents because they were aware of their parents being tired and upset. Play was an emotional outlet for them and helped to process their own feelings (Nabors et al. 2013).

Healthy siblings are often overlooked in the planning and implementation of care for a child who is unwell. This is because the unwell child is the immediate centre of concern for their parents and the focus of their attention and care. The needs of healthy siblings can be unmet, especially at the time of initial diagnosis or if a crisis

〇 ┅┅┅ in their sibling's life. Children who have burns are often cared for in hospitals far from home so siblings have no access to visit them (Lehna 2010). The needs of the sibling at home are overlooked by the family and health care professionals (HCPs) as the priority is the child who has been injured. Lehna found that healthy siblings focus on normalization of the pattern of daily life in order to minimize the effects of the chronic illness on the family. This was the focus after the initial crisis at the time of the injury for siblings. School attendance became important in the process of normalizing their daily routines as before. Lehna (2010) found that parents treated all their children the same when the initial crisis had subsided and a sense of normalcy was gained.

Healthy siblings described the novelty of their initial experience of the traumatic injury to their sibling, as they stayed with different people and were made a fuss of, and met and did new things when they visited them in the hospital. This was a protective experience for them. This initial novelty was short-lived however, as they reported that they too wanted to be noticed and have their needs understood by adults. It was important for them as they did not want to be forgotten (Bugel 2014).

OVERLOOKED MEMBER OF THE FAMILY

Siblings are a central part of the family unit but are often overlooked in spite of the FCC approach when caring for sick children (Herrman 2010; Norris et al. 2010). They have the longest relationship in terms of individual experience with their siblings, and what happens to one can influence the other. Sibling relationships are characterized by roles, responsibilities and characteristics. Support, information and balance are required when one sibling becomes unwell. This can be gained from family, school and community but should include information that is accurate, honest and timely, and given in an age-appropriate way to maximize its effect and reduce stress. This aids the adaptation of the family as it is sensitive to the family functioning.

Siblings can be affected by chronic illness such as type 1 diabetes mellitus (T1DM), from a personal and family perspective, as they need to make adaptations to their lives. Siblings have reported that negatives of diabetes were pain associated with blood sugar monitoring and insulin administration, frequency of attendance at hospital or clinic, and being teased and the amount of time taken to care for the condition (Herrman 2010). Restrictions were placed on their own activity because of the unwell siblings' requirements and risks of deterioration of control. Dietary restrictions were frustrating as they were often placed on the whole family so the unwell sibling did not feel left out, which made them different to others because of the required treatment. This could be embarrassing at times. Healthy siblings reported that they had to help their sibling keep in control of their diabetes. They worried about them in terms of hypo- and hyperglycaemic episodes. There was also jealousy at the amount of attention the unwell sibling received (Herrman 2010). Although they admitted to being jealous, siblings acknowledged the negatives of having T1DM also. They did not want the diabetes even if this meant they got more attention from their parents too. They could see that it put pressure on parental relationships due to the care burden associated with the condition, especially on mothers as they were the main caregivers. Their knowledge and skill developed over time in terms of understanding how to manage the sugars. Costs and rewards of diabetes and its management on them, the unwell child and the family were all recognized (Herrman 2010).

Siblings of children who were newly diagnosed T1DM were found to have a fear of developing the condition themselves (Wennick and Huus 2012). Everyday life was transformed due to the physiological and psychological changes in the affected sibling, which became their new normal after a while. Life became more structured around the needs of the affected child and healthy siblings had to be more patient with the child who had T1DM as they became irritated more easily. Parents changed also; even when the affected child got more attention this was understandable to the healthy siblings as they felt sorry for them. They reported that they knew little about the illness and did not envy them the physical aspects of treatment and testing. Nurses can help siblings in this situation by explaining in age-appropriate terms what is happening and why, or by using distraction techniques to reduce the discomfort associated with the process of blood glucose monitoring in order to reduce the associated fear for siblings. The protective role of siblings was enhanced as they routinely engaged in checking if the affected child felt ok. They were also active in reassuring their affected sibling that their life would get better. They understood why they had to live separate from family at the time of diagnosis, and they had to assume more responsibility, and they missed their company. It was very positive to be reunited when the whole family were all back together at home. Their role developed further at that stage as monitoring their sibling's blood sugars became part of their role now, in addition to their chores. They felt that one of the positives of the illness was that the family got closer as a result. Healthy siblings reported that they would like to participate in educational sessions but this was not feasible for them (Wennick and Huus 2012).

CHANGES IN SIBLING FUNCTIONING

Having a child with a developmental disability or chronic illness alters the family function in terms of roles typically associated within families. Because of the caregiving demands of the child with the developmental disability or chronic illness, a change in family roles can have a significant impact on the lives of well siblings (Dauz Williams et al. 2010; Graff et al. 2010). Healthy siblings can also be burdened with excessive child care and household responsibilities for their family, and miss out on relationships and experiences outside of the home, e.g. spending time with friends after school. Healthy siblings take on more of the caregiving tasks required in families the older they get (Nagl-Cupal et al. 2014).

Dauz Williams et al. (2010) found that parents of children with developmental disabilities felt that their well sibling had a greater responsibility and did more chores around the home than would be typical for a child of their age, in order to help out. They felt they were more responsible at their age than would be typical, and their social activities were curtailed both inside and outside of the home. The positive outcomes were that the family was very close and that the well sibling was very protective of their brother or sister. Parental perceptions of a great sense of togetherness and sensitivity, which compensated for the inability of the unwell child to perform tasks or fulfil expected roles, were also found. There was a greater development of personal growth and the well sibling matured because of having an unwell sibling. This enabled the well siblings to manage their emotions and develop their cognitive and personal/social attributes as a result. Similar results were found in families who had a child with cystic fibrosis or cancer (Williams et al. 2009). Nurses can assist siblings and families by discussing ways of integrating the care needs of children with disabilities into the day-to-day routines of family life, such as inclusive mealtimes and therapy sessions in playtime. Each member of the family can develop a role in such activities as they become family activities and not just for the parent–child dyad.

Siblings recognized that family roles change when a child becomes unwell or has a chronic illness because of the caregiving demands of the unwell child. Roles within the household change, chores are allocated differently and parents assume a nursing role by undertaking complex tasks for the unwell child (Dauz Williams et al. 2010). Gaining an in-depth understanding of why these changes are necessary can be problematic for healthy siblings due to a lack of communication with them. Research has shown that they experienced a lack of communication with nurses, resulting in a disconnect as they did not know what was going on with their sibling. They struggled with trying to make sense of the hospital environment and what was happening to their sibling, as nurses never communicated this to them (Bugel 2014). This lack of communication is similar to the findings of O'Shea et al. (2012), who found that healthy siblings wanted to know what was going on and what the nurses were doing with or for their sick sibling. Not being told resulted in a rise in the fear of the healthy sibling, and an increase in their self-blame. They wanted to help, so finding a role for them was very important not only for themselves but also for their sick sibling. Being left out had a negative effect on healthy siblings and they felt that they could not discuss this with their parents (Nabors et al. 2013). Healthy siblings have reported increased awareness of their protective role and responsibilities toward their sick sibling. Siblings of children with Batten disease and mucopolysaccardiosis (MPS) reported having an intuitive knowledge of their sibling and worrying about symptoms they recognized as dangerous (Malcolm et al. 2014). They had developed an understanding of the conditions and their symptoms were understood and the challenges they posed were described by the siblings. Pain was particularly commented upon as it was difficult to recognize and treat. Coughing was the most difficult symptom to deal with as their unwell sibling could not cough and this worried them as they were afraid they would die. Their protection role extended beyond their sibling however; they protected their parents by not acknowledging the full extent of their knowledge of the situation. This was protective on both sides of the relationship between parent and child, recognizing the awareness of physical, psychosocial and emotional factors in their lives. They took pride in their family and how they dealt with the impact of having a sick child as a family member. They acknowledged, however, that this did restrict their family life, which caused them sadness.

The children also experienced a range of emotions in relation to how others viewed their sick sibling, particularly when they viewed the negative reactions of some people. They did not understand how people could be so unkind. They were protective of the sick child and worried about them deteriorating, which impacted on their social relationships with others. They acknowledged the provision of additional support from their peers in coping with such instances. They wanted wider support from the community in accepting their sibling. They felt isolated at times, and organized sibling support groups were found to be beneficial in allowing them to express their emotions. The meetings were too infrequent however, and they would have liked more of them (Malcolm et al. 2014).

It is important to consider age and gender of the healthy sibling in relation to the sibling relationship when developing a plan of care (Nielsen et al. 2012). Nurses should also ask the children about their experience and family functioning, as parents may have different perceptions of their relationships when evaluating them. Parents have been found to have higher expectations of healthy siblings in order to compensate for the unwell sibling (Smith 2006). Those conditions that have more of an impact on daily functional ability have been found to impact siblings more negatively. Positive adjustment is seen in family and sibling relationships when siblings are involved. Kindness and empathy increased as well as support through kinder interactions with their unwell sibling (Nielsen et al. 2012). Nurses should make a full assessment of social and family support and behaviours when considering the needs of siblings of sick children who may be at risk of developing psychological problems (Norris et al. 2010; O'Brien et al. 2009).

CASE STUDY

Kate, aged 5, and Paul, aged 7, are in the family room of your ward waiting for their parents who are visiting their sister Alice who is in isolation. Alice is 9 and has recently been diagnosed with acute lymphoblastic leukaemia. Their mother Anne is resident with Alice, staying full-time in the hospital as it is quite far from their home. Their dad, John, is taking care of Kate and Paul and working full-time. They are in primary school and go to after school with Alice as usual every day. Kate and Paul are playing with some of the toys in the family room and as you pass you hear the interaction between them. You decide to go in and have a chat to see how they are. Kate tells you she is happy because her dada told her she is getting sweets on the way home if she is good. Paul is less excited by this and asks you if he can go in to visit Alice. Somebody at school told him that she would have no hair and he is worried that this is the case. You ask if their dad has told them what is wrong with Alice and they reply that they know she has a bug in her blood. They cannot understand why they are not allowed to visit her and think this is very unfair. After all they brought her lovely new nightclothes and slippers and lots of cards and presents from friends and family. She is having all the fun they say.

QUESTIONS

- What would you do in this situation?
- How will you discuss the care of Kate and Paul with their parents?
- Should Kate and Paul be made aware of Alice's diagnosis and what her treatment entails?

REFLECTION POINTS

- What resources do you consider are important to support siblings and families to negate the negative outcomes for siblings and build on positive attributes?
- How would you include well-being of siblings as part of the care plan for sick children?
- Think about how you would communicate effectively with siblings and parents and use available resources to support them.

PRINCIPLES FOR PRACTICE

- Nurses should alert parents to the needs of siblings and allow them to express their feelings. Spend time alone with the sibling to reduce their fears and anxieties and jealousy.
- Nurses should consider including siblings when planning family-centred care and in interactions with the family. Include fun activities for them with their sibling where possible.
- Nurses should communicate with siblings to explain in an age-appropriate manner the hospital environment and what is happening with their sibling, answering their questions. Parental consent is needed for this.
- Nurses should be aware of the changing emotional needs of siblings over time.
- Nurses should make a full assessment of social and family support and behaviours when considering the needs of siblings of sick children who may be at risk of developing psychological problems.
- Nurses should encourage parents to spend more time with the siblings and answer their questions honestly.
- Nurses should recognize the needs of healthy siblings and get them involved.
- Nurses should make and maintain connections for support, share information in an age-appropriate manner, be a resource for the healthy sibling, be consistent and give support.
- Nurses should bend the rules to allow siblings to visit at critical times in recognition of the benefits of involving them, and use all additional resources available (O'Shea et al. 2012).

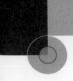

BEREAVED SIBLINGS

The finality that death of a family member brings is one of the most stressful life events. In its wake it leaves sorrow, grief and loss. While the death of a parent leaves a huge void for family members, the loss of a child or young adult can leave family members disillusioned, bewildered and distraught. Recent statistics estimate that worldwide 6.3 million children under the age of 5 died in 2013 and 1.3 million adolescents died in 2012 (World Health Organization [WHO] 2014a, 2014b). In the United Kingdom in 2012, more than 3000 babies died before age 1 and 2000 between the ages of 1 and 19 (Royal College of Paediatrics and Child Health 2015).

Childhood and young adult deaths occur worldwide for a variety of reasons. Sudden infant death, acute or chronic illness, accidents, suicide, violence, war, famine, natural disasters, neglect, drugs and alcohol misuse all contribute to the untimely death of a baby, child or young adult (WHO 2014a, 2014b).

Siblings that grow up together within a family develop a bond and experience their early life together. The death of a sibling can have a devastating effect on a family and have a lifelong impact on the lives of the surviving siblings (Davies 2006).

Research on death and loss and the effects it can have on an individual has to date mainly focused on adults. In recent years studies have emerged looking at the impact the loss of a sibling can have on a child or young adult (Foster et al. 2012; Bradley Eilersten et al. 2013; Eilegard et al. 2013b; Rosenberg et al. 2015).

As health care professionals it is important to examine the impact of sibling bereavement and the effects it has on a child or young adult. It is also necessary to discuss and examine the supports that are necessary following the loss of a sibling.

EFFECTS OF BEREAVEMENT

The death of a significant person in one's life evokes an individual response, with young people trying to make sense of this significant event within the framework of their own lives (Sharpe et al. 2005). Bowlby described grief as 'a special case of separation anxiety, bereavement being an irreversible form of separation' (Holmes 2004, p. 89). It is imperative therefore to examine the human reaction to coping with the loss of a loved one in order to be able to comprehend the components of healing and provide the support necessary to deal with this hurt (Paris et al. 2009). Children and young adults respond to the death of a loved one in different ways and their reaction and response to it depends on various circumstances. It may be the first time that a child has experienced death. A child will not deal with grief and loss as an adult would. There are many factors that need to be taken into consideration when a child or young adult has experienced the loss of their sibling. A child's age, position within the family, social circumstances, culture, religious and spiritual understanding and beliefs are influencing factors (Parkes et al. 2003; Barnardos 2007; Health Service Executive 2008; National Child Traumatic Stress Network 2009).

Many theories exist that describe the stages of loss and grief experienced when a loved one is dying and the loss that is felt following their death (Copp 1998). Kubler-Ross (1969) described the process of grief and loss as denial, anger, bargaining and acceptance. Parkes (1996) described the stages of grief and loss, underpinned by the work of Bowlby, as shock and numbness, yearning and searching, disorganization and despair, and reorganization. However, no such 'theory' exists that explains how a child can process or deal with grief or the loss of their sibling. From the literature it is clear that sibling bereavement can have both negative and positive effects on children and young adults (Foster et al. 2012). The child's developmental (cognitive and emotional) stage must be considered and may hinder the child's psychological ability to prepare for death and comprehend its finality (Paris et al. 2009). See Table 5.1.

Negative effects associated with sibling bereavement include sadness, longing for the deceased, anxiety, guilt, resentment, becoming withdrawn, maladaptive behaviours, fear of death (Foster et al. 2012), frustration, loneliness (Davies 2006), denial, crying, shivering, sleep disturbance, clinginess, regressive behaviour, insecurity, withdrawal, sleeping disturbance and lack of concentration in school (Barnardos 2007; National Child Traumatic Stress Network 2009).

Grief and trauma are two other prominent, reactive emotions associated with the loss of a sibling. The manner in which the sibling died is also a consideration when attempting to understand the reaction to death and the grieving process. Paris et al. (2009) investigated the concept of grief and trauma in children (9–18 years) following the death of a sibling. They surmised that the emotions of grief and trauma are present in children whether the death is sudden or anticipated. Participants in McNess's study (2007) of bereaved

Table 5.1 Children's and young adults' understanding of death

Children under 2	Have no understanding of death. Will seek out the deceased person. Are sensitive to parent's anxiety and distress.
Preschool (3–5 years)	A child at this stage of development has no concept of infinite time. They do not understand that death is final and thinks the person can come back. There is mystery and magical thoughts surrounding the concept. A child may believe at this age that the death was all their fault if, for example, they were cross and had secretly wished the person would die.
School-age children (6–8 years)	A child at this stage of development has more of an understanding of what death is and means. They can have fears about dying and also be pre-occupied by it. May wonder about the practicalities of it, e.g. asking, 'How you get up to heaven?' As they get closer to age 8 they will understand that death is final and the person does not come back. May learn about death through a personal experience, e.g. the loss of a pet or through the media – from television, the Internet and the movies.
Children (9–12 years)	Begin to understand that death is final. They also realize that death could include them. This can cause feelings of anxiety and fear around separation and loss. Surviving siblings feel a huge sense of loss and loneliness now that a special friendship and bond no longer exists. School work can suffer and the child can find it difficult to concentrate. Acting out in school becoming the 'class clown' or 'bully'. Children at this age may form friendships with others who have also experienced a loss.
Young adults (12–18 years)	Have a full adult understanding of death and know that it is irreversible. May display similar behaviours to school-age children. Feel sad, lonely, become withdrawn or suddenly feel very angry. Young teenagers may start engaging in more childlike behaviour in order to feel more secure. May lose interest in hobbies and activities. Can act out and engage in risky behaviour, such as alcohol or drug use, to help deal with their feelings. Will have concerns about the future and find it hard to adapt to the new family situation and their own status in the family. May now be the eldest in the family or have become an only child. May not express how upset they are to protect their parent/caregiver. More at risk of depression and may find it hard to deal with the finality of the death.

Source: Health Service Executive, *Children's grief*, 2008, available at www.healthserviceexecutive.ie/Children's Grief; 2008; National Child Traumatic Stress Network, *Sibling loss fact sheet: sibling death and childhood traumatic grief*, 2009, available at www.nationalchildtraumaticstressnetwork.org; Barnados, *Death: helping children understand*, 2007, available at http://www.barnardos.ie/resources-advice/publications/free-publications/death_helping_children_understand.html; Wender, E., *Pediatrics*, 130(6), 1164–9, 2012.

young siblings add strength to this argument, stating that the loss of a loved one rather than the manner in which they died was the primary concern for bereaved young adults as they went about their everyday lives.

Knowing that death is going to come doesn't make it any easier when it does come. Both ways are bad, but some deaths also have the trauma factor because of the suddenness.

McNess 2007, p. 14

In cases of isolated motor accidents, suicides, cause of death unknown and workplace accidents bereaved siblings' expression of grief can be curtailed as the young people experience anxiety in relation to being judged by society and stigmatized. They also exercise caution in their social interactions as a way of protecting familial standing and reputation (McNess 2007). However, the impact of multiple deaths (for example multiple suicides in a said geographic area or accidents which resulted in more than one death) is significant and led to the attainment of varied and meaningful assistance and support. Because the death was in the public domain siblings were afforded an increased level of empathy, assistance and support from members of the public (McNess 2007). An interesting finding in Paris et al.'s study (2009) study was gender reaction to death, where girls and boys experienced the same levels of trauma but girls reported higher levels of grief than boys. Paris et al. (2009) postulate that this may be due to gender stereotyping where girls are socialized to be helpers and nurturers and boys are socialized to be brave and strong.

Sibling loss can also have an impact on education and career goals. Dyregrov et al. (2015) discuss the impact of loss and trauma which negatively affect both school and work performances. Some siblings reported a higher use of alcohol and drug abuse during the first year after the death took place (Rosenberg et al. 2015).

Bereaved siblings may have used alcohol and drugs as a means of escaping the trauma, grief and loss that they were experiencing. However, in Rosenberg et al.'s study (2015) consumption levels returned to near baseline levels after the first year.

Children's reactions to sibling death are also influenced by the reactions of their significant others, for example parents, grandparents, and other siblings. Sharpe et al. (2005) propose that bereaved children and young people take their signals from those family members closest to them; this often results in avoidance of conversations related to the loss. It is imperative to also consider that these family members are struggling to deal with their own loss and emotions as well as trying to function in the parenting role of supporting and guiding. Reactions of the mother and father can differ (Sharpe et al. 2005; Wender 2012; Rosenberg et al. 2015).

In research by Barrera Alam et al. (2012) looking after the surviving siblings became an important coping stratagem for the bereaved mothers (more so than the bereaved fathers). Involvement in their child's daily activities and helping them cope with the loss of their sibling became a major focus for them.

> When you come home, you still have a three year old that still needs his mom and is bereaved and doesn't understand … but you have to comfort him and … you almost … feel like there's nothing left. But you have to find it 'cause he still needs everything … so … you pull it out and … you stay his mom but it's like you are on the surface of real and not real.
>
> *Barrera Alam et al. 2012, p. 7*

Being on the surface of real and not real as described in the above extract illustrates the surreal situation the whole family finds themselves trying to function as normal within. Some fathers in Barrera Alam et al.'s study (2012) admitted their inner struggle to bond with the remaining children, feeling unable to talk to them about their grief and loss. This exemplifies how changes in parental relationships can occur post-bereavement. These changes can add to the sense of loss and devastation for bereaved siblings.In some instances both fathers and mothers admit to being more protective of the surviving siblings, worrying about their safety and what could happen to them in the future (Barrera Alam et al. 2012).

The loss of a brother or sister can also bring about some positive outcomes. Positive effects of sibling bereavement included positive adaptation to the death, increased maturity, changes in priorities, increased compassion (Foster et al. 2012), increased spirituality, a more balanced view of life and a profound appreciation of significant relationships in their lives (Ribbens McCarthy and Jessop 2005).

REFLECTION POINTS

- Consider how a child might react to the death of a sibling.
- How might age influence a sibling's understanding of death?

SUPPORTS FOR BEREAVEMENT SIBLINGS

In recent times there has been a surge in the number of child bereavement support services available within both the community and hospital settings provided by statutory and voluntary groups. This is due to an increasing consciousness of the needs of bereaved children alongside a growing body of literature which explores the specific needs of bereaved siblings (Kammin and Tiley 2013). Cultural and religious practices may help an individual through the grieving process, and children can learn not to fear death but have a more spiritual experience and find more meaning in the death of a sibling (Parkes et al. 2003). Many cultures and religions exist in the world, and these can also affect how one copes with the loss of a loved one and how one mourns following their death. Those of Christian faith believe that following death their loved one's 'soul' will go on to heaven. Ritual practices take place following the death, such as a religious ceremony followed by burial at consecrated grounds. Those of Islamic faith undertake a ritual of washing, shrouding and anointing and burial of the deceased within a 24-hour period. Other religions such as Hinduism, Judaism, Buddhism and Islamic religions have different beliefs and burial practices following a death, and it is important to understand an individual's cultural and religious beliefs, as health care professionals, to be able to fully support them (Hedayat 2006).

Emotional support from the immediate family is paramount for the grieving sibling. Bradley Eilersten et al.'s study (2013) highlights that adolescent and young adult siblings report the importance of the caring role of parents, grandparents and siblings before and following the death of their sibling. In instances where the bereaved siblings felt uncared for or a lack of social support before or after the death, they were at higher risk for long-term anxiety. Those who felt supported were less likely to suffer from anxiety, depression and behavioural problems.

McNess (2007) speaks of the concepts of 'wide-ranging and meaning' post-bereavement support. Wide-ranging support encompasses support from individuals from a variety of social circles such as family, friends, work associates and sports groups. These groups are, in a phenomenological sense, characteristic of a caring society. The concept of meaningful support differed along gender lines. For bereaved females being listened to and being given an opportunity to reflect on, express and disclose their grief was meaningful to them. Males found support in sympathetic individuals who kept in contact and accompanied them on leisure activities such as participating in sports or going to the cinema.

McNess (2007) discusses the concept of 'social disconnect' and disillusionment in humanity within one's social life environment as a result of a lack of meaningful post-bereavement support, whether the bereaved sibling is 1 year or 10 years down the road since the sibling's demise. Social disconnect encompasses feelings of social isolation, disappointment and disconnection within ones 'social life world'. This can lead to negative inner feelings of resentment, disillusion and cynicism. On the other hand, where significant and meaningful support is available a more positive and optimistic outlook is experienced. Bradley Eilersten et al. (2013) emphasizes the essential role of the nurses in providing information regarding the role of the family as a means of social support for the bereaved sibling.

Packman et al. (2005) looked at the merits of attending of sibling camps which are now available in many countries. Sibling camps refer to a designated place where bereaved siblings come together to meet other children/young adults who are also bereaved through the loss of a brother or sister. Trained counsellors are on hand to provide support either individually or in groups. Siblings participate in many fun outdoor and indoor activities with other children who are going through the same grieving experiences as themselves.

The Rocks and Pebbles model is one sibling support group which uses music as a therapeutic medium of expression. These group sessions are facilitated by music therapists and bereavement counsellors who worked as a team providing a safe environment which enables the children to express their feelings of grief through music and create a musical masterpiece of expressions (Kammin and Tiley 2013).

CASE STUDY

Andrew was six when he attended the Rocks and Pebbles group at Christopher's. His younger sister, Cathy, has died a year previously following a cardiac arrest at 11 months. Cathy has spent long periods of her short life in hospital and so Andrew had not only experienced the separation from his only sibling but from his mother as she cared for Cathy in the hospital. Andrew's mother was struggling to cope with his anxiety and demands for attention whilst managing her own grief. The group gave Andrew an opportunity to express his feelings of loss and focus on the special memories he had of his sister. He created a piece of music around these memories including the placing of his precious Action Man toy in his sister's coffin. Developing the words and music for this piece enables Andrew to gain a sense of control over what he was expressing and a sense of pride in the finished composition which he shared with the rest of the group and with his parents.... It enabled his mother to gain an insight into Andrew's own unique experience of grief.

Kammin and Tiley 2013, p. 34

The literature illuminates the process for surviving siblings of keeping the memory of their deceased brother or sister alive. This can be done by making photograph albums or videos, and keeping clothes or other mementoes as a reminder of their loved ones. This phenomenon is described by some as 'continuing bonds' and can be beneficial, therapeutic and meaningful for some bereaved siblings (Foster et al. 2011). While grief is a very personal experience and causes of death differ, families expressed the importance of keeping the memory of their loved one alive and continuing the bond as a way of coping with their loss and being able to go on with their own lives. It helps both parents and siblings in their day-to-day lives, keeping the memory of the loved one present. Visiting the grave and leaving vestiges, placing flowers at their picture at home and holding onto their belongings are all ways of doing so (Thompson et al. 2011). Blood and Cacciatore (2014) examined how photographs following a perinatal death were invaluable keepsakes and mementoes for parents following the loss of their baby. Two Native American parents, however, found the practice distasteful and it went against their traditional beliefs. Other parents expressed regret at turning down the opportunity of having a picture of their baby taken.

Overall there is little recent research literature available on siblings bereaved by cancer when compared to the amounts of studies undertaken on non-bereaved siblings. Reasons for this may be primarily due to the increasing cancer survival rates. Other reasons may be related to ethical concerns such as imposing pain and discomfort by questioning about deceased sisters or brothers (Eilegard et al. 2013a). Eilegard et al. (2013a) in a nationwide Swedish study looked at bereaved siblings' perceptions of participating in research. Results of this research were very positive in that none of the participants envisage any long-term effects from participating in such a study. In fact most (79%) felt that it would affect them in a positive way, giving them a chance to tell their story about their brother and sister.

> Yes, it stirs up lots of thoughts and feelings, but at the same time I am glad because I feel noticed.
> I believe that being a sibling in these particular situations makes us siblings often left aside.

Eilegard et al. 2013a, p. 414

This reinforces the necessity and usefulness for future research in this area. Time, for some, is helpful in the grieving process, while for others the sorrow can resurface at significant events through the life trajectory with unexpressed grief occurring many years later. This is significant for support groups or bereavement intervention groups who need to be aware that early childhood grief emotions may not be in the past but may be bubbling beneath the surface (Sharpe et al. 2005).

In Sweden all university oncology units have a 'sibling social supporters' group whose mission it is to concentrate on siblings both throughout the illness and after the death of a brother or sister (Bradley Eilersten et al. 2013).

More research is needed in the area of sibling bereavement. The impact it has on a child or young adult and the long-term effects also need to be examined across all areas that have caused the death of a sibling, from suicide to a sudden death, natural disasters, war and so on. As health care professionals we need to fully understand the impact across all areas that have caused the death of a sibling to be able to fully support the grieving child and young adult and minimize the lifelong psychological and mental health impact it could have on them.

When a child dies siblings need to be facilitated to grieve, adapt and grow (Foster et al. 2011).

REFLECTION POINTS

- Consider the supports that are available for bereaved siblings in your health care settings.
- Can you identify some voluntary groups in your community that help support bereaved siblings?

PRINCIPLES FOR PRACTICE

When a child dies nurses, embracing a family-centred care ethos, need to be mindful of the needs of not only the bereaved parents but also the bereaved siblings.

- Nurses need to consider the age of a sibling and their understanding of death in order to help them cope with the loss of a brother or sister.
- Nurses need to be cognisant of how different religions and cultures view death and dying to be able to provide holistic care to siblings and families, following the death of a brother or sister.
- Nurses need to be aware of bereavement support groups and organizations – both locally and nationally (to refer parents and siblings to) – in order to help them cope with the death of a sibling.

Nurses need to be mindful of the long-term impact the death of a sibling can have on remaining siblings and promote both short- and long-term supports.

CONCLUSION

This chapter began by exploring the nature of sibling relationships. It highlighted the importance of the sibling relationship in terms of emotional and behavioural development while also focusing on the bonds that develop between siblings during their childhood years. FCC was discussed in detail while challenging nurses to take a more active role in including well siblings in FCC.

The needs of healthy siblings were examined, especially when their brother or sister is unwell and in need of increased parental attention. Healthy siblings' needs are often overlooked and ignored, leading to feelings of resentment, jealousy and anxiety. Nurses need to be cognisant of the impact of illness/disability on well siblings in order to fully implement a plan of care that is family centred.

The final section of this chapter explored the effects of a sudden or anticipated death on siblings. Grief, sadness and guilt are some of the emotions experienced by the bereaved which can impact on schooling and social functioning. However, it is important to note that children's understanding of death differs across the age span. Support structures for bereaved siblings were discussed and are deemed important and necessary in aiding the sibling journey through the grief process.

It is important that work continues in research with children who are siblings of a sick child in order to fully understand their experiences within the challenging health care situations that families encounter. This will ensure that their voices are heard, and their rights and views acknowledged and valued so that care can be truly family centred.

REFERENCES

Barnados (2007) Death: helping children understand. Available at http://www.barnardos.ie/resources-advice/publications/free-publications/death__helping_children_understand.html (accessed 24 March 2015).

Barrera Alam RM, D'Agostino N, Nicholas D, Schneiderman G (2012) Bereavement experiences of mothers and fathers over time after the death of a child due to cancer. *Death Studies* **36**: 1–22.

Blood C, Cacciatore J (2014) Parental grief and memento mori photography: narrative, meaning, culture and context. *Death Studies* **38**: 224–233.

Bradley Eilersten ME, Eilegard A, Steineck G, Nyberg T, Kreicbergs U (2013) Impact of social support on bereaved siblings' anxiety: a nationwide follow-up. *Journal of Pediatric Oncology Nursing* **30**(6): 301–310.

Brandon S, Lindsay M, Lovell-Davis J, Kraemer S (2009) What is wrong with emotional upset? 50 years on from the Platt Report. *Archives of Diseases in Childhood* **94**: 173–177.

Buchbinder D, Casillas J, Zeltzer L (2011) Meeting the psychosocial needs of sibling survivors: a family systems approach. *Journal of Pediatric Oncology Nursing* **28**: 123–136.

Bugel MJ (2014) Experiences of school-age siblings of children with a traumatic injury: changes, constants, and needs. *Pediatric Nursing* **40**: 179–186.

Callery, P (1991) A study of role negotiation between nurses and the parents of hospitalised children. *Journal of Advanced Nursing* **16**(7): 772–781.

Callery P, Milnes L (2012) Communication between nurses, children and their parents in asthma review consultations. *Journal of Clinical Nursing* **21**: 1641–1650.

Central Health Services Council (CHSC) (1953) *The reception and welfare of inpatients in hospital.* London: Ministry of Health.

Copp G (1998) A review of current theories of death and dying. *Journal of Advanced Nursing* **28**(2): 382–390.

Coyne I, O'Neill C, Murphy M, Costello T, O'Shea R (2011) What does family-centred care mean to nurses and how do they think it could be enhanced in practice? *Journal of Advanced Nursing* **67**(12): 2561–2573.

Davies B (2006) Sibling grief throughout childhood. *The Forum* Jan/Feb/Mar. Available at www.adec.org.

Davies R (2010) Making the 50th anniversary of the Platt Report: from exclusion to toleration and parental participation in the care of the hospitalised child. *Journal of Child Health Care* **14**(1): 6–23.

Dauz Williams P, Piamjariyakul U, Carolyn Graff J, Stanton A, Guthrie AC, Hafeman C, Williams AR (2010) Developmental disabilities: effects on well siblings. *Issues in Comprehensive Pediatric Nursing* **33**: 39–55.

Dyregrov K, Dyregrov A, Kristensen P (2015) Traumatic bereavement and terror: the psychosocial impact on parents and siblings 1.5 years after the July 2011 terror killings in Norway. *Journal of Loss and Trauma* **20**(6): 556–576.

Eilegard A, Steineck G, Nyberg T, Kreicbergs U (2013a) Bereaved siblings' perception of participating in research – a nationwide study. *Psycho-Oncology* **22**: 411–416.

Eilegard A, Steineck G, Nyberg T, Kreicbergs U (2013b) Psychological health in siblings who lost a brother or sister to cancer 2 to 9 years earlier. *Psycho-Oncology* **22**: 683–691.

Erikson EH (1995) *Childhood and society.* Rev. ed. London: Vintage.

Foster T, Gilmer M, Davies B, Dietrich M, Barrera M, Fairclogh D, Vannatta K, Gerhardt C (2011) Comparison of continuing bonds reported by parents and siblings after a child's death from cancer. *Death Studies* **35**: 430–440.

Foster T, Gilmer M, Vannatta K, Barrera M, Dietrich M, Fairclough D, Gerhardt C (2012) Changes in siblings after the death of a child from cancer. *Cancer Nursing* **35**(5): 347–353.

Graff JC, Hankins JS, Hardy BT, Hall HR, Roberts RJ, Neely-Barnes SL (2010) Exploring parent-sibling communication in families of children with sickle cell disease. *Issues in Comprehensive Pediatric Nursing* **33**: 101–123.

Hayes C, Savage E (2008) Fathers' perspectives on the emotional impact of managing the care of their children with cystic fibrosis. *Journal of Paediatric Nursing* **23**(4): 250–256.

Health Service Executive (2008) Children's grief. Available at www.healthserviceexecutive.ie/Children's Grief (accessed 24 March 2015).

Hedayat K (2006) When the spirit leaves: childhood death, grieving, and bereavement in Islam. *Journal of Palliative Medicine* **9**(6): 1282–1291.

Herrman JW (2010) Siblings' perceptions of the costs and rewards of diabetes and its treatment. *Journal of Pediatric Nursing* **25**: 428–437.

Higham S, Davies R (2013) Protecting, providing, and participating: fathers' roles during their child's unplanned hospital stay, an ethnographic study. *Journal of Advanced Nursing* **69**(9): 1390–1399.

Holmes J (2004) *John Bowlby and attachment theory.* East Essex, NY: Brunner-Routledge.

Howe N, Recchia H (2006) Sibling relations and their impact of children's development. In *Encyclopedia of Early Childhood Development.* Available at http://www.child-encyclopedia.com/sites/default/files/textes-experts/en/829/sibling-relations-and-their-impact-on-childrens-development.pdf.

Hughes M (2007) Parents' and nurses' attitudes to family-centred care: an Irish perspective. *Journal of Clinical Nursing* **16**(12): 2341–2348.

Jenkins J, Rasbash J, Leckie G, Gass K, Dunn J (2012) The role of maternal factors in sibling relationship quality: a multilevel study of multiple dyads per family. *Journal of Child Psychology and Psychiatry* **53**: 622–629.

Kammin V, Tiley H (2013) Rocks and Pebbles: a post-bereavement sibling's support group using music to explore grief. *Bereavement Care* **32**(1): 31–38.

Kilkelly U, Savage E (2013) *Child friendly healthcare: a report commissioned by the ombudsman for children.* Dublin: Office of the Ombudsman for Children.

Kirk S (2001) Negotiating lay and professional roles in the care of children with complex health care needs. *Journal of Advanced Nursing* **34**(5): 593–602.

Kramer L (2014) Learning emotional understanding and emotion regulation through sibling interaction. *Early Education and Development* **25**: 160–184.

Kubler-Ross E (1969) *On death and dying.* New York: Macmillan.

Kuo D, Houtrow A, Arango P, Kuhlthau KA, Simmons JM, Neff JM (2012) Family-centered care: current applications and future directions in pediatric health care. *Maternal Child Health Journal* **16**: 297–305.

Lambert V, Glacken M, McCarron M (2008) 'Visible-ness': the nature of communication for children admitted to a specialist children's hospital in the Republic of Ireland. *Journal of Clinical Nursing* **17**(23): 3092–3102.

Lane C, Mason J (2014) Meeting the needs of siblings of children with life limiting illnesses. *Nursing Children and Young People* **26**(3): 16–20.

Lehna C (2010) Sibling experiences after a major childhood burn injury. *Pediatric Nursing* **36**: 245–251.

MacDonald E, Hastings R (2010) Mindful parenting and care involvement of fathers of children with intellectual disabilities. *Journal of Child Family Studies* **19**: 236–240.

Malcolm C, Gibson F, Adams S, Anderson G, Forbat L (2014) A relational understanding of sibling experiences of children with rare life-limiting conditions: findings from a qualitative study. *Journal of Child Health Care* **18**: 230–240.

McNess A (2007) The social consequences of 'how the siblings died' for bereaved young adults. *Youth Studies Australia* **26**(4): 12–20.

Mikkelsen G, Frederiksen K (2011) Family-centred care of children in hospital – a concept analysis. *Journal of Advanced Nursing* **67**(5): 1152–1162.

Ministry of Health, Central Health Services Council (1959) *The welfare of children in hospital report of the committee* [Platt Report]. London: HMSO.

Nabors L, Bartz J, Kichler J, Sievers R, Elkins R, Pangallo J (2013) Play as a mechanism of working through medical trauma for children with medical illnesses and their siblings. *Issues in Comprehensive Pediatric Nursing* **36**: 212–224.

Nagl-Cupal M, Daniel M, Koller MM, Mayer H (2014) Prevalence and effects of caregiving on children. *Journal of Advanced Nursing* **70**: 2314–2325.

National Child Traumatic Stress Network (2009) Sibling loss fact sheet: sibling death and childhood traumatic grief. Available at www.nationalchildtraumaticstressnetwork.org (accessed 24 March 2015).

Nielsen KM, Mandleco B, Roper SO, Cox A, Dyches T, Marshall ES (2012) Parental perceptions of sibling relationships in families rearing a child with a chronic condition. *Journal of Pediatric Nursing* **27**: 34–43.

Norris JM, Moules NJ, Pelletier G, Culos-Reed SN (2010) Families of young pediatric cancer survivors: a cross-sectional survey examining physical activity behavior and health-related quality of life. *Journal of Pediatric Oncology Nursing* **27**: 196–208.

O'Brien I, Duffy A, Nicholl H (2009) Impact of childhood chronic illnesses on siblings: a literature review. *British Journal of Nursing* **18**: 1358–1365.

O'Shea ER, Shea J, Robert T, Cavanaugh C (2012) The needs of siblings of children with cancer: a nursing perspective. *Journal of Pediatric Oncology Nursing* **29**: 221–231.

Packman W, Greenhalgh J, Chesterman B, Shaffer T, Fine J, VanZutphen K, Golan R, Amylon M (2005) Siblings of pediatric cancer patients: the qualitative and quantitative nature of quality of life. *Journal of Psychosocial Oncology* **23**(1): 87–107.

Paris M, Carter B, Day S, Armsworth M (2009) Grief and trauma in children after the death of a sibling. *Journal of Child and Adolescent Trauma* **2**: 71–80.

Parkes MC (1996) *Bereavement: studies of grief in adult life.* 3rd ed. London: Routledge.

Parkes MC, Laungani P, Young B (2003) Death and bereavement across cultures. East Essex, NY: Brunner Routledge.

Piaget J, Inhelder B (1969) *The psychology of the child.* London: Routledge & Kegan Paul.

Ribbens McCarthy J, Jessop J (2005) *Young people, bereavement and loss: disruptive transitions.* York: Joseph Rowntree Foundation.

Rosenberg AR, Postier A, Osenga K, Kreicbergs U, Neville B, Dussel V, Wolfe J (2015) Long-term psychosocial outcomes among bereaved siblings of children with cancer. *Journal of Pain and Symptom Management* **49**(1): 55–65.

Royal College of Paediatrics and Child Health (2015) Why children die: death in infants, children and young people in the UK. Available at http://www.rcpch.ac.uk/news-campaigns/campaigns/why-children-die/why-children-die-rcpch-campaign (accessed 23 April 2015).

Savage E, Callery P (2007) Clinic consultations with children and parents on the dietary management of cystic fibrosis. *Social Science & Medicine* **64**: 363–374.

Sharpe S, Ribbens McCarthy J, Jessop J (2005) Young people's experiences of bereavement. In Ribbens McCarthy J, Jessop J (eds.) Young people, bereavement and loss: disruptive transitions. York: Joseph Rowntree Foundation, pp. 7–20.

Shaw MR, Oneal G (2014) Living on the edge of asthma: a grounded theory exploration. *Journal for Specialists in Pediatric Nursing* **19**: 296–307.

Shields L (2010) Questioning family-centred care. *Journal of Clinical Nursing* **19**: 2629–2638.

Shields L, Pratt J, Hunter J (2006) Family-centred care: a review of qualitative studies. *Journal of Clinical Nursing* **15**: 1317–1323.

Shuttleworth L (1997) Use of action research to explore the experience of being a parent living in a regional paediatric oncology unit. *Journal of Cancer Nursing* **1**(3): 119–125.

Sleeman F, Northam EA, Crouch W, Cameron FJ (2010) Psychological adjustment of well siblings of children with type 1 diabetes. *Diabetic Medicine* **27**: 1084–1087.

Smith TL (2006) *Siblings of children with autism: An investigation of sibling and parent characteristics contributing to positive and negative psychosocial outcomes.* University of Toronto (Canada).

Stuart M, Melling S (2014) Understanding nurses' and parents' perceptions of family-centred care. *Nursing Children and Young People* **26**: 16–20.

Swallow V (2008) An exploration of mothers' and fathers' views of their identities in chronic-kidney-disease management: parents as students? *Journal of Clinical Nursing* **17**: 3177–3186.

Thompson AL, Miller KS, Barrera M, Davies B, Foster TL, Gilmer MJ, Hogan N, Vannatta K, Gerhardt CA (2011) A qualitative study of advice from bereaved parents and siblings. *Journal of Social Work in End of Life & Palliative Care* **7**: 153–172.

Tong A, Lowe A, Sainsbury P, Craig J (2008) Experiences of parents who have children with chronic kidney disease: a systematic review of the qualitative studies. *Paediatrics* **121** (2): 349–360.

United Nations (1989) Convention on the rights of the child. Geneva: United Nations.

Wender E (2012) Supporting the family after the death of a child. *Pediatrics* **130**(6): 1164–1169.

Wennick A, Huus K (2012) What it is like being a sibling of a child newly diagnosed with type 1 diabetes: an interview study. *European Diabetes Nursing* **9**: 88–92.

Wilkie B, Barr O (2011) The experiences of parents of children with an intellectual disability who use respite care services. *Learning Disability Practice* **11**(5): 30–36.

Williams PD, Ridder EL, Setter RK, Liebergen A, Curry H, Piamjariyakul U, Williams AR (2009) Pediatric chronic illness (cancer, cystic fibrosis) effects on well siblings: parent's voices. *Issues in Comprehensive Pediatric Nursing* **32**: 94–113.

Wilkins KL, Woodgate RL (2005) A review of qualitative research on the childhood cancer experience from the perspective of siblings: a need to give them a voice. *Journal of Pediatric Oncology Nursing* **22**: 305–319.

World Health Organization (2014a) Maternal, newborn, child and adolescent health. Available at www.worldhealthorganisation.int/maternal-child-adolescent/topics/child/mortality/en/ Maternal, newborn, child and adolescent health (accessed 7 May 2015).

World Health Organization (2014b) Children: reducing mortality. Available at http://www.who.int/mediacentre/factsheets/fs178/en/ (accessed 7 May 2015).

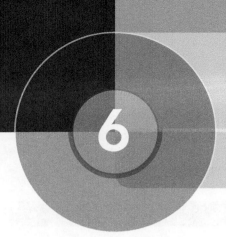

The need for a culturally sensitive approach to care

PAT COLLIETY AND VASSO VYDELINGUM

OVERVIEW

This chapter focuses on contemporary issues of growing up as a member of a minority in a predominantly white majority culture for children and young people who may perceive themselves as not belonging to the mainstream culture. The chapter starts with an explanation of terms such as *culture, race, ethnicity* and *whiteness*, and a discussion of terminologies such as *black* and *Asian*, and factors affecting child-rearing practice are considered. Using a rights-based approach, the chapter then addresses issues affecting caring for children and young people from ethnic minorities in community, school and health care settings. The chapter seeks to engage the reader with contemporary issues that affect the provision of culturally sensitive care such as safeguarding children; health problems such as sickle cell disease, thalassaemia and diabetes; health inequalities; and talking to children about death and grieving. Within school settings, issues such as bullying, school uniforms, teenage pregnancy, obesity, mental health issues and arranged marriages are discussed. The last section of the chapter addresses the implications for practice through the development of cultural competence and the provision of antidiscriminatory practice.

INTRODUCTION

From the early age of 6 months children are able to differentiate colours and shapes, and by the age of 3 years children certainly can recognize differences, including skin colour differences, long before they go to school. They are clearly learning to recognize the colours of the objects around them. Dunham et al. (2015) argue that for younger children, recognition of 'race' is based on skin colour rather than any other characteristic. However, Ouseley and Lane (2008) argue that children are not born with attitudes that view colour necessarily in negative terms. They are reflecting the attitudes and values derived from their parents and significant others. This is particularly true of both black and white children, although some black children may also be carrying the burden of learning that they are the objects of racism or negative experiences. It must be noted that children do not live in a colour-blind environment.

How far children and young people 'participate' varies enormously within and between societies, and the ratification of the United Nations (UN) Convention on the Rights of the Child (1989) by many countries, including the UK, should demonstrate a change in the approaches that such countries have toward children's rights. This is particularly important in relation to children and young adults from minority ethnic groups.

CULTURE, ETHNICITY AND RACE

The aim of exploring definitional aspects of current terms is to provide readers with a critical overview of terminology and discuss some of the theoretical concepts, which affect the way children and young people from ethnic minorities are viewed. The following sections will explore definitions of culture, ethnicity and race.

CULTURE

Culture refers to habits of thought, beliefs, diet, dress, music and art and reflects ethnicity. Helman (2007) refers to culture as a set of guidelines which an individual inherits as a member of a particular society that tells him or her how to view the world and how to behave in relation to other people, through a cultural lens. It also provides him or her with a way of transmitting these guidelines to the next generation through the use of symbols, language, art and rituals. McNeely (1996) suggests that it is more a set of belief systems which form an ideology. Thus culture could be seen as lens through which the child views the world, shaping their perception and understanding.

It is important for children and young people's nurses and other practitioners to recognize the value of language and the socialization process in the way children and young people learn about culture, as it is a way of life that is shared by all members of that particular group. There is a danger of viewing culture as static with frozen attributes about people; culture is constantly evolving and people respond to the technological developments in a dynamic fashion. Box 6.1 summarizes the key characteristics of culture.

ETHNICITY

Ethnicity, on the other hand, refers to social groups who often share a cultural heritage with a common language, values, religion, customs and attitudes. Members are aware of sharing a common past, possibly a homeland, and experience a sense of difference. An 'ethnic person' may be used to refer to a foreigner or member of an immigrant community, whereas an 'ethnic minority' is used to describe someone related to a group of people having common racial, national, religious or cultural origins, existing within a majority culture. Such a person may belong to an ethnic group that is a group of people whose members identify with each other, through a common heritage that is real or presumed.

The classification of ethnicity in the UK, as shown in Table 6.1, has attracted controversy in the past, particularly at the time of the 2001 census, when the existence and nature of such classifications, which appeared on the census form, became public. If one goes by the above definitions of *ethnicity*, the labels included in the census form were not really seeking ethnic identities of people as labels, such as white and black, African, Caribbean, Asian, Indian and Chinese, will do very little to reveal the ethnic identities of people. Africa and Asia are vast continents with such a diversity of people that to classify oneself as Asian or African might suggest no more than a desire, from the authorities, to count the number of non-white people in the UK rather than truly reflecting the ethnicity of the population. The self-defining nature of ethnicity,

> ### BOX 6.1: Key points of culture
>
> Culture is learned through both language acquisition and socialization.
> - The individual is fitted into the way of life.
> - Culture is shared by all members of the group – it gives group identity.
> - Culture responds to factors such as technology and the environment.
> - Culture is dynamic and evolving.

Table 6.1 Pre-defined categories used in 2011 census

White	1. English/Welsh/Scottish/northern Irish/British
	2. Irish
	3. Gypsy or Irish Traveller
	4. Any other white background; please describe
Mixed/multiple ethnic groups	5. White and black Caribbean
	6. White and black African
	7. White and Asian
	8. Any other mixed/multiple ethnic background; please describe
Asian/Asian British	9. Indian
	10. Pakistani
	11. Bangladeshi
	12. Chinese
	13. Any other Asian background; please describe
Black/African/Caribbean/black British	14. African
	15. Caribbean
	16. Any other black/African/Caribbean background; please describe
Other ethnic group	17. Arab
	18. Any other ethnic group; please describe

Source: ONS, *Census general report*, Full report, 2014, available at http://www.ons.gov.uk/ons/guidemethod/census/2011/uk-census/index.html

the basis for categorization in the UK, lacks objectivity as the classification is centred on the self-report of how subjectively meaningful the label is to that person, unlike the data for age and gender.

The use of the term *ethnicity* in common usage and in academic literature is not without controversy, as the term is more often used to describe non-white groups, which assumes that there is no ethnicity in the white population, when there clearly is. In addition, ethnicity may be inaccurately used to describe other objects such as ethnic food, ethnic décor or ethnic vegetables, which can mean nothing more than foreign or non-European. Such an approach often ignores ethnicity in white majority groups.

Mathur et al. (2013) argue that while concepts of race, which are discussed below, were imposed by those in power, ethnicity is defined by an individual to reflect their own identity and how they choose to identify themselves. It involves a broad range of characteristics that are socially constructed, which means that they are influenced by social and political factors and can change over time.

It is now widely recommended that the concept of ethnicity replaces the unscientific concept of race in all spheres of research as it is a more individualized concept and is a more meaningful way of grouping individuals with some shared identity – encompassing, but not limited to, country of birth, language, religion, culturally determined practices and where they live. As Britain becomes an increasingly diverse society, this flexible and constantly evolving approach to defining and grouping people becomes more important. It is interesting to note that a question on ethnicity was only introduced in the 1991 census and respondents defined themselves. There were seven pre-defined categories with a possibility of ticking more than one box to provide a further 28 categories; 98.6% of respondents used a pre-coded category and only 1.4% defined themselves using free text. By the 2011 census there were 13 pre-defined and 5 'other – please describe' categories (National Statistics 2006; Office for National Statistics [ONS] 2014).

REFLECTION POINTS

- Looking at these categories, how easy do you find it to define your ethnic background?
- What, if anything else, do you think needs to be added?

RACE

Use of the term *race* has been controversial as the term is a social construct to refer to genetic or biological differences (usually skin colour), without scientific basis. The idea of race has developed from evolutionary theories and also physical differences, based on geography, such as skin colour or hair colour and type, but no other corresponding variation in other human characteristics (Appiah 1996). Steer (2014) argues that the concept of race was discredited by its association with the eugenics movement, particularly within Nazi Germany. These concepts of race need to be differentiated from the large biomedical literature which focuses on studying conditions which are more prevalent among groups from a similar background, for example the prevalence of diabetes among people of South Asian origin (Ramachandran et al. 2014).

While it is recognized in academic circles that race per se does not exist, as there is only one human race, Appiah (1996) also suggests that it is important to understand how people think about race and how such concepts, ideas and definitions of the term vary in time and place.

MIXED-RACE CHILDREN AND YOUNG PEOPLE

Children and young people with mixed parentage, however, often seem to be excluded in any discourse about categorization, and in both the UK and the US a major factor of differentiation is based on whites in an epicentre of swirling colours. In effect, to be 'mixed' is a function of coloured realities, not white ones, as some people of mixed race may feel that the blanket use of the term *black* often robs them of the pride of their mixed parentage.

Data from the 2011 census show that people with mixed parentage are a fast-growing group in the UK, so what are the implications for children and young people in this group? Song and Aspinall (2012) discussed 'racial assignment' by families and others, describing how one of their respondents had found this irritating at times because she did not see herself in that way. Song and Gutierrez (2014a) are currently undertaking a 2-year study into how children from a mixed parentage background are socialized. Their interim report categorizes socialization approaches into:

- Raised as British
- Mostly British with ethnic symbolism
- Emphasis on minority heritage
- Cosmopolitanism
- Missing data or did not know

Cosmopolitanism was the most common response; this incorporated concepts such as acceptance of diversity and difference, open-mindedness to others and multiculturalism. Some respondents valued their specific ethnic backgrounds, while others did not want to stress alignment with any particular background (Song and Gutierrez 2014b). Emery (2014) argues that it is easy to apply labels to people from mixed race and that these labels do not reflect their particular identity and heritage. She also argues that there is a danger that they may face social exclusion and discrimination, particularly young people at secondary school.

A report by the National Children's Bureau (Morley and Street 2014) found that children from mixed-race backgrounds were potentially at much higher risk of having mental health problems, possibly as a result of experiencing discrimination from both white and black peers or having low self-esteem, and were overrepresented in the youth justice system. The report also concluded that public services in general, and schools in particular, were not sensitive to their needs.

WHITENESS

While 'white' is always in the list of categories for ethnicity classification, there is a dearth of definitions about what it is. It is assumed to be a neutral category against which all other classifications are measured. However, Puzan (2003) argues that 'white' is about white privilege, conferring certain indelible and undeniable advantages to those who fit that category. Such a view is supported by Marx and Pennington (2003), who suggest that whiteness is a highly privileged social construction rather than a neutral racial category. King (no date) discusses the inherent white perspective in a range of resources available for teachers in the US and how some did not see that there was any perspective bias and that the viewpoint presented was monocultural, e.g. white. In her book King (2015) takes this discussion further, presenting a range of evidence and research to inform the debate.

Within health care, this is also relevant as practitioners need to be aware of their conscious or unconscious biases and what these are based on. For example it could be that the practitioner assumes that everyone will conform to the behaviours, values, beliefs and practices of the dominant culture. Children and young people's nurses and other health and social care practitioners should be aware of this assumption when dealing with children and young people from ethnic minorities as this inherent power difference may be the cause of friction and resentment.

WHAT'S IN A NAME? (NOTE ON TERMINOLOGY)

Vydelingum (1998) suggested that whatever label or name is used for members of the diverse minority ethnic population in Britain, it is problematic and changes over time. Often, practitioners can be reluctant to use terms which might cause offence, whereas other people might quite rightly reject terms used to describe them, especially when such terms are no more than euphemisms for inferiority. Some terms may do no more than emphasize a minority ethnic's differentness, which in turn may lead to the legitimation of discrimination against them.

Permissible nomenclature is transitory and writers are often guilty of using currently in-vogue words which may in later years invite criticism. For example, just over three decades ago, 'coloured' was polite common currency in describing non-whites in the UK and the US, except for Orientals and American Indians, notes Gaine (1987). 'Coloured', until the dismantling of apartheid, remained a legal category, though a controversial one, in South Africa. The Black is Beautiful movement by people of African origins in the US assisted them tremendously in ridding themselves of the negative connotations of the word *black*, and for African Americans, which now seems to be the currently preferred term in the US, the term *coloured* is a euphemism – an apology for a skin colour socially defined as undesirable. 'Black' has gained new meaning, suggestive of political identity and ethnic pride. Table 6.2 illustrates which words are currently acceptable and those which are deemed offensive.

OBJECTIONS TO THE 'BLACK' LABEL

In Britain, young South Asians may object to the term *black* to describe them as this may appear to conflate a variety of ethnic groups which should be treated separately, e.g. African Caribbeans, Bangladeshis, Indians, Pakistanis, Sikhs, Hindus and Muslims, and which may relate to their parents' country of origin. Within the sociology of race, Modood (1994) argues that the term *black* and its concept are harmful to British Asians. The reason why many young South Asians continue to reject the label 'black' lies in the attempts to impose it on them by the advocates of 'black' rather than being actively sought by them. 'Black' has limited applicability as it has to do with socially defining a group of people not by themselves but by the majority (white, dominant) group.

Modood (1994) suggests that 'black' evokes a false essentialism: that all non-white groups have something in common other than how others treat them. 'Black', being evocative of people of African

Table 6.2 Key points for practitioners on the current terminology to use

Acceptable usage	Not acceptable as likely to cause offence
African: Often used as a prefix, e.g. African Caribbean and African American, to denote the origins. Some early literature still refers to West Indian for people from the Caribbean.	Afro-Caribbean Nigger Negro
Black: Political category to denote all non-whites; children and young people may wish to be identified as black British.	Negroid Wog
Mixed race: Children and young people with mixed parentage such as a black father and a white mother or vice versa.	Coloured Half-caste
South Asian: People who hail from or who descend from people from the Indian subcontinent such as India, Pakistan, Sri Lanka and Bangladesh. Some may prefer to be called Hindu, Muslim or Sikh. Children and young people may wish to be identified as British Muslim, British Hindu or Sikh.	Paki Coolie Ethnics Ethnic minorities
White: Political category to denote people from a European origin.	
Minority ethnic group: Denotes people who are minorities, but also indicates that there is a majority ethnic group.	

origins, understates the size, needs and specific concerns of Asian communities. However, Modood fails to recognize that 'black' also treats people of African origins as a homogeneous group, which they are not, with the resultant underemphasizing of the multiplicity of cultures and the diversity of languages among the African Caribbeans too (Figueroa 1991). Modood (1994) further argues that while African Caribbeans can use the concept for the purposes of ethnic pride, for South Asians it can be no more than 'a political colour', leading to a politicized identity, consequently resulting in a smothering of Asian ethnic pride. The smothering of ethnic pride created by the use of the blanket term *black* is also true of people of African Caribbean origins whose tribal, ethnic and cultural identities are denied.

WHAT IS AN ASIAN CHILD OR YOUNG PERSON?

The term *Asian* is misleading as it was a colonial invention used to describe people of Indian descent who had been either transported as indentured labourers or encouraged to settle as traders in the British colonies, suggest Westwood and Bachu (1988). Few young Asians in Britain identify with the term or attach great meaning to it. 'Asian' refers to people who were either born in or whose forebears originated from the Indian subcontinent, often living as ethnic minorities in Britain, excluding the Japanese, Chinese or Southeast Asians. Just like the use of the term 'black' discussed earlier, utilization of the catch-all *Asian* term also suppresses cultural diversity and tends to mask the many types of family structures, specific religions, culture and migratory patterns of the Asian people.

Under some circumstances, there may be objections to bracketing together a wide variety of cultural ethnic groups often with different positions within British society, argues Vydelingum (1998). Young Asians would prefer to be seen as people of Indian, Pakistani, Bangladeshi or Sri Lankan origins. However, some young people may prefer to be identified as black British; this has the advantage of stressing the fact that the people are referred to first as British. Other young people might prefer use of the term *British Asians* or *British Hindu*, *Muslim* or *Sikh*.

CULTURAL CONFLICTS

Children and young people's nurses and other health and social care practitioners must note that the contemporary issue here is that children and young people from minorities may not always assign the same ethnic identities as their parents to themselves. Such children growing up in the UK may be experiencing conflict about straddling two or more cultures and also speaking more than one language. For example, a child born to Asian Bangladeshi parents may speak Sylheti or Bengali. Children born of Bangladeshi parents will probably enter the school with a degree of fluency in Sylheti, but with a very limited knowledge of Bengali and, often, with little exposure to the written word. Through exposure to the British school system and meeting children from other cultures and backgrounds the child will learn English and may later wish to self-identify as both Bangladeshi and British or a British Bangladeshi.

ETHNOCENTRISM AND RACISM

Far too many practitioners are unsure when dealing with cultural aspects of care as a high level of confusion exists about ethnocentrism and racism. Ethnocentrism is the tendency to use one's own group as the basis for all comparison, and to view one's own group as the norm (Bizumic and Duckitt 2012).

Racism is more about discriminating and providing a less favourable service to someone on the basis of race or racial features and can prevail as part of the ethos or culture of the organization. It is a corrosive disease, suggests Macpherson (1999), who believes that institutional racism can be the most difficult organizational process to tackle. Concluding from the Stephen Lawrence Inquiry, MacPherson (1999) suggested that institutional racism is the collective failure of an organization to provide an appropriate and professional service to people because of their colour, culture or ethnic origin. It can be seen or detected in processes, attitudes and behaviour, which amount to discrimination through the unwitting prejudice, ignorance, thoughtlessness and racist stereotyping which disadvantage ethnic minority people.

In the following case study we will illustrate the meaning of ethnocentrism, and we believe that this is far more common in practice, especially when dealing with children and young people from ethnic minorities.

CASE STUDY

This incident occurred in a children's ward and relates to Ahmad, a young Muslim boy of 8 with physical disabilities, admitted for assessment and fitting of prosthesis, as he had poliomyelitis. He was about to be discharged. As part of the discharge planning meeting, the nurse in charge said: 'We can send him home tonight. There is no need to arrange social services or organize any homecare as Asians are very good and usually look after themselves and do not like to accept help from us'. All staff present agreed with the staff nurse and nobody felt it necessary to check that the father, an accountant, worked away from home a lot, and the mother, a school teacher, did not have any relatives living nearby, as they had moved to the area recently and did not know anybody in the community.

Ethnocentrism is problematic as just because something appears 'normal' and familiar does mean that it is. Ethnocentric practices prevent health care practitioners from respecting one another and understanding the 'other'. Although the views expressed above might seem complimentary to Asians, at the same time they are judgements made by the nurse's own cultural standards, with the consequence of rationing or denying services to patients or clients.

Children and young people's nurses and other health care practitioners should be aware of their own stereotypical views and the impact such views might have on the care for sick children.

REFLECTION POINTS

Can you recall times in practice when obvious ethnocentric views have been expressed?

- Describe what happened.
- Were the views of individuals challenged in any way?
- How do you handle people who hold strong stereotypes?

STEREOTYPING

Ethnocentric approaches in care provision can be the result of stereotyping, which assumes that cultures are static, homogeneous and have a biological basis (Schneider 2004). This may have a detrimental impact on health; for example Perkins (2014) argues that black women in the US underutilize health care compared with white women, and he suggests that one reason for this may be that they have experienced stereotyping leading to a negative health care experience.

Stereotyping in turn may lead to pathologizing of culture, meaning the locating of people's health problems in terms of their pathological culture; for example, children from South Asian parents tend to be submissive because of the oppressive patriarchal family relationships, and children from west Indian families tend to lack discipline as they come from single-parent families with matriarchal relationships. Other examples include Asian rickets in children, Asian tuberculosis and self-harm in young female Asians. Rickets is a disease of calcium deficiency, which can occur in any child who has calcium deficiency, and low calcium serum levels do not have an Asian marker; similarly, the tubercle bacillus that infects Asians does not have a specific biological marker and is the bacillus that would infect anyone (black or white) who was malnourished and living in overcrowded conditions. The use of such terms would lead practitioners to believe that these were new diseases. Such an approach, argues Ahmad (1993), not only pathologizes minority cultures but also ignores issues of power, deprivation and racism and distracts from putting more resources into exploring such diseases. The end result is a black family pathology; i.e. problems with children and illnesses are due to the nature of black families. Further examples of stereotyping and ethnocentric approaches in care can be found in Vydelingum (2006).

CULTURAL DIVERSITY AND TRANSCULTURAL NURSING

In a critical review of concepts and definitions, Kroeber et al. (1963) explained that cultural diversity in nursing practice derives its conceptual base from nursing, other cross-cultural health disciplines and the social sciences, such as anthropology, sociology and psychology. Culture is conceptualized broadly to encompass the belief systems of a variety of groups. Cultural diversity refers to the differences between people based on a shared ideology and valued set of beliefs, norms, customs and meanings, evidenced in a way of life. However, the term *transcultural nursing*, coined by Dr Madeleine M. Leininger in the mid-1950s, began to attract more widespread interest and concept development in the 1970s and 1980s. A comparatively new and marginal discipline in the UK, transcultural nursing refers to a specialty within nursing focused on the comparative study of different cultures and subcultures (Papadopoulos 2006).

What is important when dealing with children and young people from minority ethnic groups is that the values and beliefs of the practitioner, more often white middle class, may not be convergent. For example, the values of nursing in the US or the UK are embedded in the values of a Western culture placing stress on self-reliance and individualism – beliefs that 'individuals have the ability to pull themselves up by their bootstraps' and that an individual's rights are more important than a society's. However, many cultures, especially Asian and African cultures, do not share the primacy of the value of individualism. It is worth noting that the majority of cultures around the world are in essence collectivistic, meaning that the loyalties of a person to a group exceed the rights of the individual, rather than individualistic, in which the rights of the individual supersede those of the group. In many cultures, health decisions are not made by an individual but by a group – family, community or society – and this is a very important point to remember when dealing with sick children.

FACTORS AFFECTING CHILD REARING

The immigration process is a change agent in family life and affects people's roles, expectations and obligations; however, children born to immigrants are UK citizens and are as entitled to all rights and entitlements as any other child. It should be noted that the worst affected are asylum seekers and refugee families, because of government dispersal policies.

The relationship between family and society is dynamic, and rapid changes in family structure, values, customs and systems of obligations are major catalysts for social change, as noted by Wilmot and Young (1957). Family reproduces culture, through ideological, structural and personal factors, but what is important is that the rate of social change for immigrants may be faster than for 'natives', and differences between generations may be greater at the level of both assumptions and behaviour. The contemporary issue here is that external social, economic and legal constraints may exert greater pressure for change in children born to minority ethnic families. The current issues about migration into western Europe (Adams 2014) bring into sharper focus the effects of migration on children. According to the World Development Report (UNICEF 2007), the focus on children and migration has been neglected in the past. This is an area that is underresearched. Children are the most vulnerable to risks when being left behind by one or both parents, migrating with the family or alone. Harttgen and Klasen (2008) have conducted some preliminary research and note that children's habits may have to change when moving to a host country and the language barrier causes constraints, and they are consequently at greater risk of poor health outcomes. Children learn the foreign language faster than their parents; the latter will urge their children to communicate with the authorities. Sometimes this responsibility is given into the hands of very young children, imposing pressure upon them. Migration also has a serious effect on the mental health of the children with regard to the process of migration. They argue that migration causes stress due to the loss of family, friends and habitual surroundings; questions about their identity and sense of belonging; the fear of deportation; and discrimination, all of which can cause problems that can be taken into adulthood.

ROLE OF THE FAMILY

The family reproduces values and behaviours, e.g. honour, shame, identity, religion, obligations and expectations, and these are often seen as the prime responsibility of parents. Religious and cultural institutions assist the family in cultural retention.

Concerns about the values and institutions of the wider society and external hostility may reinforce encapsulation. Hence in addition to going to a British school, some children may attend afternoon or evening classes at their local religious centres, such as Madrassahs (for Muslims) or Gudwarahs (for Sikhs), to learn about their language, religion or culture. Here, gender differences in childhood upbringing, as seen by that particular culture, may also be reinforced. This may be a cause for conflict in children and young people growing up in the UK, particularly if such differences are in conflict with the wider values of British society.

For example, if some girls are brought up in such a way that they are not able to participate as equal citizens, they may resent such gender stereotypes, leading to generational conflicts. Such demands on young people about roles, obligations, honour and respect may set some of them on a collision course with their parents, when taking the 'personal choices' route can lead to personal rejection by family and local community.

CULTURAL INFLUENCES ON CHILD REARING PRACTICES

Most Southeast Asian groups (Vietnamese, Cambodian and Laotian) share cultural values that influence parental socialization practices. Confucian principles of filial piety, ancestral unity and lineage are the most crucial of these, according to Vernon (1982), Yamamoto and Kubota (1983) and Morrow (1989). A central principle – 'pride and shame', in which an individual's action reflects either positively or negatively on the entire family – is inherent within each culture. From an early age, children are taught to respect their parents, older siblings and other adults in positions of authority, and individual family members are made aware of their place in the vertical hierarchy. The fostering of mutual interdependence is started from an early age, such that obligation to parents and family is expected to outweigh personal desires or needs (Morrow 1989). Such an upbringing may be in stark contrast to Western values of assertiveness and independence and raises questions about children's rights in the context of childhood. Morrow (1999, 2011) draws from her extensive research on children's perspectives on their rights and decision making, and indicates that children from minority ethnic groups are very aware that their parents make decisions in their household and that as children it is their duty to listen to their parents.

Children and young people's nurses and other practitioners should be cognizant of the fact that, although such practices may infringe on the rights of the young people, the wider role of the family should be acknowledged, especially in relation to the education of children and young people from minority ethnic groups.

PRACTICE

SAFEGUARDING CHILDREN FROM MINORITY ETHNIC GROUPS

The common core set of knowledge and skills required to practice at a basic level in six areas when dealing with safeguarding children is shown in Box 6.2.

The Children Act 1989 (s. 22 (5)) (Office of Public Sector Information 1998) states that local authorities have a duty to give due consideration 'to the child's religious persuasion, racial origin and cultural and linguistic background' in decision making, and under the UN convention (UN Convention on the Rights of the Child 1989), all children have the right to be protected from harm. Boushel (2000) suggests that there are only a small number of studies that incorporate race and ethnicity in social welfare research and children from minority ethnic groups are disproportionately represented both in child protection registrations and in the looked after population (Barn et al. 1997). The Social Services Inspectorate (2000) has noted that disparities have been found to be particularly pronounced in local authorities that have a small proportion of ethnic minority families. Stereotyping, colour blindness, cultural deficit and inadequate training of professionals lead to failures in the statutory processes designed to protect children, according to Webb et al. (2002). More children from minority ethnic groups were permanently placed away from their birth parents than their white peers, although they were more likely to be placed with relatives. Such placements may reflect stereotypical views concerning the family support available to minority ethnic groups, for example that minority ethnic groups receive additional support from their extended family. As within all groups, there will be a wide diversity of support available to families in different circumstances, and basing decisions on erroneous assumptions about different cultures can have grave consequences.

Using such an uncritical approach may lead to dire consequences, as seen in the Victoria Climbié case. Professionals' perceptions of respect and obedience in African Caribbean families were cited as reasons why they failed to note or act on signs of ill treatment in the case of Victoria Climbié (Laming 2003, p. 16).

BOX 6.2: Core knowledge and skills

- Effective communication and engagement
- Child and young person development
- Safeguarding and promoting the welfare of the child and young person
- Supporting transitions
- Multiagency working
- Sharing information

> **BOX 6.3: Assessment of abuse in children from minority ethnic groups**
>
> - Dark skin complexions may mask evidence of bruising.
> - Some children from minority ethnic groups may show dark patches on their lower back known as 'Mongolian blue'; this is normal.
> - Female genital mutilation may be seen as normal practice in some cultures, although it is illegal in the UK.
> - Language barriers may prevent children and young people from expressing their wishes and views or disclosing abuse.
> - Some children and young people may not view corporal punishment as abuse if it is perceived as endemic in the household, and such practice may be viewed as 'normal' child-rearing practices.
> - Professionals may be reluctant to express concerns for fear of being viewed as racist.

The report states 'cultural norms and models of behaviour can vary considerably between communities and even families' (Laming 2003, p. 345).

Large numbers of children and young people arrive into this country from overseas every day. Many of these children do so legally in the care of their parents. However, many children are arriving into the UK who may be in the care of adults who, although they may be their carers, have no parental responsibility for them, and some may be in the care of adults who have no documents to demonstrate a relationship with the child (Connolly 2014). Evidence from the Inter-Agency Protocol on Safeguarding Children from Abroad shows that unaccompanied children or those accompanied by someone who is not their parent are particularly vulnerable. The children and many of their carers will need assistance to ensure that the child receives adequate care and accesses health and education services. There is also a need to ensure that these children receive culturally appropriate care (Miller et al. 2013). A small number of these children may be exposed to the additional risk of commercial, sexual or domestic exploitation.

ASSESSMENT FOR SAFEGUARDING CHILDREN AND YOUNG PEOPLE FROM MINORITY ETHNIC GROUPS

Harran (2002, p. 413) emphasizes the importance of recognizing 'that professionals and clients are not culturally neutral but a product of their own cultural conditioning and life experiences'. Practitioners do not necessarily have sufficient understanding of cultural diversity, which may lead to a failure to conduct 'culturally competent assessment and intervention'. It may also undermine the emphasis placed on the child's or young person's rights and needs and cause delays in the decision-making process.

There are also specific issues relating to assessing the risk and presence of abuse in children from minority ethnic groups, which are summarized in Box 6.3.

> **REFLECTION POINTS**
>
> - What are the developmental needs of black children and their families?
> - In what ways are these similar to, and in what ways do they differ from, the developmental needs of white children and families?
> - How can these developmental needs be responded to in work with black children and families?
> - When considering the points in Box 6.2, have you ever experienced any of these challenges? What happened?

WHEN IS ABUSE NOT ABUSE?

Cultural differences in the way families rear their children should be respected, but when child abuse does occur it should be understood that this particular family has gone beyond what is acceptable not only in their own and British culture (Chand 2000, cited in Harran 2002, p. 411) but also in the law of the land. In the US, statutes specify exemptions regarding abuse thresholds, most commonly in relation to religious belief (e.g. concerning withholding medical treatment on religious grounds) or cultural practice; such considerations do not operate in the UK. As Chand points out, extensive recruitment from overseas into the health and welfare services may increase the diversity of cultural norms and expectations. Health and social care practitioners need to be aware that their beliefs may affect the decisions they make.

Female genital mutilation (FGM) is one of the troubling issues relating to culture and ethics argues Gallagher (2006), who cites the British Medical Association's (2001) definition of *female genital mutilation* as

> a collective term used for a range of practices involving the removal of parts of healthy female genitalia, from the removal of the head of the clitoris to the total amputation of the clitoris and labia minora and part of the labia majora, the remainder of which is stitched together leaving a matchstick-sized opening for the passage of urine and menstrual blood.

FGM is still a widely used traditional practice in northern Africa, and the World Health Organization (2010) estimates that more than 2 million girls have this operation every year and the UN Secretary General, speaking in 2014, estimated that by 2030, 86 million young girls will have been victims of FGM and be suffering the consequent physical and mental trauma (Winter 2014). Winter also quotes UK government statistics which suggest that there are 66,000 women in the UK living with the aftermath of FGM and that 20,000 girls under the age of 15 years are at high risk of FGM.

Reasons for such social, cultural and religious practices are put forward as the preservation of chastity and the restoration of family honour in that the woman remains a virgin until she has intercourse with her husband. However, Lindroos and Luukkainen (2004), in a study in Nigeria, found that this practice was more a matter of male domination and a convenient way of controlling sexual behaviour in women. They also found that FGM was a significant factor in maintaining high numbers of maternal mortality because of the associated pain, infections and haemorrhage during labour. Practitioners should keep in mind that FGM is illegal in the UK, whatever the cultural reasons behind it. There is a clear need for increased awareness and understanding of the criminal law sanctions for FGM among the communities where it is practiced as well as among the professionals most likely to come into contact with women and girls at risk. Clearer protocols for the identification and reporting of suspected cases of FGM are vital to ensure that they are appropriately investigated and ultimately prosecuted, as recommended by the Multi-Agency Practice Guidelines (HM Government 2011, p. 5).

OTHER HEALTH ISSUES FOR CHILDREN AND YOUNG PEOPLE

INFANT MORTALITY

Hollowell et al. (2011) found that within the UK there were clear differences in infant mortality between social groups. Additionally they found that there were significant differences between ethnic groups. For example the highest rates for infant mortality were found in Caribbean and Pakistani infants and the lowest in Bangladeshi and white infants. They concluded that although it is possible to identify individual risk factors, the reasons why certain groups are more at risk are less clear.

SICKLE CELL DISEASE AND THALASSAEMIA

In England, sickle cell disease (SCD) is more common than cystic fibrosis, and NHS Choices (2013) states that thalassaemia and sickle cell are two of England's most common inherited serious genetic disorders. They estimate that sickle cell affects approximately 13,500 with a further 240,000 people being carriers. Sickle cell is most prevalent among black British, black Caribbean and black African communities in the UK. Thalassaemia major affects approximately 950 people in the UK with an estimated 214,000 carriers. As with sickle cell, there is a higher prevalence in particular groups, in this case Chinese, Bangladeshi, Cypriot, Indian and Pakistani communities.

Implications for practice involve adequate screening programmes such as the NHS Sickle Cell and Thalassaemia Screening Programme, which was set up in England in 2001 (NHS England 2015). Early detection and adequate management of the condition can improve quality of life. For SCD, this enables parents/guardians to learn to recognize certain risk factors in their child, to avoid those that can trigger painful 'crisis' attacks and to administer antibiotics each day to prevent infections. Children with thalassaemia major will require blood transfusions every 4–6 weeks and can suffer from chronic diseases (such as diabetes) and growth or puberty failure.

HEALTH INEQUALITIES WITHIN BLACK AND MINORITY ETHNIC COMMUNITIES

There are also significant health inequalities within black and minority ethnic communities. Public Health England (2013) argues that across nearly all measurements of health, compared with the health of the majority white British population, the health of the UK's minority ethnic populations is worse. They also argue that even where these inequalities are not present, there is still inequality in terms of access to preventive services, health care and patient experience.

Health inequalities are linked to socio-economic status and poverty, and Public Health England (2013) points out that people from minority ethnic backgrounds are generally more deprived in terms of poverty and socio-economic status. This makes it very difficult to determine what the root cause of the health inequality is. For example, in addition to lower socio-economic status, and in some cases poor education, people from minority ethnic groups may be unaware of lifestyle issues such as smoking and unhealthy diets, have poor access to health services and have limited social networks leading to social isolation. Thus poorer health outcomes may be the result of health inequalities that influence people's behaviours and increase risk of illness.

TALKING TO CHILDREN ABOUT DEATH

In a multicultural society, each culture has its own way of dealing with death and dying, and aligned with this are rituals and practices that may be very dear to the people concerned. While today's diversity adds to the richness of British culture, misunderstandings by health and social care practitioners may lead to accusations of insensitivity and ethnocentric approaches. Grief and bereavement are emotions that are experienced by all people, but these are expressed differently in different communities. For example, both Christians and Muslims believe that death is a transition to a more glorious place, and in the sovereignty of God or Allah. However, Hindus and Buddhists both believe that death is not the end of life, but merely the end of the body. The spirit is believed to remain and will seek attachment to a new body and a new life.

When children and young people from such communities are dying, their parents often want certain religious rituals and practices to be carried out properly. Although it is not expected that health and social practitioners will be aware of all the rituals, parents of children and young people would expect a degree of sensitivity. In such circumstances, it is better to ask rather than show ignorance; respect should be shown for the body as it is almost a universal practice to treat the dead body with reverence, rather than just a dead body. Some guidelines for practitioners are summarized in Box 6.4.

The following case study raises questions about the standards of care for a young Muslim man.

CASE STUDY

A young male Asian patient (teenager) had died in a ward in a general hospital. His mother was called in to see the body. She was horrified to find him in a smelly side room, on a bed lying in a pool of vomit. She was very distressed and the picture of her son, in such a disgusting state in that bed, had been haunting her ever since. She complained to the hospital authorities and said that, in her mind's eye, the only picture she could see of her son was the last time she saw him lying in that bed. The nursing staff's comments were that, as he was a Muslim, they did not think they were allowed to touch the body: 'We usually let the family deal with the body'. The staff nurse said that the nurses were just following the guidelines.

REFLECTION POINTS

- What about the rights of the teenager whose body was left in a pool of vomit?
- Were nurses providing culturally sensitive care?
- Could the nurses have used gloves to wash the body to make it presentable to the mother?
- What were the nurses' responsibilities under their professional code of conduct?
- Is it right to follow guidelines to the letter even if these could lead to insensitive and poor practice?

- Ask the family if there are specific things in their culture that they do when someone is dying.
- Ask whether there are specific rituals or customs that they use to recognize death.
- Do they have certain traditions surrounding the disposal of the body?
- Ask about their beliefs regarding what happens after death.
- Explore what their feelings are about mourning after death.
- Ask whether there are any social stigmas associated with certain types of deaths.
- Ask how important is a transition death of a child or young person.
- What are their views on post-mortem and tissue donation?

HELPING CHILDREN AND YOUNG PEOPLE COPE WITH LOSS AND GRIEF

While grieving processes may appear to be generic, the way children and young people from minority ethnic groups cope will be shaped by their religious upbringing and socialization and acculturation into their own cultures. Children's coping with grief may be affected by the way they are brought up, and is influenced by the values and beliefs enshrined in their culture, such as respect, honour, responsibility and caring for others.

There are a range of resources available for professionals, parents and carers working with children and young people who are bereaved, for example Child Bereavement UK, Winston's Wish and Barnardos. Sandra Fox, from the Boston Medical Center (Fox 1985), has developed a framework outlining four psychological tasks that children and adolescents must accomplish if their grief is to be 'good grief', i.e. a grief that promotes coping skills and prevents future mental health problems. They are understanding, grieving, commemorating and going on.

UNDERSTANDING

Children and young people need honest, age-appropriate information to make sense of death, and need to know what happened and why and that the person is no longer alive and will never be part of their lives in the way he or she used to be. Children go through 'magical thinking', which is especially true when death occurs because it is so hard to make sense out of death. Therefore children often feel that the death must be the result of something they did or said or failed to do or say. Magical thinking must be challenged, so as not to leave them with lifelong guilt.

GRIEVING

While the style of grieving will differ depending on the age of the child, the relationship with the person who died, and perhaps the suddenness of the death, may involve many feelings such as sadness, anger, abandonment and ambivalence. There is no one way or right way to grieve. All feelings must be validated as children grieve in spurts. They will re-grieve through adolescence. It is important to be aware of the anniversary date of the death and other significant dates to the bereaved child.

COMMEMORATING

Commemorating is done both formally and informally, remembering the person who died and confirming the reality of the death and the value of human life. In this stage, friends, fellow students and teachers may be involved in the planning of the commemoration.

GOING ON

During this phase children and young people are expected to be returning comfortably to regular activities. This process becomes easier and healthier after the tasks of understanding, grieving and commemorating have been gone through, although all tasks are spiral and not linear. Pain should be anticipated at anniversaries and special times of remembering as 'going on' is not about forgetting or loving that person any less but about the reality of moving on in life.

STEPS NURSES AND OTHER PRACTITIONERS CAN TAKE TO HELP BEREAVED CHILDREN

Outlined below are the ways that nurses can help bereaved children according to the four steps suggested by Fox.

SHARE THE FACT OF THE DEATH WITH CHILDREN AND PARENTS

Explain to children what has happened in an age-appropriate way, but share only the information that is public knowledge. Explain to younger children that a person dies when his or her body stops working totally. Communicate to parents or send a letter home telling them what has happened, what you have discussed at the clinic, ward or nursery, and encourage them to listen to their children's reactions to the death and to talk with them about it.

RECOGNIZE YOUR OWN FEELINGS

Particular events or anniversaries of losses in our own lives can make it difficult to talk with children about death. It is all right to tell children how hard it is for you to talk about what has happened, and it is all right to cry. If your own grief makes it impossible for you to talk to children or young people, find someone who can. Stay in the room during the discussion, however, so you will know which children still have questions or concerns. Be authentic.

WATCH PARTICULARLY VULNERABLE CHILDREN CAREFULLY

Be aware of children who may be 'at risk' for later emotional problems as a result of the death, for example close friends or enemies of a child who died or children whose parents or siblings have illnesses similar to the one that caused the recent death. When someone's parent dies, all children worry about the mortality of their own parents. The death of a friend or classmate raises similar fears, particularly if one has the same symptoms or has done the same things as the child who died. Remind children that most people live a long time.

ADDRESS THE CHILDREN'S FEARS AND FANTASIES

Children's active imaginations sometimes lead them to think something they have done or not done has caused a death. Give them accurate information about the cause of the death and allow them to talk about what they think happened.

ISSUES FACING SCHOOL NURSES AND COMMUNITY CHILDREN'S NURSES

All children within the UK are required by law to be in full-time education between the ages of 5 and 16. There is, however, a huge range of settings within which this education can occur, including state schools, both selective and comprehensive entry, and those that are private (fee paying), single sex, mixed and affiliated with a religious group. Being at school is a central part of a child or young person's life as they spend a large proportion of their time there. As well as the more obvious learning that occurs in school, such as literacy, numeracy and science, more subtle learning occurs, for example secondary socialization, which imparts the morals of the school and the society within which it is located, and peer learning, which involves the child or young person in discovering the culture of their peer group and deciding to accept it or reject it.

REFLECTION POINTS

- What was the ethnic mix in your school?
- Was one ethnic group in the majority?
- Did this have an influence on the culture of the school?
- How did it affect those from other ethnic groups?

BULLYING

Schools are also communities that, as with any community, can be either nurturing or destructive. Bullying, both face-to-face and cyber bullying, is a worldwide phenomenon that is gaining an increasing amount of attention (Ybarra and Mitchell 2004; Cowie and Jennifer 2007; David-Ferdon and Hertz 2007; Huesmann 2007; Byron 2008; Cowie and Colliety 2010a, 2010b). Much of the literature on bullying suggests that one of the factors involved is a perception of being different (Kowalski and Limber 2007; Williams and Guerra 2007; Wolak et al. 2007; Ybarra et al. 2007; Cowie and Colliety 2010a, 2010b). The UK has a very diverse ethnic mix, which suggests that bullying is an issue that needs to be considered in relation to children and young people from diverse backgrounds.

Ethnic diversity within the UK population is increasing; between 2001 and 2011 the percentage of the population who defined themselves as white fell from 92.12% to 87.17% while the percentage of the population defining themselves as Asian rose from 4.39% to 6.92%, the percentage defining themselves as black rose from 1.95% to 3.01%, the percentage defining themselves as British mixed rose from 1.15% to 1.98% and the percentage of the population defining themselves as 'other' rose from 0.39% to 0.92% (ONS 2012).

Country of birth does not necessarily correlate to ethnicity; for example, the high numbers born in Germany can be attributed to the UK military bases in the country. However, for the other groups, the country of birth tends to correlate with ethnicity.

There also tend to be clusters of people from different ethnic groupings in the UK. For example, those of Polish origin tend to settle in the east of England and Scotland; those of Pakistani origin in the northwest of England, Yorkshire and Humberside; and those of Indian origin in the Midlands and the southeast of England (ONS 2012). London and other UK cities have large numbers of ethnic groups, with 2.3 million (32%) of Londoners being born outside the UK compared with 7% of the rest of the population. Outside London, the southeast and West Midlands have the highest migrant populations (ONS 2012).

REFLECTION POINTS

- Think about your own educational experience. Did you or anyone you know experience bullying?
- What form did this bullying take?
- What was done about it? By whom?
- Can you identify any factors that led to this bullying?
- What would you do about it now?

SCHOOL UNIFORMS AND RIGHTS OF MINORITY ETHNIC CHILDREN

Eason (2005), a BBC Education editor, reported on the Court of Appeal ruling that a Muslim girl's human rights were violated by a school's insistence on its dress code. The court called on the Department for Education and Skills (DfES) to give schools more guidance on how to meet their obligations under the Human Rights Act 1998 (Office for Public Sector Information 1998).

He outlined the case of Shabina Begum, aged 15, who had accused Denbigh High School in Luton, Bedfordshire, of denying her the 'right to education and to manifest her religious beliefs' over her wish to wear a full-length jilbab gown.

The school, where most pupils were Muslim, had consulted Islamic scholars for advice, and had argued that Ms Begum had chosen a school with a uniform policy and, if she did not like it, could move to another school. However, Lord Justice Brooke, vice president of the Civil Division of the Court of Appeal, ruled that her exclusion was unlawful and that the school had unlawfully denied her 'the right to manifest her religion'.

A representative for the DfES had reported that school uniform guidance states that governors should bear in mind their responsibilities under sex and race discrimination legislation and the Human Rights Act, be sensitive to pupils' cultural and religious needs and differences, and give high priority to cost considerations.

Eason reports that, currently in the UK, there is no legislation that deals specifically with school uniforms, and that individual schools, their governing bodies and the head teacher enforce the policy as part of day-to-day discipline. However, the DfES 'does not consider that exclusion from school would normally be appropriate where a pupil fails to comply with the school's rules on uniform'. The guidelines say schools must be 'sensitive to the needs of different cultures, races and religions' and accommodate those needs within their general uniform policy, such as allowing Muslim girls to wear appropriate dress and Sikh boys to wear traditional headdress.

REFLECTION POINTS

- Consider whether members of other religious groups might wish to wear clothing not permitted by a school's uniform policy, and the effect this might have on its inclusiveness.
- Is it appropriate to override the beliefs of very strict Muslims, when liberal Muslims have been permitted the dress code of their choice?
- Is it appropriate to take into account concerns about such things as other pupils feeling intimidated or coerced by the presence of very strict Muslim garb?
- Could schools do more to reconcile their wish to retain a uniform policy with the beliefs of those who think it exposes too much of their bodies?
- Could schools apply a policy without considering the individual child or young person?

PRINCIPLES FOR PRACTICE

- The culture within the family, the school and the peer group may not be compatible.
- Practitioners need to be aware that any child or young person may be being bullied, and that any child or young person who may be perceived as different is particularly vulnerable.
- Many people from the same ethnic groups live in the same area. This may result in cultural and social isolation for those who live in other areas.
- For some children and young people, English may not be the language that is used at home.

PUBLIC HEALTH PRIORITIES

The UK government has put public health high on the policy agenda, and a number of reports have been published on the state of the nation's health and identifying the public health priorities arising from it (Department of Health 2003, 2004, 2010a; Public Health England 2014).

In relation to children and young people the priorities are focused around obesity, mental health, sexual health and teenage pregnancy. Here, we will consider teenage pregnancy and obesity.

TEENAGE PREGNANCY

Although improving, the UK still has one of the highest teenage pregnancy rates in the world and the highest rate in Europe. However, the rates of teenage conception in 2013 were at their lowest since records began in 1969 (ONS 2013).

REFLECTION POINTS

- Why do you think that the UK has one of the highest rates of teenage pregnancy in the world?
- Why do you think that it is falling?
- Why do you think that it matters?

In the UK, reducing the number of teenage pregnancies (those ending in a live birth or a termination) is a priority (Department of Health 2010b). There is a link between social deprivation and the rates of teenage pregnancy, with girls from socially deprived backgrounds being more likely to become pregnant than others (ONS 2015). There is also a link between the age of the mother at the time of conception and the socio-economic outcomes for the mother and child, which tend to be worse for mothers and children when the mother was younger at the time of conception.

Crawford et al. (2014) reviewed a number of studies in a report for the Institute for Fiscal Studies and found that girls who were born of teenage mothers came from disadvantaged families, had low educational

Table 6.3 At the end of year 11, compared with white British girls

Girls of South Asian ethnic origin	85% less likely to conceive	Girls of black Caribbean ethnic origin	33% more likely to conceive
Girls of black African ethnic origin	36% less likely to conceive	Girls of mixed ethnic origin	25% more likely to conceive

attainment or came from black Caribbean, Pakistani and Bangladeshi ethnic origin, and those who had low educational attainment were more likely to give birth as a teenager.

When looking at conception rates, Crawford et al. (2014) found that there were differences in rates of conception at the end of year 11, between different ethnic groups, as shown in Table 6.3.

What the statistics do not explain, however, is the possible cultural influences on these rates. For example, within some cultures it is the norm for women to marry and have babies much younger than in other cultures. In addition, the statistics do not differentiate the ethnic groups which make up the UK as their country of origin. As has been discussed, the UK is an ethnically diverse population with many people from different ethnic groups describing themselves as British, and they, their parents, grandparents and previous generations were born there.

REFLECTION POINTS

- Why is it important to differentiate between teenage pregnancy and planned pregnancy and birth among young people under the age of 20?
- What other factors do you need to take into consideration when assessing the possible impact of pregnancy on a young woman?

Another contemporary issue is sexual health. In 2008, the UK government began immunizing girls against the human papilloma virus, which has been linked to the development of cervical cancer. It has been estimated that this immunization campaign will prevent thousands of deaths from cervical cancer per year. As with any immunization, parental consent is sought. Some parents have refused consent as they believe that their daughters are not sexually active and therefore their daughters do not need it; others believe that having the immunization may encourage promiscuity. Some Hindu, Muslim and Catholic parents may find the suggestion very offensive that their teenage schoolchildren might be considered sexually active and that they need to be protected against what could be considered a sexually transmitted disease.

REFLECTION POINTS

- If you were the parent of a teenage girl who was offered the human papilloma virus vaccine, what might your concerns be?
- What cultural or religious issues do you think there might be in relation to this?

OBESITY

Obesity is another public health priority for the government, and it has initiated a number of strategies to try to halt the year-on-year increase in the incidence of obesity. The National Child Measurement Programme (Department of Health 2006) involves all children in reception and year 6 having their height and weight recorded. The exercise will take place in schools every year. Primary care trusts coordinate the exercise with the support and cooperation of schools, and the exercise allows collection and monitoring of information about children's health to inform local planning and targeting of resources and to enable tracking of local progress against government targets on childhood obesity.

Public Health England (2015) statistics suggest that obesity rates are levelling out from a peak in 2004, although the levels are still high.

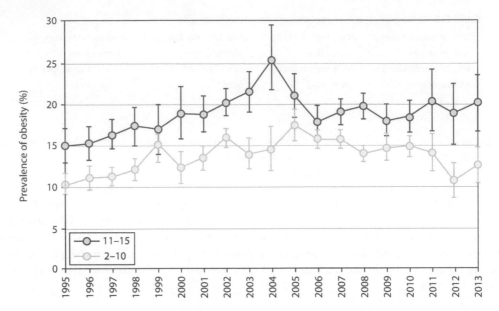

(From Public Health England, About obesity: UK prevalence, 2015, available at http://www.noo.org.uk/NOO_about_obesity/child_obesity/UK_prevalence.)

MENTAL HEALTH ISSUES

SELF-HARM

Promoting positive mental health among children and young people has been identified as a priority (Department of Health 2015); however, there are some specific challenges when looking at mental health issues among some children and young people from ethnic minority groups.

The term *self-harm* refers to a range of motives or reasons for behaviour which includes several non-suicidal intentions. Although young people who self-harm may claim that they want to die, the motivation in many is more to do with an expression of distress and desire for escape from troubling situations. Even when death is the outcome of self-harming behaviour, this may not have been intended (Mental Health Foundation 2006). Hawton and James (2005) found that young South Asian females in the UK seem to have a raised risk of self-harm. Intercultural stresses and consequent family conflicts may be relevant factors. Hicks et al. (2003), in a study on perceived causes of suicide attempts in 180 ethnic South Asian women living in the London area, found three factors which were endorsed most frequently and strongly as causes of suicide attempts: violence by the husband, being trapped in an unhappy family situation and depression.

The evidence for conflicts between teenage girls and their families is provided by the Asian Family Counselling Service's (2011–2012) annual report, which highlights not only intergenerational conflict but also issues surrounding forced marriages.

ARRANGED AND FORCED MARRIAGES

Children and young people's nurses and other practitioners must not confuse an arranged marriage and a forced marriage. Arranged marriages have been common practice in the UK, especially among the nobility. Forced marriage is where either participant is doing so against their will.

The government's Forced Marriage Unit (FMU) says it gave advice or support in 1302 cases in 2013 (FMU 2014). Of those, where the age was known, 15% of cases involved children under the age of 16 years and 25% victims aged 16–17. Eighty-two percent of the victims were female, with 18% being male. A range of countries were involved, the most common being Pakistan (42.7%), India (10.9%) and Bangladesh (9.8%).

There is evidence to suggest that the peak risk time for children and young people to be taken out of the country to be subjected to a forced marriage is in the school summer holidays. Guidance published by the FMU (2014) urges those who work in schools to be aware of signs of a possible forced marriage because school or college is often the only place where the potential victim can speak freely.

Forced marriages are not something that practitioners must be culturally sensitive about as such an act could be seen as a child abuse issue, and practitioners must treat it in that way and follow child protection procedures.

PRINCIPLES FOR PRACTICE

- Be aware of links between social deprivation and rates of teenage pregnancy.
- The statistics for higher rates of teenage pregnancy among some ethnic groups do not account for the cultural trends of younger age of marriage in such ethnic groups.
- Human papilloma virus vaccination may be an emotive or inappropriate topic for discussion in some ethnic and cultural groups.
- Levels of obesity are increasing, but the data are not detailed enough to make links to socio-economic status, ethnic origins or culture.
- Nurses working with teenage girls must be aware of the possibility of forced marriage and the peak risk times for girls to be taken out of the country.

IMPLICATIONS FOR PRACTITIONERS

Health and social care practitioners should respond to ethnic diversity by recognizing and acknowledging the continuing and contextual nature of culture and ethnicity. There is a need to critically reflect on personal values and beliefs, relating these to professional understanding within the wider ideological and policy contexts. More importantly, practitioners must develop cultural competence. Murphy (2011) argues that in order to be culturally competent, the practitioner must develop in three areas: knowledge, skills and attitude.

Murphy argues that knowledge covers information about the culturally diverse groups in the practice area and knowledge about cultural practices and observances in relation to health care practices and beliefs. Knowledge can help promote understanding between cultures, and practitioners must deliberately seek out various worldviews and explanatory models of disease. Although it is essential to gather cultural knowledge, it is an equally important, but sometimes neglected, culturally competent skill to be humble enough to let go of the security of stereotypes and ethnocentric views and remain open to the individuality of each client or patient. Central to the development of cultural knowledge lies the ability for health and social care providers to have an educated knowledge base about various cultures to better understand children and young people who may come from a culture different from their own.

Murphy discusses culture in terms of avoiding stereotypical assumptions about individuals and being aware of one's own biases and prejudices, appreciating and accepting differences, and the ability of health and social care providers to appreciate and understand their clients' values, beliefs, practices and problem-solving strategies. Self-awareness is also a vital part of this construct. This allows practitioners to analyze their own beliefs to avoid bias and prejudice when working with clients. On cultural awareness of the 'other', Duffy (2001) argues that there are more similarities than differences between cultures; therefore it is important to celebrate the similarities and acknowledge the differences.

Skill is vital as an adequate effective assessment, whether for educational or health and social care intervention, and it rests on the centrality of effective communication. Far too often practitioners complain of language barriers as obstacles to their ability to conduct an accurate and culturally competent history taking and physical examination. Most children or young people from a minority ethnic group may be able to speak English and may be either bilingual or even trilingual. In the event that a child or young person does not speak English, unless you are thoroughly effective and fluent in the target language, always use a professional interpreter, preferably of the same sex. Plan what needs to be said ahead of time and always address the client/patient directly when talking.

ANTIDISCRIMINATORY PRACTICE

Antidiscriminatory practice is an approach to working with people that promotes diversity and self-esteem, positive group identity, fulfilment of the individual and full participation of all groups in society. Practitioners need to explore their own work setting to consider whether it values people for their individuality and ensures a sense of belonging that promotes self-esteem. Does the setting respect where people come from, what they achieve and what they bring to the learning situation?

There is so much discrimination and inequality that seemingly go unchallenged by our institutions, despite legislation to the contrary.

REFLECTION POINTS

- Should a disabled child who is not ready to be toilet trained be prevented from attending a local playgroup because there is a shortage of staff and no convenient changing area?
- Should a traveller child never get to go to a nursery because he or she is always at the bottom of the waiting list because of first come, first served admission policies?

CONCLUSION

This chapter has provided an overview and explanation of the various terminologies about culture, race and ethnicity, and discussed the problematic nature of using such labels and definitions uncritically. Contemporary issues such as obesity, bullying, sexual health, human papilloma virus vaccination, the contentious issue of wearing uniforms and arranged marriages have been considered.

Issues around practice have engaged the reader on aspects that affect the provision of culturally sensitive care, such as safeguarding children, as well as health issues, such as SCD, thalassaemia and diabetes; health inequalities; talking to children about death; grieving; and developing cultural competence. Finally, the chapter addressed the implications for children and young people's nurses and other health and social care practitioners using a cultural competency framework.

Children and young people are entitled to culturally sensitive care, and children and young people's nurses have a moral, ethical and professional duty to ensure this is respected in practice.

SUMMARY OF PRINCIPLES FOR PRACTICE

- Children and young people's nurses must ensure that children and young people from ethnic minorities receive the culturally sensitive care they are entitled to.
- Children and young people's nurses must take into account cultural diversity and develop cultural competence.
- Children and young people's nurses must meet their moral, ethical and professional obligations to provide care that is culturally sensitive for every child and young person.

REFERENCES

Adams P (2014) Migration surge hits EU as thousands flock to Italy. BBC News. Available at http://www.bbc.co.uk/news/world-europe-27628416.

Ahmad WIU (1993) 'Race' and health in contemporary Britain. Milton Keynes: Open University Press.

Appiah KA (1996) Race, culture and identity: misunderstood connections. In Appiah KA, Gutman A (eds.) *Color conscious, the political morality of race*. Princeton, NJ: Princeton University Press.

Asian Family Counselling (2011–2012) Annual report. Available at http://www.asianfamilycounselling.org/sites/default/files/Annual%20Report%202011-2012.pdf.

Barn R, Sinclair R, Ferdinand D (1997) *Acting on principle: an examination of race and ethnicity in social services provision to children and families*. London: BAAF.

Bizumic B, Duckitt J (2012) What is and is not ethnocentrism? A conceptual analysis and political implications. *Political Psychology* **33**(6): 887–909.

Boushel M (2000) Childrearing across cultures. In Boushel M, Fawcett M, Selwyn J (eds.) *Focus on early childhood: principles and realities*, pp. 65–77. Oxford: Blackwell Science.

British Medical Association (2001) *The medical profession and human rights: handbook for a changing agenda*. London: Zed Books in association with the BMA.

Byron T (2008) *Safer children in a digital world: the report of the Byron Review*. Available at http://www.dcsf.gov.uk/byronreview/.

Connolly H (2014) 'For a while out of orbit': listening to what unaccompanied asylum-seeking/refugee children in the UK say about their rights and experiences in private foster care. *Adoption & Fostering* **38**(4): 331.

Cowie H, Colliety P (2010a) Cyberbullying: the situation in the UK. In Mora-Merchán JA, Jäger T (eds.) *Cyberbullying – a cross-national comparison*. Landau: Verlag Empirische Pädagogik.

Cowie H, Colliety P (2010b). Cyberbullying: sanctions or sensitivity. *Pastoral Care in Education* **28**(4): 261–68.

Cowie H, Jennifer D (2007) *Managing violence in schools: a whole school approach to best practice*. London: Sage.

Crawford C, Cribb J, Kelly E (2014) *Teenage pregnancy in England*. CAYT Impact Study Report No. 6. Available at http://www.ifs.org.uk/caytpubs/caytreport06.pdf.

David-Ferdon C, Hertz M (2007) Electronic media, violence, and adolescents: an emerging public health problem. *Journal of Adolescent Health* **41**(6): S1–5.

Department of Health (2003) *Tackling health inequalities: a programme for action*. London: DH.

Department of Health (2004) *Race equality action plan*. Available at http://webarchive.nationalarchives.gov.uk/+/www.dh.gov.uk/en/Publicationsandstatistics/Bulletins/DH_4072494.

Department of Health (2006) *National child measurement programme 2006/07*. Available at www.dh.gov.uk/en/Publichealth/Obesity/DH_083093.

Department of Health (2010a) *The Marmot review. Fair society healthy lives*. Available at http://www.instituteofhealthequity.org/projects/fair-society-healthy-lives-the-marmot-review.

Department of Health (2010b) *The Public Health White Paper 2010*. Available at https://www.gov.uk/government/publications/the-public-health-white-paper-2010.

Department of Health (2015) *Future in mind. Promoting, protecting and improving our children and young people's mental health and wellbeing*. Available at https://www.gov.uk/government/uploads/system/uploads/attachment_data/file/414024/Childrens_Mental_Health.pdf.

Duffy ME (2001) A critique of cultural education in nursing. *Journal of Advanced Nursing* **36**(4): 487–95.

Dunham Y, Stepanova EV, Dotsch R, Todorov A (2015) The development of race-based perceptual categorization: skin color dominates early category judgments. *Developmental Science* **18**(3): 469–83.

Eason G (2005) School uniforms needs a review. BBC News Online 2 March.

Emery H (2014) *The specific challenges facing students with mixed race*. Available at http://www.magonlinelibrary.com/doi/full/10.12968/bjsn.2014.9.4.197.

Figueroa P (1991) *Education and the social construction of 'race'*. London: Routledge.

Forced Marriage Unit (2014) *Statistics January to December 2013*. Available at https://www.gov.uk/government/uploads/system/uploads/attachment_data/file/291855/FMU_2013_statistics.pdf.

Fox S (1985) *Boston Medical Center: Good Grief Program*. Available at http://ebookyes.info/download/good-grief-pdf-online.

Gaine C (1987) *No problem here: a practical approach to education and 'race' in white schools*. London: Hutchinson Radius.

Gallagher A (2006) The ethics of culturally competent health and social care. In Papadopoulos I (ed.) *Transcultural health and social care*. Edinburgh: Churchill Livingstone, chap. 5.

Harran E (2002) Fragile: handle with care – protecting babies from harm. *Child Abuse Review* **11**(1): 65–79.

Harttgen K, Klasen S (2008) *Well-being of migrant children and migrant youth in Europe*. Available at http://globalnetwork.princeton.edu/publications/interest/34.pdf.

Hawton K, James A (2005) Suicide and deliberate self harm in young people. *British Medical Journal* **330**: 891–4.

Helman CG (2007) *Culture, health and illness*. 5th ed. London: (Hodder) Arnold.

Hicks M, Hsiao-Rei M, Bhugra D (2003) Perceived causes of suicide attempts by U.K. South Asian women. *American Journal of Orthopsychiatry* **73**(4): 455–62.

HM Government (2011) *Multi-agency practice guidelines: female genital mutilation*. Available at http://tinyurl.com/nhh7qdl.

Hollowell J, Kurinczuk JJ, Brocklehurst P (2011) Social and ethnic inequalities in infant mortality: a perspective from the United Kingdom. *Seminars in Perinatology* **35**(4): 240–4.

Huesmann LR (2007) The impact of electronic media violence: scientific theory and research. *Journal of Adolescent Health* **41**(6): S6–13.

King JE (2015) *Dysconscious racism, Afrocentric praxis, and education for human freedom*. New York: Routledge.

King JE (No date) *A moral choice*. Available at http://www.pps.k12.or.us/files/district-leadership/A_Moral_Choice_Dr_Joyce_King.pdf.

Kowalski RM, Limber SP (2007) Electronic bullying among middle school students. *Journal of Adolescent Health* **41**(6): S22–30.

Kroeber AL, Kluckhohn C, Untereiner W, Meyer AG (1963) *A critical review of concepts and definitions*. 2nd ed. New York: Vintage Books.

Laming W (2003) *The Victoria Climbié Inquiry: summary report of an inquiry by Lord Laming*. London: HMSO.

Lindroos A, Luukkainen A-R (2004) Antenatal care and maternal mortality in Nigeria. *Public Health Programme-exchange to Nigeria*. Available at www.uku.fi/kansy/eng/antenal_care_nigeria.pdf.

Macpherson W (1999) *The Stephen Lawrence Inquiry*, p. 28, para. 6.34. London: Home Office.

Marx S, Pennington J (2003) Pedagogies of critical race theory: experimentation with white pre-service teachers. *International Journal of Qualitative Studies in Education* **16**(1): 91–110.

Mathur R, Grundy E, Smeeth L (2013) *Availability and use of UK based ethnicity data for health research*. National Centre for Research Methods Working Paper 01/13, Available at http://eprints.ncrm.ac.uk/3040/1/Mathur-_Availability_and_use_of_UK_based_ethnicity_data_for_health_res_1.pdf.

McNeely CL (1996) Understanding culture in a changing world. A sociological perspective. *Journal of Criminal Justice and Popular Culture* **4**(1): 2–11.

Mental Health Foundation (2006) *The truth hurts*. Report of the National Inquiry into Self Harm among Young People. London: MHF.

Miller K, Irizarry C, Bowden M (2013) Providing culturally safe care in the best interests of unaccompanied humanitarian minors. *Journal of Family Studies* **19**(3): 276–84.

Modood T (1994) Political blackness and British Asians. *Sociology* **28**(4): 859–76.

Morley D, Street C (2014) *Challenges face mixed raced children and young people in the UK today*. Available at http://www.ncb.org.uk/news/challenges-face-mixed-raced-children-and-young-people-in-the-uk-today.

Morrow R (1989) Southeast Asian parent involvement: can it be a reality? *Elementary School Guidance and Counseling* **23**: 289–97.

Morrow V (1999) 'We are people too': children's and young people's perspectives on children's rights and decision making in England. *International Journal of Children's Rights* **7**: 149–70.

Morrow V (2011) *Understanding children and childhood*. Lismore, Australia: Centre for Children & Young People, Southern Cross University.

Murphy K (2011) The importance of cultural competence. *Nursing Made Incredibly Easy!* **9**(2): 5. Available at http://journals.lww.com/nursingmadeincrediblyeasy/Fulltext/2011/03000/The_importance_of_cultural_competence.1.aspx.

National Statistics (2006) *A guide to comparing 1991 and 2011 census ethnic group data*. Available at http://www.ons.gov.uk/ons/search/index.html?pageSize=50&sortBy=none&sortDirection=none&newquery Focus+on+Ethnicity+and+Identity+-+Comparing+1991+and+2001+Census+ethnic+group+data.

NHS Choices (2013) *Inheriting sickle cell anaemia disorder*. Available at http://www.nhs.uk/Livewell/Blackhealth/Pages/Sicklecellanaemia.aspx.

NHS England (2015) *NHS sickle cell and thalassaemia screening programme*. Available at http://sct.screening.nhs.uk/statistics.

Office of Public Sector Information (1998) Human Rights Act 1998. London: OPSI. Available at http://www.opsi.gov.uk/acts/acts1998/ukpga_19980042_en_1.

ONS (2012) *Ethnicity and national identity in England and Wales 2011*. Available at http://www.ons.gov.uk/ons/rel/Census/2011-census/key-statistics-for-local-authorities-in-england-and-wales/rpt-ethnicity.html.

ONS (2013) *Teenage pregnancies at lowest level since records began*. Available at http://www.ons.gov.uk/ons/rel/vsob1/conception-statistics--england-and-wales/2013/stb-conceptions-in-england-and-wales-2013.html.

ONS (2014) *Census general report. Full report*. Available at http://www.ons.gov.uk/ons/guide-method/census/2011/uk-census/index.html.

Ouseley H, Lane J (2008) Nipping prejudice in the bud. *Guardian* 7 August. Available at www.guardian.co.uk.

Papadopoulos I (ed.) (2006) *Transcultural health and social care*. Edinburgh: Churchill Livingstone.

Perkins R (2014) Racial stereotypes linked to health care disparity. University of Southern California. Available at http://www.futurity.org/race-stereotypes-health-care-735192/.

Public Health England (2013) *Ethnic minority health*. Available at http://www.apho.org.uk/resource/view.aspx?RID=78571.

Public Health England (2014) *From evidence into action: opportunities to protect and improve the nation's health*. Available at https://www.gov.uk/government/publications/from-evidence-into-action-opportunities-to-protect-and-improve-the-nations-health.

Public Health England (2015) *About obesity: UK prevalence*. Available at http://www.noo.org.uk/NOO_about_obesity/child_obesity/UK_prevalence.

Puzan E (2003) The unbearable whiteness of being (in nursing). *Nursing Inquiry* **10**(3): 193–200.

Ramachandran A, Snehalatha C, Ching Wan Na R (2014) Diabetes in South-East Asia: an update. *Diabetes Research and Clinical Practice* **103**(2): 231–7.

Schneider D (2004) *The psychology of stereotyping*. New York: Guildford Press.

Social Services Inspectorate (2000) *Excellence not excuses: inspection of services for ethnic minority children and families*. Available at http://webarchive.nationalarchives.gov.uk/+/www.dh.gov.uk/en/Publicationsandstatistics/Publications/PublicationsInspectionReports/DH_4009334.

Song M, Aspinall P (2012) Is racial mismatch a problem for young 'mixed race' people in Britain? The findings of qualitative research. *Ethnicities*. Available at http://etn.sagepub.com/content/early/2012/02/09/1468796811434912.

Song M, Gutierrez C (2014a) *Mixed race parents*. University of Kent. Available at http://www.kent.ac.uk/mrp/about.html.

Song M, Gutierrez C (2014b) *Mixed race parents and the socialisation of their children – summary of key findings* Available at http://www.kent.ac.uk/mrp/files/socialisation.pdf.

Steer PJ (2014) Race and ethnicity in biomedical publication. *BJOG 2015* **122**: 464–7.

United Nations (1989) *Convention on the Rights of the Child*. Adopted under General Assembly Resolution 44/25. Geneva: UN.

UNICEF (2007) *Child poverty in perspective: an overview of child well-being in rich countries – a comprehensive assessment of the lives and well-being of children and adolescents in the economically advanced nations*. UNICEF Innocenti Research Centre Report Card 7. Florence: UNICEF.

Vernon P (1982) *The abilities and achievements of Orientals in North America*. Calgary: Academic Press.

Vydelingum V (1998) 'We treat them all the same'. Nurses' and South Asian patients' experiences of care. Unpublished PhD thesis, University of Southampton, Southampton.

Vydelingum V (2006) Nurses' experiences of caring for South Asian minority ethnic patients in a general hospital in England. *Nursing Inquiry* **13**(1): 23–32.

Webb E, Maddocks A, Bonglli J (2002) Effectively protecting black and minority ethnic children from harm: overcoming barriers to the child protection process. *Child Abuse Review* **11**: 394–411.

Westwood S, Bachu P (1988) *Images and realities*. 6th ed. Gabriola Island, BC: New Society.

Williams KR, Guerra NG (2007) Prevalence and predictors of Internet bullying. *Journal of Adolescent Health* **41**(6)(suppl.): S14–21.

Wilmot P, Young M (1957) *Family and kinship in East London*. London: Routledge & Kegan Paul.

Winter G (2014) Female genital mutilation. *British Journal of Midwifery* **22**(4): 38–44.

Wolak J, Kimberley JD, Mitchell J, Finkelhor D (2007) Does online harassment constitute bullying? An exploration of online harassment by known peers and online-only contacts. *Journal of Adolescent Health* **41**(6): S51–8.

World Health Organization (2010) *Female genital mutilation*. Geneva: WHO. Available at http://www.who.int/mediacentre/factsheets/fs241/en/.

Yamamoto J, Kubota M (1983) The Japanese-American family. In Powell GJ (ed.) *The psychosocial development of minority group children*. New York: Brunner/Mazel.

Ybarra M, Diener-West M, Leaf P (2007) Examining the overlap in Internet harassment and school bullying: implications for school intervention. *Journal of Adolescent Health* **41**(6): S42–50.

Ybarra M, Mitchell K (2004) Online aggressor/targets, aggressors, and targets: a comparison of associated youth characteristics. *Journal of Child Psychology and Psychiatry* **45**(7): 1308–16.

PART **3**

CARE DELIVERY ACROSS A RANGE OF SETTINGS

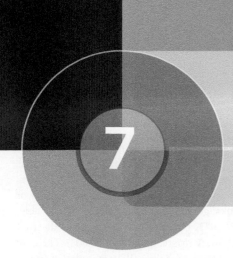

Neonatal care: Provision, nursing and challenges

7

ELISABETH PODSIADLY

OVERVIEW

This chapter explores the provision of neonatal care, particularly that of the preterm baby, from a global and national perspective. Service delivery from the four countries of the United Kingdom is compared and contrasted to neonatal provision in four economically similar countries: Canada, the US, Australia and Sweden. Key neonatal documents which not only define the organization of UK neonatal care but also influence the shape of current and future nursing practice, education and role development are discussed. Finally, because the provision of neonatal care is a societal issue, the ongoing challenges of providing inclusive neonatal care to the family and the impact of neonatal outcomes on ethical dilemmas are considered.

INTRODUCTION

Infants born too soon, too small and too sick are society's most vulnerable and smallest members and until recently have been invisible, as care and care issues have been dealt with behind the closed doors of the neonatal unit. Prematurity is a global issue. Efforts to reduce mortality rates in children under 5 have shifted the world's focus to the preterm infant. Global strategies, such as improving newborn resuscitation or attending to the infant's thermal needs at birth to improve morbidity and mortality, are now in place. Whether one is working within a low-resource/low-income country or high-resource/high-income country, the neonatal nurse plays an important front-line role in improving infant and family outcomes for this group.

In highly resourced countries advances in neonatal care, organization and provision have resulted in the boundaries of viability pushed to as early as 22 weeks' gestation. These advances have impacted neonatal outcome and in particular resulting disability. Neonatal nurses have been key players in the bedside delivery of these advances, providing care to both the infants and their families.

Neonatal organization and service provision has undergone many changes which have predominantly been medically led. Historically neonatal nurses have had limited roles in these changes, although both nursing and parental participation in these developments have increased. Neonatal units, unlike many other areas of paediatrics, are very structured as a result of both professional and governmental documentation including guidance on types of units, categories of care, nurse–patient ratios, educational expectations and service standards to ensure safe and high-quality care. Despite increased involvement in later organizational developments many neonatal nurses' view of neonatal care is restricted to the delivery of day-to-day care. Neonatal nurses, regardless of position or grade, need to become more politically aware of current organizational issues and service provision so they can shape their own future and voice their needs and those of the infants and families in their care. The aims of this chapter are to increase the children and young people's nurses' and neonatal nurses' understanding of organizational and service provision from a national and international perspective.

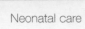

HISTORY AND DEVELOPMENT OF NEONATAL CARE

Neonatology, caring for the newborn in the first 4 weeks of life, is an evolving and relatively new speciality or branch of paediatrics. The term *neonatology* was coined as recently as 1960 (Brennan 1988). In the history of medicine, neonatology is considered to still be in its infancy. Midwives, the first neonatal nurses, were responsible for the development of early neonatal facilities and care. They converted ward broom or store cupboards to care for infants, the majority premature (<37 weeks' gestation) and considered non-viable. The initial neonatal care was provided with limited resources. In 1931, Dr Mary Crosse opened the first neonatal unit in the UK at the Sorrento Maternity Unit in Birmingham (Christie and Tansey 2001). The care provided at this time could only be described as basic, but it followed the principles still used today of trying to keep the infant pink, warm and sweet (Glasper et al. 2015). The development of neonatal care and units has been predominantly outside of the public eye. Initially parents were felt to be a major source of infection, and therefore access to their infants and opportunities to interact and partake in any caregiving was extremely limited. Parents were only allowed to visit briefly, but were not really welcomed into units or encouraged to be part of the 'care team' as they are today. It was not until discharge that the premature infant was integrated into the family unit and visible to society (Podsiadly 2008).

Initially advancements in neonatal care were slow. In the early 1980s cutting-edge neonatal care was given to infants of gestations between 28 and 29 weeks. As our understanding of fetal and neonatal anatomy, physiology and pathophysiology has developed, so has our ability to provide evidence-based care through the development of innovation, technology and research. We are now caring for infants at and just below the age of viability (24 weeks' gestation). Table 7.1 captures the key milestones in the development and delivery of neonatal care.

Neonatal units traditionally sat within midwifery and then women and children or paediatric directorates, which made it difficult for the midwife to maintain their 'intention to practice' or midwifery registration. Today, the majority of neonatal units employ predominantly neonatal nurses from an adult and children's nursing background. Their varied experiences, knowledge and skills collectively ensure the needs of the infants and families in their care are met. The development of the Neonatal Nurses Association in 1977 has played a significant role in giving the neonatal nurse a voice in the organization of neonatal care and the education of neonatal nurses (Christie and Tansey 2001).

CASE STUDY

The following letter, from 1 January, 1890, was written in response to an earlier enquiry from a reader requesting information on the management of premature infants:

Dear Madam,

Within the last few months I have attended several cases of premature births – two sets of twins – one of each set died within the three days, the other two survived and are still doing well. Also four other single premature infants have come under my notice, all about the seven months, each mother having a history of continued miscarries and premature births, the infants not living beyond two or three days.

My system of managing such cases is thus: – After separating the mother and child, to carefully handle the latter, putting it into a warm bath, well sluicing, but not turning it over in the water. After softly wiping, wrap in warm cotton wool – having first rubbed the baby all over with cod-liver oil, to which add a few drops of brandy.

Cut a little jacket of cotton wool to put on next the skin, over which dress the infant in the ordinary clothes, then place in the mother's arms to procure animal heat. Continue this treatment every other day, and the same process for a week or ten days, after which it can have its daily bath.

With regard to feeding: – a premature infant is not strong enough to draw the breast for the first two or three days, consequently about every six hours feed it with one-third of *new* cow's milk to two-thirds of *boiling* water, add a small quantity of moist sugar. To each teaspoonful of fluid put one drop of brandy and give through the feeding bottle. This continue night and morning for six weeks.

Under this system the little ones are generally found to be in a satisfactory condition, and, it is hoped grow to maturity, and become useful members of society.

Yours truly,
G. W. (*Midwife L.O.S*)

Source: WG, Nursing notes. From the past, *Midwives Chronicles and Nursing Notes*, March 1987.

Table 7.1 Key developments and milestones in neonatal care

Date	Development
1958	Phototherapy reported from England
	Improved survival of premature infants by increasing environmental temperatures
1959	Surfactant deficiency associated with respiratory distress syndrome (RDS)
1960	The term *neonatology* is coined
1963	Intrauterine transfusion of the fetus in haemolytic disease described in New Zealand
	Early feeding begun in premature infants
1965	Reports of successful use of assisted ventilation to treat respiratory disorders in newborn infants
1966	Use of Rh immune globulin (anti-D) to prevent Rh incompatibility
1967	Chronic lung disease following ventilator therapy described in the US and England
	Growth classification for birthweight described: small, appropriate and large for gestational age
1969–1973	Continuous positive airway pressure (CPAP) introduced and developed to treat RDS
1970s	Introduction of family-centred care and developmental supportive care into neonatal units
1971	American Academy of Pediatrics reports a causal relationship between PaO_2 and then retrolental fibroplasias (now retinopathy of prematurity)
	High caloric peripheral intravenous alimentation described in premature infants
1972	Use of prenatal corticosteroids to prevent RDS from New Zealand
	Use of negative-pressure ventilation for the treatment of RDS
1973	First report of anomalies in infants born to alcoholic mothers in France
	Methylxanthines introduced for the treatment of apnoea of prematurity
1975	The US reports on the first successful use of extracorporeal membrane oxygenation (ECMO) to successfully treat neonates with severe respiratory distress
1976	Pharmacological closure of the ductus arteriosus in the preterm by prostaglandin inhibition described
1980	First report of the use of human surfactant on a premature baby to treat RDS in Japan
1981–2004	Development and trials of synthetic/artificial surfactants and natural surfactants
1987	Development of trigger ventilation, the first synchronous ventilation strategy to treat RDS
1988	Development of nasal CPAP with fluidic flip (Infant Flow Driver in UK, Aladdin in the US)
1989	High-frequency oscillation ventilation (HFOV) trials on premature infants commence in the US
1990s	Re-emergence of volume ventilation in neonatal units
1992	*Science* magazine names nitric oxide (NO) 'molecule of the year'; the US reports of the benefits of inhaled NO in infants with persistent pulmonary hypertension
1994	Liquid ventilation trials to treat RDS set up in the US
2003	Re-organization of neonatal service to manage clinical networks
2003–2004	Introduction of humidified high-flow nasal cannula (HHFNC) into neonatal units

Source: Compiled from Brennan, C., History of neonatology, unpublished attachment prepared for presentation to the South West Thames Regional Health Authority Working Party on Neonatal Nursing and Education, London, 1988; Podsiadly, E., Portrayal of the premature baby in the *Times* newspaper from 1930–2008, MSc dissertation, University of Surrey, Guildford, 2008; Donn, S., Boon, W., *Respiratory Care*, 54(9), 1236–43, 2009.

REFLECTION POINTS

- What strategies has this midwife used to keep the preterm infants in her care 'pink, warm and sweet'?
- Are any of these strategies used or modified in practice today?

PROVISION OF NEONATAL CARE

GLOBAL PERSPECTIVE

Prematurity is a global issue. Worldwide the incidence of prematurity is 1 in 10 births (World Health Organization [WHO] 2012a). To quantify, this is the equivalent of 15 million infants born too soon, of which 1 million will die (WHO 2012a, 2014). Prematurity, defined as birth prior to 37 completed weeks of pregnancy, is a leading cause of death for children and only comes second to pneumonia in children under 5

(Liu et al. 2015; United Nations [UN] 2015b) The WHO definitions of prematurity can be found in Table 7.2. Forty percent of these deaths occur in the first 4 weeks of life, or what is defined as the neonatal period. On closer examination of this period, 75% of neonatal deaths occur in the first week of life and a staggering 25%–40% occur in the first hours of life (WHO 2012b).

In 2000, the United Nations held the Millennium Summit and launched eight Millennium Development Goals (MDGs), as illustrated in Box 7.1, to unite worldwide effort to meet the needs of the world's poorest by 2015. Unlike children born into wealthier families, children born into poverty are nearly twice as likely to die before the age of 5 (UN 2015a). MDG 4 aims to decrease childhood mortality by two-thirds and increase childhood survival in the under-5 age group between 2010 and 2025. Current and predicted trends indicate that some countries have made great strides in reducing childhood mortality in the under-5 group. Countries that have made great strides in reducing their under-5 childhood mortality include Bangladesh, Ethiopia, Liberia, Malawi, Nepal, Timor-Leste and the United Republic of Tanzania (UN 2015b). The number of deaths in children under 5 has decreased from 12.7 million in 1990 to 6.3 million in 2013, despite an increase in population (UN 2015b). Unfortunately this trend is not seen in every country, specifically those in sub-Saharan Africa and Southern Asia, with currently 80% of deaths in children under 5 (Liu et al., 2015). Liu et al. (2015) predict that sub-Saharan African countries by 2030 will be responsible for a third of the world's live births and unless effective measures are taken to decrease cases of malaria, HIV/AIDS, pneumonia and complications of prematurity, they will in fact see a continued increase in under-5 deaths.

The overall rate of under-5 deaths in children has decreased as reductions in pneumonia, diarrhoea and measles rates have taken place in response to improved immunization programmes in low-resource countries (Liu et al. 2015). As a result of this decrease the proportion of deaths occurring in the neonatal period is increasing. Causes include prematurity and low birthweight, infections, asphyxia and birth trauma. Collectively these causes account for 80% of the deaths occurring in the neonatal period, with the

Table 7.2 WHO definitions of prematurity

Preterm	<37 completed weeks of gestation
Moderate or late preterm	32–37
Very preterm	28–32
Extremely preterm	<28

Source: Reprinted from *The Lancet*, 379, Blencowe H, Cousens S, Oestergaard M, Chou S, Moller A, Narwal R, Adler A, et al. National, regional, and worldwide estimates of preterm birth rates in the year 2010 with time trends since 1990 for selected countries: a systematic analysis and implications, 2162–72, Copyright (2012), with permission from Elsevier.

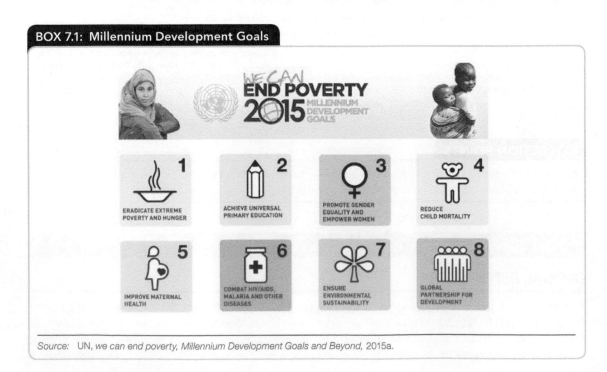

BOX 7.1: Millennium Development Goals

Source: UN, *we can end poverty, Millennium Development Goals and Beyond*, 2015a.

leading cause being prematurity (WHO 2012b). The causes of prematurity are varied. The majority of preterm birth occurs spontaneously and unexpectedly with no causative factors identified. However, there are some known risk factors and these include multiple pregnancies, maternal infections and chronic conditions like diabetes and high blood pressure (WHO 2012b). A better understanding of the known causes can hopefully result in strategies to prevent or limit the effects of these conditions. Twelve percent of preterm deliveries occur in the poorest or low-resource countries compared to 9% in countries with higher incomes or better healthcare resources (Blencowe et al. 2012). Therefore the delivery of neonatal care and services and its impact on outcome is very much determined by where you live in the world. Neonatal provision varies considerably worldwide, and clearly those countries which have greater resources generally speaking have better mortality and morbidity outcomes. Africa and South Asia account for 60% of preterm deliveries (Blencowe et al. 2012). Surprisingly, the United States is ranked within the top 10 countries noted to have the highest number of premature deliveries (Blencowe et al. 2012). Low-resource and poor countries not only experience greater prematurity rates but also experience considerably lower survival rates. Nine out of 10 babies at a gestation of less than 28 weeks will die in low-income countries compared to 1 out of 10 in high-income countries (Blencowe et al. 2012). WHO (2012b) suggests that up to two-thirds of newborn deaths could be prevented by basic strategies including resuscitation, attending to thermal needs, basic umbilical cord care and promotion and support of early and exclusive breastfeeding, to name a few. Many of these interventions are taken for granted as they are standard in developed mid- to high-resource countries. Neonatal inequalities need to be addressed and strategies which include pre-conceptual care, quality maternity care, education in maternal health and basic, low-cost interventions to keep the neonate pink, warm and sweet are urgently required (Murray 1997; WHO 2012a).

In order to reduce prematurity, considering the neonate in isolation will not be effective. The eight MDGs are inter-related; a success in one will lead to successes in others. For example, it has been noted that children of educated mothers with as little education as primary schooling are more likely to survive than children whose mothers had no education at all (UN 2015b). In September 2010, the United Nations Foundation launched a programme to further support the MDGs, entitled 'Every Woman Every Child', a global strategy for women and children's health. This programme is committed to continuing the global effort to address the MDGs, particularly MDGs 4 and 5, by addressing the maternal and child health of those most vulnerable, and in turn reducing the numbers of premature infants and improving the neonatal care provided, especially in low-resource countries. Although the MDG project ended in July 2015, the United Nations and governments of member countries, as well as national and international public and private organizations, will continue to support transforming women and children's health as the MDGs become Sustainable Developmental Goals (SDGs).

A key resource to ensure delivery of safe and effective neonatal care is appropriate and adequately trained staff. High-resource countries can identify their levels and needs, but on a global level Eklund (2014) notes a lack of data to quantify neonatal nurses. She goes on to state that 'the lack of data translates to invisibility of the neonatal nurses on the global front' (p. 166). Neonatal nurses and those healthcare workers involved in front-line mother–baby care have a responsibility to advance the achievement of the MDGs 4 and 5. Membership in local, national and international neonatal organizations to network and collectively voice the needs of and increase the public awareness of the premature infant is one way to advance these MDGs. The Council of International Neonatal Nurses (COINN) represents 60 countries, sharing the world's neonatal expertise and disseminating important information to those countries that have little or no access by organizing conferences, international work experiences and projects promoting education/training, research and care improvement (Kenner et al. 2011; Anonymous 2015).

REFLECTION POINT

What can you do to advance the achievement of MDGs 4 and 5?

World Prematurity Day: 17 November

Beresford (2015, p. 1) describes World Prematurity Day as a 'global movement to raise awareness about prematurity highlighting the burden of premature birth, informing on simple, proven cost effective solutions, and evoking passion for families who have experienced preterm birth'.

How can you or your unit participate?

For information and ideas on World Prematurity Day, see http://www.efcni.org/.

COMPARISON OF PROVISION: UK VERSUS NON-UK

In 2007, the National Audit Office (NAO) commissioned the RAND Corporation to undertake an objective analysis of whether the re-organization of England's neonatal service in 2003 was value for money. In order to make this comparison, the completed report compared neonatal care in four economically comparable high-resource countries: Canada, the United States, Australia and Sweden. In addition a comparison was made of the four countries within the United Kingdom.

A comparative analysis using the following five themes was made:

1. Trends in high-risk births and related outcomes to include review of mortality and co-morbidities
2. Organization and scale of provision of neonatal services
3. Transport services
4. Costs of neonatal services
5. Best practices for infants and their families (Hallsworth et al. 2007)

A discussion using these five themes will be made to compare the UK to the non-UK countries, by an exploration of the individual UK countries – England, Scotland, Wales and Northern Ireland.

Overall, the rate of preterm births across all countries (with the exception of Northern Ireland) in 2004 over a 10-year period appeared to have remained steady (Hallsworth et al. 2007). A review of recent data from 2010 suggests some improvements in preterm birth rates have been made (March of Dimes 2015). Please note it is not possible to comment on preterm birth rates in Northern Ireland as they do not currently collect this data (Tommy's 2015). Neonatal mortality rates have generally decreased with improvements in maternal and neonatal care. The rates in the US continue to exceed those of Canada, Australia and UK, which are on a par. Swedish rates continue to fall and in fact are half of those in the US, predominantly due to high-quality peri-natal care resulting in a decrease in intrapartum and postnatal deaths (Hallsworth et al. 2007).

The provision of healthcare is either publically funded, as in Canada and Australia, or funded by private healthcare companies, as in the US. Sweden's healthcare is nationally funded, but the delivery of healthcare is decentralized to politically elected county councils. In Canada, Australia and Sweden, as in the UK, health-care is available to all and free at the point of service (Health Canada 2014; Australian Institute of Health and Welfare 2014; Swedish Institute 2013–2015). In the US, healthcare is available to those with appropriate health insurance, or for those in poverty there may be free or low-cost care offered by individual states (USA.gov 2015). In terms of monies for neonatal care, the US has more neonatal intensive care resources per capita than Canada and Australia (Hallsworth et al. 2007). Despite this the US data demonstrate higher mortality rates for preterm and low birthweight babies (Gallagher et al. 2004; March of Dimes 2015). Therefore it is not just how many resources you have, but how you use them (Hallsworth et al. 2007).

Provision or organization of a neonatal service across the countries is very much determined by its geography, population, funding and resources, including staff. Canada, the US and Australia are, respectively, the second, third and sixth largest countries in the world and are divided up into states and provinces or territories (UN 2006). Regionalized neonatal care is then provided by the states and provinces/territories, which reflects the needs and locations of the population. Sweden has in comparison to other countries a considerably lower rate of low birthweight births and therefore is moving to a more centralized provision of care (Hallsworth et al. 2007), thereby maintaining expertise for its neonatal population.

Neonatal transport services in the non-UK countries use a variety of coordinating mechanisms and types of transport. In the US, the type of transport service offered changes from state to state. Transport could be a centralized service or organized by the main Level III Unit. A third of dedicated teams responsible for transport are neonatal, while half service both neonates and paediatrics. The majority of transports are made by road with a small number provided by helicopter and fixed-wing aircraft. In Canada two options are provided. Transport is provided by either a single provincial/territorial transport coordinating service or the regional Level III Unit. Australia has a highly developed and managed transport service which despite the geographical distances utilizes effectively a newborn transport system via road, fixed-wing aircraft and helicopter. In Sweden, transport teams are organized regionally, not nationally. Ambulance services are locally based and organized closely with local healthcare centres. In mid- and northern Sweden, fixed-wing aircraft are used for neonatal transport (Hallsworth et al. 2007).

As in Canada and the US, transport services across the four UK countries are varied. Since 2003, Scotland has led the way and has provided a national and integrated neonatal transport network with dedicated teams, ambulances for road transfer and a publically funded air ambulance service. England at the time of the report was still striving to achieve 24-hour dedicated transport teams for all its networks. Northern Ireland and Wales had at this time no recognized network transport service but were dependent on transport teams arising from inpatient services to undertake transfer. This service arrangement runs the risk of compromising care for inpatient services. Since this report, the NHS England Neonatal Critical Care Clinical Reference Group has adopted service specifications for critical care retrieval transport to ensure all transport services deliver high-quality care and 24-hour service (NHS England 2013). In 2011, Wales had developed a part-time service. Cymn Inter Hospital Acute Neonatal Transport Service (CHANTS) is delivered rotationally by three neonatal units in South Wales and to one North Wales unit with support from the Cheshire and Merseyside Neonatal Network Transport Service (CMNNTS) (Wales Neonatal Network n.d). In 2014 Northern Ireland expanded its retrieval services to include a central service known as Child or Neonate Need Emergency Critical Care Transport (CONNECT) (Northern Ireland Executive 2014).

Neonatal care has vastly improved as a result of growing knowledge and advancements in technology. The result has been a greater survival of infants previously not considered viable, which have impacted healthcare costs. Birth rates of preterm babies across these countries averaged 7.5 per 1000 births. These numbers have a significant impact on how a country manages its healthcare resources (Canadian Institute for Health Information 2006). Hallsworth et al. (2007) considered comparing costs of neonatal service provision but due to the country-specific variables in the delivery of healthcare, direct comparisons were possible but meaningless. Rogowski (1999) explored and compared costs across 25 nationally representative neonatal intensive care units in the US. As healthcare costs in the US are itemized, she was able to compare treatment costs per infant, ancillary costs (to include respiratory therapy, laboratory, radiology and pharmacy costs, to name a few), accommodation costs and comment on length of stay. Costs were categorized in a variety of ways. In the UK we cost by identifying the category of care received, while costs in the US were identified based on birthweight and gestation. Not surprisingly, the lower birthweight or gestation had the greatest impact on the cost of the care provided. In the case of the preterm low birthweight baby this relationship also exists. The smaller and preterm babies are more likely require intensive care. The time periods relating to the data available vary from country to country, which make direct comparisons of costs difficult as does currency exchange rates when trying to work out costs in one currency. In 2008–2009 the national average cost per day for special care was £476, high dependency £759 and intensive care £1081 (National Institute for Health and Clinical Excellence [NICE] 2010).

Hallsworth et al. (2007) also explored the mechanisms that non-UK countries use to ensure best practice. Guidelines developed at the national or regional level, audit tools and input from medical and nursing associations/organization also play a role in setting and achieving best practice.

In the UK each country has its own best practice guidelines specific to its needs. In addition all four countries operate using the British Association of Perinatal Medicine (BAPM) guidelines as starting standards (Hallsworth et al. 2007). Many changes have taken place in the four UK countries since Hallsworth et al.'s (2007) review was completed. Commonalities and differences will be explored.

KEY POINTS

- Rates of prematurity in the UK, Canada, US, Australia and Sweden have remained steady.
- Provision or organization of services is determined by a network's geography, population, funding and resources.
- Neonatal transport services are determined by size of country, province, state or network.
- Birthweight and gestation impacts cost of neonatal care.
- Neonatal mortality rates have generally decreased with improvements in maternal and neonatal care.

ORGANIZATION OF UK NEONATAL CARE

Key documents which nationally currently or potentially shape the delivery of neonatal care include the BAPM guidelines *Categories of Care* (2001, 2011) and *Service Standards for Hospitals Providing Neonatal Care* (2010) and definitions for levels of neonatal care (Department of Health [DH] 2009; AAP 2012). In addition the Department of Health (2009) *Toolkit for High-Quality Neonatal Services* and *Specialist Neonatal Care Quality Standards* (NICE, 2010) documentation are central to the provision of care. Each document will be discussed briefly in turn.

BAPM plays an enormous role in both the shape and delivery of neonatal care across the four countries of the UK. They represent all players involved in the delivery and education of neonatal care. Membership includes paediatricians involved in neonatal care, neonatal nurses and midwives and professionals allied to neonatal care such as pharmacists, speech and language therapists, occupational therapists, physiotherapists and dieticians, to name a few (BAPM 2010). BAPM is responsible for defining the categories of care which play a vital role in ensuring adequate funding for neonatal services, documentation of activity and development of standards appropriate to level of care, which in turn will enable research comparisons of service delivery, costs and outcome. The categories of care were most recently updated in 2011 to reflect changes that occurred in the delivery of care, changing complexities of neonatal care ensuring the service provision is fit for purpose. However in practice, due to a variety of issues, mainly staffing and financial, some units continue to use the 2001 edition. The categories identify four levels of care and more explicit definitions are now provided for intensive care (IC), high dependency (HD) and special care (SC), and for the first time transitional care (TC) is included. These can be seen in Table 7.3.

BAPM also provides service standards for hospitals providing neonatal care within a managed clinical network (MCN). These were last updated in 2010 in response to changes in neonatal organization and workforce developments and to support a variety of documentations produced by government organizations and professional bodies. For example, the *Toolkit for High-Quality Neonatal Services* (DH 2009) talks broadly about key staff delivering care as being qualified in speciality (QIS). BAPM has expanded this and focused particularly on care delivered by nurses and provided a working definition. A neonatal nurse QIS would hold a first-level qualification with the Nursing and Midwifery Council (NMC) and would, following completion of introductory learning, complete a university accredited post-registration programme which enables them to care for an infant and family regardless of category of care and to be assessed competent by a nurse already QIS. The service standards make recommendations for the pattern of service, care at the point of delivery and if ongoing, staffing of nursing and non-nursing care roles, medical staff and allied health professionals.

Although originally intended for neonatal service in England and written in response to the issues identified by the NAO (2007) when undertaking a review of the 2003 re-organization, the *Toolkit for High-Quality Neonatal Services* (DH 2009) has informed the standards developed in Scotland and Wales. The toolkit does, as its name suggests, provides eight detailed principles to ensure a quality neonatal service which is equitable, transparent and auditable (Table 7.4). A framework for commissioning a neonatal service and range of resources which include best practice examples of care pathway, parental support and recruitment/retention strategies, to name a few, is also provided. In addition for each principle measurable indicators have been provided for use in benchmarking.

The delivery of neonatal care provision across the four countries is currently in a fluid state as each country tries to address its various populations and geographical limitations. Service provision in each country will be discussed individually.

ENGLAND

In 2001, a national review of neonatal care was undertaken on behalf of the Department of Health with recommendations made in 2003, followed in 2004 by the implementation of MCNs (Marlow and Gill 2007; NAO 2007). Demands for neonatal care were on the increase. Care could be provided long distances from home as a result of underfunded regional organization, leading to a number of neonatal units delivering some intensive care, thereby diluting the expertise (NAO 2007). Marlow and Gill (2007, p. F137) define a MCN:

> Networks are linked groups of health professionals and organisations from primary, secondary and tertiary care working together in a coordinated manner across organisational boundaries to ensure equitable provision of high quality clinically effective services, unconstrained by existing professional and Health Board boundaries.

Table 7.3 Categories of care and recommended nurse staffing levels for levels of dependency

	Intensive care (IC)	High dependency (HD)	Special care (SC)	Transitional care (TC)
General principles	This is care for babies who are the most unwell or unstable and have the greatest needs in relation to staff skills and staff-to-patient ratios.	This is care provided for babies who require highly skilled staff but where the nurse-to-patient ratio is less than that for IC.	Special care is provided for babies who require additional care delivered by the neonatal service but do not require either IC or HD care.	TC can be delivered in two service models, within a dedicated TC ward or within a postnatal ward. Care above that needed is normally provided by the mother with support from a midwife/healthcare professional who needs no specialist neonatal training

Definition of care day	• Any day where a baby receives any form of mechanical respiratory support via a tracheal tube
	• *Both* non-invasive ventilation (e.g. nasal CPAP, SIPAP, BIPAP, HHFNC and PN)
	• Day of surgery (including laser therapy for ROP)
	• Day of death
	• Any day receiving any of the following:
	  • Presence of an umbilical arterial line
	  • Presence of an umbilical venous line
	  • Insulin infusion
	  • Presence of a chest drain
	  • Exchange transfusion
	  • Therapeutic hypothermia
	  • Prostaglandin infusion
	  • Presences of a Replogle tube
	  • Presence of epidural catheter
	  • Presence of silo for gastroschisis
	  • Presence of external ventricular drain
	  • Dialysis (any type)
		• Any day where a baby does not fulfil the criteria for intensive care where any of the following apply:
		• Any day where a baby receives any form of non-invasive respiratory support (e.g. nasal CPAP, SIPAP, BIPAP, HHFNC)
		  – Any day receiving any of the following:
		  – Parenteral nutrition
		  – Continuous infusion of drugs (except prostaglandin or insulin)
		  – Presence of a central venous or long line (PICC)
		  – Presence of a tracheostomy
		  – Presence of a urethral or suprapubic catheter
		  – Presence of trans-anastomotic tube following oescphageal atresia repair
		  – Presence of NP airway/nasal stent
		  – Observation of seizures/CFM
		  – Barrier nursing
		  – Ventricular tap
			• Any day where a baby does not fulfil the criteria for IC or HD and requires any of the following:
			• Oxygen by nasal cannula
			• Feeding by nasogastric, jejunal tube or gastrostomy
			• Continuous physiological monitoring (excluding apnoea monitors only)
			• Care of a stoma
			• Presence of IV cannula
			• Baby receiving phototherapy
			• Special observations of physiological variables at least 4 hourly	

Nurse-to-patient ratio	Due to the complex needs of both the baby and family the ratio of neonatal nurses QIS to baby should be 1:1	The ratio of neonatal QIS responsible for the care of babies requiring high dependency should be 1 nurse to 2 babies	The recommended nurse-to-baby ratio is 1:4 Registered nurses and non-registered clinical staff may care for these babies under the direct supervision and responsibility of a neonatal nurse QIS	Mother must be resident with her baby and providing care

Source: British Association of Perinatal Medicine, *Service standards for Hospitals providing neonatal care*, 3rd ed., BAPM, London, 2011.

Note: BIPAP: Bi Level or Biphasic Positive Airway Pressure; CFM: Cerebral Function Monitoring; CPAP: Continuous Positive Airway Pressure; HHFNC: Humidified High Flow Nasal Cannula; PN: Parenteral Nutrition; ROP: Retinopathy of Prematurity; SIPAP: Bi Level Nasal CPAP (Trade name). British Association of Perinatal Medicine, *Categories of Care*, 3rd ed., BAPM, London, 2010;

Table 7.4 Comparison of neonatal standards

England	Scotland	Wales
Toolkit for High Quality Neonatal Service (DH 2009)	National Care in Scotland: A Quality Framework (NEAG 2013)	All Wales Neonatal Standard (Welsh Assembly Government 2013)
Organization of neonatal services	Person centred	Access to neonatal care
Staffing of neonatal services	Safe	Staffing of neonatal services
Surgical services	Efficient	Facilities for neonatal services including equipment
Care of the baby and family experiences	Effective	Care of the baby and family/patient experience
Transfers	Equitable	Transportation
Clinical governance	Timely	Clinical pathways, protocols and guidelines/clinical governance
Professional competence, education and training		Education and training/clinical governance
Data requirements		

Table 7.5 Levels or designation of units

Numbered levels of care have been replaced by designation for simplicity and to improve understanding

Levels of units	Designation
Pre-2011	From 2011
Level 1	Special care (SC)

Units provide special care but do not aim to provide any continuing high dependency or intensive care

Level 2	High dependency (HD)

Units provide high dependency care and some short-term intensive care as agreed within the network

Level 3	Intensive care (IC)

Units provide the whole range of medical neonatal care but not necessarily all specialist services, such as neonatal surgery

Source: British Association of Perinatal Medicine, *Categories of Care*, 2nd ed., BAPM, London, 2001; British Association of Perinatal Medicine, *Categories of Care*, 3rd ed., BAPM, London, 2011.

By 2007 when the re-organization was reviewed by the NAO, England had 180 neonatal units structured into 23 regional networks. Neonatal units within each network were identified as delivering care at Levels 1, 2 or 3. In 2011 these numbered levels of care were replaced by designation for simplicity and to improve understanding (BAPM 2011). This designation is now used by all four UK countries (Table 7.5). The *Toolkit for High-Quality Neonatal Services* (DH 2009) now designates neonatal units within an MCN to improve understanding of each unit's role to that network: special care units (SCUs), local neonatal units (LNUs) and neonatal intensive care units (NICUs) (Table 7.6). NAO's (2007) review findings were encouraging, acknowledging that improvement in neonatal re-organization continues as the NHS continues to re-structure, resulting in amalgamations of some networks into larger networks or organizational delivery networks (ODNs) as part of wider maternity and children strategic networks (Beresford 2013). Gale et al. (2012) also confirmed some service improvement in achieving re-organizational aims. Poor coordination between maternity and neonatal units appears to be an ongoing problem in spite of an increase in babies of 27–28 weeks being delivered in appropriate centres; 50% of these infants were delivered in non-specialist centres. An improvement in early transfers (<24 hours) was also reported; however, a shortage of neonatal cots in specialist centres was noted as a third of infants were transferred to a unit offering comparable or a lower level of care and multiple births were often separated. Ongoing changes to the networks are intended to ensure the delivery of high-quality neonatal care, although funding to deliver and maintain a high-quality service continues to be an ongoing issue. In England there are currently 160 neonatal units within 14 neonatal networks/ODNs. Table 7.7 provides an overview of these networks for Scotland, Wales and Northern Ireland as well.

Table 7.6 Types of neonatal units

Names of neonatal units that make up a managed clinical network (MCN) have been redefined to improve understanding

Special care units (SCUs)
- Provide SC for local population
- May provide some HD
- Provide stabilization for babies who need to be transferred to a NICU
- May receive transfers from other network units for continuing special care

Local neonatal units (LNUs)
- Provide neonatal care for own catchment (usually >27 weeks) with the exception of the sickest babies as agreed by the MCN
- Provide all categories of care, but transfer complex or long-term IC to a NICU
- May receive transfers from other neonatal services as agreed by the MCN

Neonatal intensive care units (NICUs)
- Sited along other specialist obstetric and feto-medicine services
- Provide the whole range of medical neonatal care for local population and those babies and families referred from the MCN
- May provide additional neonatal or specialist services, e.g. surgery
- Medical staff have no responsibility outside the neonatal and maternity services

Source: Department of Health, *Toolkit for high quality neonatal services*, 2009, available at http://www.dh.gov.uk/

SCOTLAND

In 2008, Scotland's Maternity Services Action Group completed its review of neonatal services, and in May 2009 the Scottish government decided the best way to develop neonatal services was to create three regional MCNs for the west of Scotland, southeast and Tayside, and north of Scotland (North of Scotland Planning Group). The aims of the networks are similar to those identified by the English review in 2003, although much simpler and more clearly expressed. The Neonatal Expert Advisory Group (NEAG 2013) published the document 'Neonatal Care in Scotland: A Quality Framework' which was informed by key documents already discussed as well as the Bliss Baby Charter. The standards are easy to read and will ensure the 'delivery of high quality evidence-based, safe, effective and person-centred neonatal care' (NEAG 2013, p. 5). Currently within the three regional MCNs are 17 neonatal units.

WALES

The provision of neonatal services in Wales is very much challenged by its geography and population characteristics. The Welsh government's *All Wales Neonatal Standards for Children and Young People's Specialised Healthcare Services* (Welsh Assembly Government 2013) was initially developed in 2008 in response to the National Assembly for Wales proposal for Welsh neonatal care to be delivered in MCNs. Currently the country serves as one network but clearly has a north and south divide. Provision in South Wales appears further developed but still is in a state of flux with many local and political issues outstanding. The decision for multiple centres rotationally contributing to a part-time transport service is one example of the issues still unresolved.

North Wales is very rural and due to its geography has many transport issues. The population of North Wales is comparatively lower than that in South Wales, with a delivery rate that falls short of the numbers needed to justify the development of neonatal intensive care facilities within North Wales itself (Royal College of Paediatrics and Child Health [RCPCH] 2013). A review of North Wales' neonatal services was undertaken by the RCPCH at the Welsh government's request from a range of options. North Wales now sends their infants requiring neonatal intensive care out of country to Arrowe Park Hospital, a bordering NICU in England. Although this solution serves the needs of the very preterm infant and parts of North Wales well, there are still issues with providing intensive care for late preterm and term infants, travel and, for many families, language (RCPCH 2013). In an effort to address some of these concerns in 2014, the Welsh government announced the development of a sub-regional neonatal unit in mid–North Wales to serve rural

Table 7.7 Neonatal networks in Scotland, England, Wales and Northern Ireland and number and types of cots

Country	No.	Name of network/organizational delivery network (ODN)	Number of units		
			SCU	LNU	NICU
Scotland	1	North of Scotland Neonatal Network	1		2
	2	South East Scotland and Tayside Neonatal Network	2		4
	3	West of Scotland Managed Clinical Network		3	5
England	4	Central Newborn Network	4	2	2
	5	East of England Neonatal ODN			
		• Norwich Cluster	1	2	1
		• Cambridge Cluster	2	4	1
		• Luton Cluster	1	2	1
		• Essex Cluster	0	2	0
	6	North Central and East London ODN	2	6	3
	7	North West London Neonatal ODN	2	3	2
	8	South London Neonatal ODN	3	4	3
	9	North West Neonatal ODN			
		• Cheshire and Merseyside	0	6	2
		• Greater Manchester	0	5	3
		• Lancashire and South Cumbria	1	2	2
	10	Northern Neonatal Network	7	0	4
	11	Southern East Coast Neonatal ODN	6	3	4
	12	South Western Neonatal ODN	2	7	3
	13	South West Midlands Maternity and Newborn Network	6	2	2
	14	Staffordshire, Shropshire and Black Country Newborn and Maternity Network	2	3	2
	15	Thames Valley and Wessex Neonatal Network			
		• Wessex	0	8	2
		• Thames Valley	1	4	1
	16	Trent Perinatal Network	1	3	2
	17	Yorkshire and Humber Neonatal ODN	2	12	5
Wales	18	Wales Neonatal Network	1	7	3 + 1[a]
Northern Ireland	19	Northern Ireland Network	2	4	1

Source: Data collated from British Association of Perinatal Medicine, *Networks information*, 2016, available at www.bapm.org/networks_info

[a] In North Wales, neonatal intensive care is provided by Arrowe Park Hospital (Cheshire and Merseyside) in England's North West Neonatal ODN.

and deprived areas of North Wales. Although all four UK countries experience issues with recruitment and retention, Wales in particular, especially North Wales, has difficulty recruiting both nursing and appropriate medical staff (Bliss 2010a).

NORTHERN IRELAND

As with the other three UK countries, Northern Ireland continues to see an increasing demand on its neonatal services. The Department of Health, Social Services and Public Safety (DHSSPS) has responded to this demand by ordering a review of the country's neonatal services. A position paper on neonatal services was published by the Neonatal Services Working Group Northern Ireland (NSWG) in 2006. At this time neonatal services were delivered by means of an informal network and the report suggested that the neonatal care needs of the Northern Ireland population could be met by neonatal units working closely and effectively together. In December 2011 and January 2012 four out of five neonatal units reported outbreaks of *Pseudomonas aeruginosa* resulting in four neonatal deaths. The DHSSPS commissioned a full enquiry into the deaths and the final report by the Regulation and Quality Improvement Authority was submitted in 2012. A key recommendation from this report was to move from an informal neonatal network to an MCN. In September 2013, the Northern Ireland health minister announced at the COINN conference held in Belfast that an MCN was to become operational (Northern Ireland Executive 2013). This network now consists of seven neonatal units offering a range of service provisions.

KEY POINTS

- BAPM plays a key role in the shape and delivery of neonatal care across all four countries of the UK.
- Documents produced by BAPM, NICE and the Department of Health (e.g. *Toolkit for High-Quality Neonatal Services* 2009) are used and inform service provision across the UK.
- In response to increasing neonatal demands, neonatal care has been re-organized within each UK country.
- Neonatal care across all the UK countries is now delivered using managed clinical networks or organized delivery networks. Services provided by each country are in different stages of development.

DEVELOPING NEONATAL NURSING AND CARE SERVICES FOR THE TWENTY-FIRST CENTURY

Service provision is not only in its infancy but also in a constant state of flux. This creates uncertainty and puts demands on neonatal services and their staff. The largest staffing component of any neonatal unit is its nurses. The recruitment and retention of qualified neonatal nurses is an ongoing global and national issue (Bliss 2010b; Eklund 2014). Bliss (2010b) reported that only 4% of neonatal units within England were able to meet the BAPM (2010) standards for staffing. If we wish to develop a first-class neonatal service, then the issues of recruitment and retention need to be addressed. Factors influencing recruitment and retention are many and complex. Neonatal unit culture and resulting job satisfaction play a role in both the retention and loss of staff. Exposure to neonatal nursing during training for a pre-registration qualification may also play a role in recruitment and career progression, which includes issues of competency, education and training.

WORKING IN A NEONATAL UNIT

Neonatal units, like many areas of nursing, are female-dominated environments with male staff predominantly represented in medical roles. Although the bedside workforce of neonatal units is changing in that special care can be provided by non-registered healthcare staff, provided they are supervised by a neonatal nurse QIS, neonatal nurses/midwives can be found at the bedside in high dependency and intensive care (Royal College of Nursing [RCN] 2015). For many neonatal nurses, remaining at the bedside to provide care to vulnerable infants and supporting the family is what neonatal nursing is about and delivers considerable job satisfaction. Carter et al. (2014) note that working with children and families can be stressful but can be rewarded with the development of supportive and beneficial relationships. Discussions with colleagues in practice reveal high levels of stress are experienced on a daily basis, often due to being short staffed. They regularly deliver excellent care above and beyond the call of duty and only continue to come back to the bedside

Table 7.8 Issues and concerns for neonatal nursing

Unit organization	Aspects of caring for babies
Cutting corners to get work done	Infant pain and suffering
Shortage of skilled nursing staff	Infant death after prolonged treatment
Working with nurses of unknown ability	Nursing a baby with multiple abnormalities
Pressured to accept babies when unit full	Making a mistake in caring for a baby
Nursing responsibility for new medical staff	Caring for a terminally ill baby
Lack of clear-cut policy	

Source: Redshaw, M., et al., *Delivering Neonatal Care: The Neonatal Unit as a Working Environment: A Survey of Neonatal Unit Nursing*, HMSO, London, 1993.

because of that direct care and relationships with infants and families in their care. Mills and Blaesing (2000) identify that this 'patient-care reward' is what has drawn them to and keeps them in nursing. Redshaw et al. (1993) identified two main areas which create stress within the neonatal working environment in England (Table 7.8). Stress can be generated by unit organization-related issues and care-related issues that arise from caring for sick and vulnerable babies and their families. Organization and staffing issues identified included staff shortage, poor skill mix, rotation of new junior doctors, exceeding bed occupancy, working within a hot and noisy environment and finally, efforts to maintain educational or self-development while trying to support a range of pre- and post-registration learners. Care-related issues identified were linked to the emotional costs of caring for very ill infants and supporting parents in crisis. These care issues could include anticipated and unexpected bereavements, ethical dilemmas, making clinical errors and working with a range of staff and parental personalities and coping mechanisms in a closed environment, often over long shifts. It is not surprising then that neonatal nurses experience frequent burnout which can affect both their professional and personal lives and lead to decreased job satisfaction (Oates and Oates 1995). Discussions with colleagues and neonatal nursing students suggest that despite the passage of time and changes in service provision and nurse education, the issues and concerns identified by Redshaw et al. (1993) are relevant today.

Job satisfaction is key to successful recruitment and retention of staff (Roberts et al. 2004). Archibald (2006) cites the American report from the Federation of Nurses and Health Professionals (2001) which identifies factors such as staffing levels, inclusion in decision making, administrative support and respect, career opportunities, salary and benefits and working conditions as contributors to nurse job satisfaction. These American findings were also supported by nursing research from Lebanon (Yaktin et al. 2003). Research specific to job satisfaction in paediatric settings suggests that salary, skills confidence and role expectations particularly in the novice and less experienced nurse were significant contributors to job satisfaction (Ernst et al. 2004). Archibald (2006) undertook a small-scale study of experienced neonatal nurses and found them to be career committed to neonatal nursing. What she found was that neonatal nurses achieve satisfaction through 'compensation, team spirit among nurses, support from physicians and advocacy' (p. 2). Compensation or reward for what one does was given in a variety of ways. They found the greatest reward for the neonatal nurse was good patient outcome and those good days when babies and their families make progress. Neonatal nurses also appreciate simple and well-meaning compliments from families and managers. Financial reward is important, although salaries widely vary globally for the delivery of the same service. Although nursing salaries in the UK have improved, colleagues in Canada and the US continue to earn more for providing the same service. Another reward which added to job satisfaction was the opportunity for and recognition of personal learning. As no two babies are the same and their response to care will vary, the informal opportunities for learning in the neonatal unit are endless. Team spirit is also important. In neonatal nursing, unit design and staffing levels result in individual patient allocation. However, the job satisfaction that is created by supporting each other creates a positive work environment that staff, babies and parents benefit from.

Neonatal units tend to be medically led and so how the medical team works with its nursing team can play a large role in job satisfaction. This support can be manifested in a number of ways, from valuing one's contribution or opinion on clinical care issues or being allowed to make 'nursing' decisions. Mulchay and Betts (2005) found in their busy Australian neonatal unit that one of the issues creating considerable friction and affecting team working was 'who should make decisions and be accountable and responsible for access and care delivery' (p. 520). Oates and Oates (1995) noted that neonatologists' perceptions of their interaction and involvement of nurses were very different to those of the nurses. Brown et al. (2003, p. e482) state, 'A collaborative NICU environment cannot exist without trust and respect among and between all team members' (p. e482). Mulchay and Betts (2005) saw improvements in nursing recruitment and retention once the unit established strategic and organisation guidelines. The guidelines include policies and guidance on individual responsibilities and teamwork-related behaviour. Ward rounds were inclusive of nursing staff and the unit explored educational opportunities, all which had the impact of creating a 'contemporary workplace culture' which 'fostered respect, value and congeniality' (p. 522).

REFLECTION POINT

We need to stop blaming the culture of the establishment for stifling motivation because each and every one of us is the culture and responsible for the culture we accept. It is well known that 'culture eats strategy for breakfast' and yet we all want to be part of the culture that is dynamic, motivated, supportive, receptive to innovative ideas and caring about nurses as well as those we care for.

Karen New
President of COINN, Council of International Neonatal Nurses, 2015

What strategies can be employed to develop a positive culture in your workplace?

Not only is the relationship between all team members important, but how we relate to infants and families in our care is essential to creating a healthy environment for infants, parents and all staff. In 2012 the Department of Health published a vision and strategy entitled *Compassion in Practice*. It outlined the six fundamental values of care (6C's) that ensure that compassion is central to our practice. The 6C's are care, compassion, competence, communication, courage and commitment. Although the 6C's have been developed for use by nursing, midwifery and care staff, the values should be embraced by the entire multidisciplinary team. Staff development, education and training are essential to ensure neonatal staff are in the best position to meet the 6C's.

REFLECTION POINT

Identify examples of how each of the 6C's can be demonstrated in neonatal care.

NEONATAL NURSE EDUCATION

As previously discussed the delivery of neonatal care suitable for the twenty-first century requires a sufficient number of adequately trained neonatal nurses. In the UK the *Toolkit for High Quality Neonatal Services* (DH, 2009), *Specialist Neonatal Care Quality Standards* (NICE, 2010) and more recently the *Service Standards for Hospitals Providing Neonatal Care* (BAPM, 2010) not only identify the nurse-to-baby ratio for each level of care, but also note that nurses providing high dependency or intensive care or overseeing other healthcare workers delivering special care need to be QIS.

The *Toolkit for High Quality Neonatal Services* (DH 2009, p. 90) defines QIS as a 'course of specialised training undertaken after initial or post registration training'. BAPM (2010) has gone a step further in their definition and have made recommendations for the achievement of this qualification in speciality. Today, what determines which course is QIS or what knowledge and skills a QIS nurse should have is the subject of much discussion.

In 1979 four national statutory nursing and midwifery bodies were established in the UK with the remit to approve educational institutions and pre-registration and post-qualifying courses for nurses, midwives and health visitors for their respective country, based on the United Kingdom Central Council for Nursing, Midwifery and Health Visiting (UKCC) standards. In 2002 the UKCC ceased to exist and was replaced by the Nursing and Midwifery Council (NMC). As result of this, the four national boards – the English National Board (ENB) for Nursing, Midwifery and Health Visiting, the National Board for Nursing, Midwifery for Scotland (NBS), the Welsh National Board for Nursing, Midwifery and Health Visiting (WNB) and the National Board for Nursing, Midwifery and Health Visiting for Northern Ireland (NBNI) – were abolished and all educational and quality assurance responsibilities were undertaken by the NMC (Wild 2014). The national boards provided a standardization for post-qualifying education, so that wherever one undertook a specialist neonatal programme each programme had the same learning outcomes (ENB 1990). Despite the national board standardization, considerable variations in the final end product – the trained neonatal nurse – were seen.

Factors which influenced quality of training were dependent on the theoretical content of the course, assessment strategies used and the quality of clinical placement. From the mid-1990s nurse education migrated into higher education institutions (HEIs) and all courses became subject to the rigours of each institution's validation process and quality assurance agency. The NMC continued to oversee the validation of pre-registration nursing and midwifery training and a few post-registration courses like Mentorship and Practice Teacher (NMC Mentor Stages 2 and 3), Return to Practice for Midwives/Nurses, Oversees Nursing and Midwifery, Preparation of Supervisors for Midwives and Prescribing for Nurses (V300). The NMC does not otherwise validate, monitor or advise on the standards of post-training courses. As a result, there is great variation within each UK country and across the countries as to the standard for neonatal nurse education.

Scotland has led the way in developing neonatal nurse competency levels in an effort to achieve standardization (Scottish Neonatal Nurses' Group, 2005). These standards are currently suggested as the core skill set used in BAPM's (2010) definition of QIS (Box 7.2). In 2012, BAPM published the document *Matching Knowledge and Skills for Qualified in Speciality (QIS) Neonatal Nurses: A Core Syllabus for Clinical Competency*. This document has served as a guide to HEI neonatal programmes and hopefully informed module and course content and assessment. Unfortunately, programmes of study of the individual universities dictate assessment tools used and until there is a professional governing body, as recommended by BAPM (2010) in their definition of QIS, neonatal programmes are required to follow the assessment strategies of their validating institution. Health Education England (HEE 2015) has the remit of providing leadership for new education and training and has taken on the role to work closely with the commissioners of health training and education to ensure neonatal nurses QIS are

BOX 7.2: Definition of neonatal nurse QIS

- Registered nurse (adult or children's) or midwife
- Period of preceptorship including defined foundation learning within the speciality
- Completion of a programme of post-registration education, which links the theory and practice elements

Theory and practice elements
- Theory modules relating to the care of the neonate and their family within special care, high dependency and intensive care, delivered and assessed within a higher education institution
- Achievement of core skills set undertaken with supervision of an experienced qualified neonatal nurse, assessed in practice and supported by evidence of learning
- Clinical decision-making skills

Core skills set
- Respiratory and cardiovascular management
- Fluid, electrolyte, nutrition and elimination management
- Neurological and pain management
- Skin and hygiene, and infection prevention management
- Temperature management
- Supporting the family
- Investigations and procedures
- Management of health, safety and security for neonates and their families, to include complex medicine management
- Breastfeeding support

Specific skills acquisition and assessment in practice to include:
- Gestational ages of neonates from extremely preterm to post-term
- Birthweight ranges: ELBW, VLBW, LBW, normal birthweight, IUGR, LGA
- Physical condition, identification of continuing improvement or deterioration
- Surgical infants with differing conditions
- Infants with congenital abnormalities
- Infants preparing to be discharged home

ELBW: Extremely Low Birth Weight, weight <1kg; IUGR: Intrauterine Growth Restriction; LBW: Low Birth Weight, weight <2.5kg; LGA: Large for Gestational Age; VLBW: Very Low Birth Weight, weight <1.5kg.

Source: British Association of Perinatal Medicine. *Service standards for Hospitals Providing Neonatal Care*, 3rd ed., London: BAPM, 2010.

fit for purpose (Turrill 2015). In March 2015, the HEE commenced a national review of neonatal training in order to collect data on current and future educational places for QIS, ascertain current educational provision and create a criteria-based audit tool that can be used to develop and validate QIS programmes (Turrill 2015). The aim of the review is to standardize the education and qualification of specialized neonatal nurses in England. In 2015 the document *Career, Education and Competence Framework for Neonatal Nursing in the UK, RCN Guidance* was published. This document includes but goes beyond what is needed for a nurse to be QIS. It also considers a competence and education framework to support career progression for non-registered healthcare staff and for registered nurses and midwives within the neonatal unit using Benner's (2001) novice-to-expert approach.

A number of neonatal courses around the UK offer the neonatal modules which lead to QIS at levels 5, 6 and 7. The argument for developing master-level modules is to accommodate the academic need of our new degree-level graduates. Children's nurses are not all allocated neonatal placements during their training and adult nurses recruited have no experience or theoretical knowledge of caring for neonates, which leaves them ill-prepared for a course which by level is intended to advance rather than develop competence.

The use of competency to standardize knowledge and skill itself is subject to much debate. Petty (2014) argues the need for neonatal nurses to be competent is a global issue and that the achievement of MDG 4 can only be realized in neonatal care, whether delivered in a low- or high-resource country, if the caregivers are competent. The ideal of all carers being competent is worthy, but the difficulty lies in both the definition and its assessment. Bromley's (2014) review of the literature suggests that assessing competence can be undermined for a variety of reasons including poor assessor preparation, reluctance to fail, potential bias of assessing a work colleague and expertise of the assessor. All of these can contribute to a competency assessment which is neither valid nor reliable. She further suggests that the three most common tools used to assess competency: direct observation, self-assessment and practice portfolios, have not been proven to be valid or reliable. These issues bring into question whether the current attempts to standardize programmes leading to QIS will in fact deliver the desired standardization.

CAREER OPPORTUNITIES IN NEONATAL NURSING

Neonatal career opportunities have been limited to staff nurse, sister, practice educator and neonatal tutor, but as the speciality has developed along with the reduction in junior doctors' hours, new opportunities have developed. Probably the most significant of these role developments has been the introduction of the advanced neonatal nurse practitioner (ANNP) in 1992. Although this role development was initially received with mixed opinion across both the nursing and medical neonatal communities, clearly the delivery of neonatal service across all levels of units would now struggle to function without ANNPs. The recent RCN document (2015) not only identifies levels of practice that are linked to the skills for a health career framework but also identifies competency levels and broad descriptions of level of practice or role and competencies based on the *NHS Knowledge and Skills Framework* (DH 2004) which are fundamental to career development (Box 7.3). The levels of competence include novice/advanced beginner, competent, proficient and expert. The document suggests that a nurse may choose to remain at their chosen level of competence, but in keeping with meeting personal and organizational goals needs to be encouraged and provided both educational opportunities and funding to develop. The roles of a proficient neonatal nurse could include neonatal transport, shift management, developmental care lead, lactation support, enhanced neonatal nurse practitioner, community outreach

---

BOX 7.3: Core competencies for neonatal practice

- Communication and interpersonal relationships
- Personal, professional and people development
- Health, safety and security
- Service development
- Quality
- Equality, diversity and rights
- Responsibility for patient care

Source: Royal College of Nursing, *Career, Education and Competence Framework for Neonatal Nursing in the UK, RCN Guidance for Nursing Staff*, RCN, London, 2015.
Note: Family-centred and developmental care are threads that run through each core competence.

nurse and practice development/clinical educator. Expert neonatal nurse roles include neonatal unit manager, neonatal practice development, family support/safeguarding lead, researcher, advanced neonatal nurse practitioner and finally nurse consultant (RCN 2015). Local career strategies to recruit and retain neonatal nurses within a specified geographical area are also being developed to enable staff mobility and recognition of acquired competencies while remaining within neonatal nursing.

CASE STUDY

The Pan London Educators Group has developed a Band 5 competency document that will serve as a passport between the neonatal units in London, allowing the neonatal nurses mobility and the opportunity to maintain their career development without interruption.

REFLECTION POINT

What local strategies are employed within your network to recruit and retain both new nurses and neonatal nurses QIS?

CHANGING PERCEPTIONS OF THE NEONATE

The public's changing perceptions of the neonate, particularly of the premature infant, provide those who provide neonatal care many challenges and responsibilities. Content analysis of 80 years of news stories and photographs demonstrates that the media portrayal to the public has served the wider community well, as the articles published have been overall timely, consistent and representative of the key developments in neonatology (Podsiadly 2008). Over the same time period, interpretative analysis of the same articles/photographs demonstrates the evolution of a human specimen to a human baby (Podsiadly 2008). This humanizing relates to the welcome of the parents into the neonatal unit, which took place in the 1970s in response to work by Klaus and Kennel (1976) on the role of early bonding. The media have also provided stories and photographs that define the premature baby as an understandable form and, by identifying potential, define human value (Podsiadly 2008). Articles and photographs identify two key themes: the premature baby as a person and the premature baby's potential as a member of society (Podsiadly 2008). Pre-1980, the premature baby was portrayed as part of an event but not the central focus of a story. Articles tended to be very factual and used few descriptive or emotive adjectives to describe the baby. From the early 1980s articles provided not just a greater insight into the event or issue, but also a sense of who and what the baby was and perhaps even what the baby was experiencing. The premature baby was personalized in three ways: identifying the baby by physicality, personality and behaviour (Podsiadly 2008). This reinforces the baby as a central member of a family, which in turn has played a role in the development of family-centred care (FCC).

The second theme, the premature baby's potential as a member of society, considers the unrealized potential on the neonatal unit and the potential in the ex-premature baby. These themes have a strong correlation between the degree of prematurity and outcome. Mortality and morbidity increase as gestational age decreases (Wilson-Costello et al. 2007). As the boundary of viability continues to be challenged, society must decide when those limits have been reached and whether the material and emotional cost of care for the pre-viable infants should continue.

The next sections will explore the role of family in the delivery of neonatal care and the role of society in deciding the ethical dilemmas that arise from the provision of neonatal care.

ROLE OF THE FAMILY

"You shouldn't be here little one. You should be warm and cosy inside me, letting me do all this hard work for you – breathing and feeding. You should be nestling down in your pool, growing and preparing yourself for this world – but not now. Why so soon? You've given us a glimpse of something we shouldn't see – Life newer than new. I can't bear it when you cry out silently. You look in such anguish. All those lights and tubes and bleeps and no soft Mum Mum to comfort you. You shouldn't be there and I don't know what to do." (Collard 1986)

The birth of a preterm or critically ill infant or an infant with an abnormality is often the beginning of a long and stressful journey for the family. Kaplan and Mason (1960), Caplan et al. (1965) and Wigert et al. (2006) suggest that this experience precipitates a crisis for the parents and family. According to Wigert et al. (2006), in order for the parents to manage this crisis they need to cope with their loss, overcome the many barriers to bonding and obtain adequate information about their infant's current and future needs. A 40-year review of literature indicates a plethora of research which identifies unchanging feelings and needs of parents, but an increased understanding and fine-tuning of strategies and interventions to help parents effectively deal with their feelings and needs from admission to discharge, enabling a seamless transition from hospital into the community (Podsiadly 2008; Baker and McGrath 2011). Historically, research has been labelled as parental, but in reality it very much addresses the feelings and needs of mothers. There is now acknowledgement that father's feelings and needs can be similar but also different (O'Shea and Timmins 2002; Lindberg et al. 2007; Fegran et al. 2008; Hollywood and Hollywood 2010). Research exploring fathers' experiences and needs during the neonatal journey is an increasing area of interest. Admission of an infant to a neonatal unit creates a wide range of feelings in parents. In addition to the feelings of elation and joy on becoming parents, Franck et al. (2005) and Wigert et al. (2006) report parents can also feel a sense of loss or grief, guilt, sadness, anger, hostility, depression, helplessness and fear, which can all lead to an overwhelming sense of failure and low self-esteem. Many describe the parental experiences as a roller coaster ride, as feelings often relate to the ups and downs in their infant's progress (Hummel 2003; Gavey 2007). The neonatal experience results in the loss of the expected or normal role transition, leaving parents frustrated and disappointed as events unfold outside of their control (Franck et al. 2005; Shin and White-Traut 2007). The neonatal nurse plays a key part helping mothers make the transition to a mothering role (Fenwick et al. 2000; Aagaard and Hall 2008).

Parents on a neonatal unit have many needs. As suggested by Miles and Holditch-Davis (1997) parents must come to terms with their loss of not having an 'ideal baby' and must bond or attach to this infant whose future may be precarious and who may be too ill to interact in a positive way. De Rouck and Leys (2009) identify that the most important need of parents is to receive adequate information and communication regarding the well-being and changing status of their infant. Bialoskurski et al. (2002, p. 62) suggest that 'it may not always be feasible to prepare the parents for a premature birth, but effective communication may reduce the impact of the crisis'. Effective communication can enable parents a modicum of control over their situation and will enable the parents to adapt and cope with their situational crisis (De Rouck and Leys 2009). This communication can be delivered by many and in many different ways. Jones et al. (2007) identify that the neonatal nurse can be an effective communicator and can play a pivotal role in helping parents with role transition and cope with stressors of the neonatal experience. De Rouck and Leys (2009) identify a range of information sources which help parents make sense of their experience. These sources could be internal or externally provided. The key sources of information come from the doctors and nurses involved in their infant's care, and printed literature which is often produced directly by the neonatal unit or provided by national charities such as Bliss (for babies born too soon, too small or too sick). Recently a series of DVDs has been developed such as 'Bump to Breastfeeding' or 'Small Wonders'. These are designed for parents to view at their leisure and re-enforce the information and parent-craft received mainly from neonatal nurses. The media portrayal through newspapers and television programmes also provide parents with an insight into other parents' experiences, as do in-house and external parental groups. A growing source of information, albeit not always reliable, is the Internet.

The admission of an infant to the neonatal unit is in reality the admission of the whole family (Baker and McGrath 2011). This acknowledgement is recognized as the cornerstone to the delivery of FCC. FCC is defined by Griffin (2006, p. 98) as 'an approach to the planning, delivery, and evaluation of healthcare that is based upon a partnership between healthcare professionals and families of patients'. Unlike paediatrics, where upon admission the parents are deemed the 'authority', in the neonatal unit the parents are challenged by the environment, technology and complex needs of their infant; they have not yet formed that 'authoritative' attachment/relationship with their infant. FCC is an attempt to ensure that parents are fully participative in care and care decisions made for their infant. Strategies to provide FCC include effective communication as key (Cockcroft 2012), creating a neonatal environment that not only meets the technological needs of the infant but also is conducive to open visiting and caregiving opportunities, and provides support (e.g. breastfeeding, transport, transition, parent to parent, emotional and bereavement), parent education and full participation in care-making decisions (Griffin 2006; Gooding et al. 2011; Cockcroft 2012).

FCC can meet the needs of the family with associated benefits to the infant. However, it does not always put the needs of the infant first. In order to ensure that care is baby centred, there is a movement to ensure that infants are provided with individual developmental supportive care. With this approach, care intends to optimize infant's potential by modulating the infant's environment and responding to behaviour cues from the infant to the delivery of care (VandenBerg 2007). Central to developmental care is the family. There is now a move within neonatal units to promote FCC as an essential and key component to developmental care. For example, Bliss, the main UK organization which supports parents in the neonatal unit, has identified seven chartered principles with standards and criteria to ensure that the essential rights of every sick and preterm infant are met by neonatal care providers (Bliss 2011) (Box 7.4). The first principle and accompanying standards reflect family-centred developmental care. Similarly, the Parents of Premature Babies Project (POPPY Steering Group 2009) undertook a systematic review of parental communication, support and information and identified the inter-relationship between FCC and developmental care strategies central to its summary.

| | Goals of developmental care | | Developmental care |
Definition	Baby	Parents	interventions
'Developmental care is a broad category of interventions designed to minimise the stress of the neonatal environment and to support the behavioural organization of each individual infant. Interventions are designed to enhance physiological stability, protect sleep rhythms and promote growth and maturation'	• ↓ stress • Conserves energy • Enhances recovery • Promotes growth • Promotes well-being • Supports developing behaviours at each stage of brain development	• Encourages and supports parents to be the primary caregiver • Develops and strengthens family emotional and social well-being	• Cue-based care • Optimal handling and positioning • ↓ noise and light • ↓ stressful/painful procedures • Appropriate pain relief interventions • Cluster care • Rest periods/quiet hour • Feeding support • Non-nutritive sucking • Kangaroo care

Source: South West Neonatal Network, *Developmental care*, 2015, available at http://www.swneonatalnetwork.co.uk/parents-families/developmental-care/

PRINCIPLES FOR PRACTICE

- The admission of an infant to a neonatal unit can precipitate a crisis for parents and family.
- Parents have many needs. Neonatal nurses play a key role in helping parents meet these needs by using a developmental family-centred care approach.
- The neonatal nurse must be an effective communicator.

NEONATAL ETHICS

A chapter on neonatal care would not be complete without briefly discussing the ethical issues that arise from the advances made in neonatal care and service provision.

Technological advances in incubator care, ventilation and therapeutic cooling, combined with pharmacological developments such as antenatal steroids, surfactant, total parental nutrition and nitric oxide have resulted in increased survival rates in neonatal care. Preterm infants, at or just below the age of viability, are now more able to survive, although the rate of neurodisability among this group remains a concern (Wilson-Costello et al. 2007). Neurodevelopmental disability can range from mild to severe. Preterm infants less than 29 weeks' gestation have increased risk of cerebral palsy (Surman et al. 2009), potential visual impairment from retinopathy of prematurity and a range of learning and behaviour difficulties, all of which affect their educational and adult potential (Hack et al. 1994, 2002). These outcomes raise a number of ethical questions and dilemmas for all those involved in the care of these vulnerable infants with uncertain futures. Who to treat, who decides to treat, what is the role of the parents in such decisions, when to withhold or provide alternative care and what is an acceptable outcome are just a few considerations.

Rijken et al. (2007) support the use of guidelines, as provided by the Dutch Paediatric Association, to aid the neonatal healthcare team and parents in deciding whether to provide palliative care or active

BOX 7.4: Bliss baby charter standards

Charter principle 1

Every baby should be treated as an individual and with dignity, respecting their social, developmental and emotional needs as well as their medical and surgical needs. This includes respecting the baby and family's right to privacy, time to make attachments and referring to the baby by name.

Standards: Dignity and privacy, comfort, touch, positioning, light, sound

Charter principle 2

Neonatal care decisions are based on the baby's best interest, with parents actively involved in their baby's care. Decisions on the baby's best interest are based on evidence and best practices, and are informed by parents who are encouraged and supported in the decision-making process and actively participate in providing comfort and emotional support to their baby.

Standards: Decision making, care plans, psychosocial support, sensitive news, palliative/end of life care

Charter principle 3

Babies receive the nationally recommended level of specialist care in the specialist unit nearest to the baby's family home.

Standards: Trained specialist staff, multidisciplinary team, near to home, consistency across the neonatal network

Charter principle 4

Units encourage parents to be involved in plans and processes for continuous service improvement, and outcomes of care are benchmarked against local and national standards.

Standards: Monitoring and benchmarking, service improvement

Charter principle 5

Parents are informed, guided and supported, so that they understand their baby's care processes and feel confident caring for them. Information provided to parents should cover clinical conditions, tests and treatment, as well as practical issues such as breastfeeding, financial support and transferring between units and local facilities.

Standards: Introduction to the unit, facilities, support networks, consistent information, use of data, daily cares

Charter principle 6

Breast milk expression and breastfeeding are actively promoted, and mothers receive practical support to achieve successful lactation. Relevant health professionals are equipped with appropriate knowledge and skills to facilitate and support lactation following a preterm birth.

Standards: Promote and support breast milk expression, breastfeeding, alternatives to maternal breast milk

Charter principle 7

Discharge planning is facilitated and coordinated from initial admission to discharge date, to ensure both the baby and their family receive the appropriate care and access to resources.

Standards: Coordinated discharge planning, rooming in, meeting the baby's needs at home

Source: Bliss, *The Bliss Baby Charter Standards*, 2nd ed., Bliss, London, 2011.

resuscitation at birth and subsequently provide 'parent centred comfort-care' if ongoing care is considered futile (p. 61). They go on to note that well-resourced countries such as Canada and the majority of Europe follow guidelines which recommend resuscitation at 25 to 26 weeks' gestation and provide active intervention at delivery for infants 23 to 24 weeks' gestation if they are born in good condition. Guidelines from the US do not recommend resuscitation if an infant is less than 23 weeks' gestation or weighs less than 400 g (Rijken et al. 2007).

Ethical decision making is guided by the four ethical principles of beneficence, nonmaleficence, respect for autonomy and justice (Beauchamp 2007). In addition to these, neonatal decisions are informed by mortality and outcome data (Miljeteig et al. 2009). In resource-scarce countries, such as India, additional factors other than what is in the infant's best interest play a role in determining how the infant is treated. These factors include avoiding financial stress, family motivation and interest, family wealth, obstetric history and hospital resources (Miljeteig et al. 2009). Clearly what is perceived as an acceptable outcome can be influenced by wide-ranging factors and is very much determined by the medical, social and cultural resources available.

The impact of new technology continually challenges existing boundaries, outcomes and therefore decision making. Expectations of neonatal units to achieve the unachievable or unexpected are high. As our expectations and successes increase and are portrayed for all to see through various media formats, so do those of our parents and ultimately society. Neonates do not have a voice in determining their care (Smith 2005) and are dependent upon the healthcare team and parents to make decisions in their best interest. Good communication between the healthcare team and parents is therefore essential. Howell and Graham (2011) surveyed parents from across England neonatal networks using the Bliss Baby Charter (2011), *Specialist Neonatal Care Quality Standards* (NICE 2010) and *Toolkit for High-Quality Neonatal Services* (DH 2009) to measure parent experiences. When asked about their involvement in decision making 55% said 'always', while the remaining parents answered 'sometimes' or 'not at all'. It is unclear from these finding as to whether the decisions made pertained to day-to-day care or ethical issues concerned with protecting or prolonging life. Decision making requires the individual to have knowledge, reasoning and reflective skills. The stress parents must be experiencing when ethical decisions are required may limit their ability to substantially contribute to any discussions. Regardless, parents must be encouraged to express any views they may have and these in turn need to be acknowledged (Smith 2005). To be fully participative in the decision-making process, parents are dependent upon the neonatal team to provide them meaningful information, time to reflect and support to be empowered to participate.

KEY POINTS

- What is ethical may not be legal.
- What is legal may not be ethical.
- What is possible may not be desirable.
- What is desirable may not be possible.

As the boundary of viability continues to be challenged, not only those who provide neonatal care, but also society must decide when those limits have been reached and whether the material and emotional cost of care for extremely premature infants should continue.

CONCLUSION

This chapter provided an overview of the developments in neonatal care including the current organization and provision of care from a global and national perspective. Neonatal care in the four UK countries is structured by a range of organizational and governmental documents to provide practitioners with clear standards to deliver high-quality care. However, care provision continues to be in a constant state of change as healthcare resources are rationalized. Re-organization of neonatal care has resulted in some improvements; however, as demand for cots outweighs availability and a national shortage of neonatal nurses QIS continues, the neonatal unit is often a stressful work environment. Critically ill infants require complex care. It is essential that neonatal nurses are adequately trained in order to deliver this care. This chapter identified some of the educational issues that resulted when neonatal nurse education transferred into higher education with the demise of the four national boards. Neonatal nurse education leading to QIS has come under scrutiny as there is currently no uniformity, resulting in nurses deemed QIS with varying levels of knowledge and skills. Recruitment and retention of neonatal nurses is essential to maintain high-quality service provision. Addressing issues relating to a neonatal career pathway, personal development, education and competence is key to job satisfaction and staff retention.

Also within this chapter the family experience of neonatal care has been explored. Parents are in crisis and mothers and fathers have similar yet different needs. To meet both the needs of the infant and those of the family, neonatal units are moving to deliver family-centred developmental care. Parents need to be fully participative in their infant's care and care decisions. Neonatal nurses play a key role in both supporting and educating parents in the care of their infant. Parent organizations play a valuable role in support but also provide the parental perspective in the development of care provision and standards. Finally this chapter has considered neonatal outcomes and the resulting ethical dilemmas that have arisen from challenging the boundaries of viability.

SUMMARY OF PRINCIPLES FOR PRACTICE

- All newborns wherever born are entitled to high-quality neonatal care. Neonatal nurses must understand service organization and delivery from both a national and international perspective and ensure that they play a role in shaping neonatal care and neonatal unit culture.
- Educational programmes that lead to a neonatal nurse QIS must be standardized to ensure high-quality neonatal care is provided in all units regardless of their designation or type.
- All neonatal nurses, regardless of role, must engage in 'lifelong learning' in order to meet service standards and deliver evidence-based high-quality neonatal care to infants and families in their care.
- Neonatal nursing provides adult and children and young people's nurses challenging career opportunities to care for those babies born too sick, too small and too soon.
- Neonatal care needs to be collaborative. Neonatal nurses are key to the facilitation of family-centred developmental care.
- The impact of new technology continually challenges existing boundaries, outcomes and therefore decision making. Neonatal nurses need to be able to reflect, demonstrate reasoning skills and have sound knowledge of issues in order to be active participants in ethical decision making.

REFERENCES

Aagaard H, Hall E (2008) Mothers' experiences of having a preterm infant in the neonatal care unit: a meta-synthesis. *Journal of Pediatric Nursing* **23**(3): 26–36.

American Academy of Pediatrics (2012) Levels of neonatal care. *Pediatrics* **130**(3): 587–97.

Anonymous (2015) Letter from New Zealand, Christchurch neonatal conference 2014. *Journal of Neonatal Nursing* **21**(1): 7–10.

Archibald C (2006) Job satisfaction among neonatal nurses. *Pediatric Nursing* **32**(2): 176–9.

Australian Institute of Health and Welfare (2014) *Australia's health 2014*. Available at http://www.aihw.gov.au/australias-health/2014/health-system/.

Baker B, McGrath J (2011) Parent education: the cornerstone of excellent neonatal nursing care. *Newborn & Infant Nursing Reviews* **11**(1): 6–7.

Beauchamp T (2007) The 'four principles' approach to healthcare ethics. In Ashcroft RE, Dawson A, Draper H, McMillan J (eds.) *Principles of healthcare ethics*, 2nd ed., pp. 3–10. Chichester: Wiley.

Benner P (2001) *Novice to expert: excellence and power in clinical nursing practice*, commemorative ed. Upper Saddle, NJ: Prentice Hall Health.

Beresford D (2013) More reorganisation – senates, SCNs and ODNs. *Journal of Neonatal Nursing* **20**(1): 1–2.

Beresford D (2015) World prematurity day – a voice for premature infants. *Journal of Neonatal Nursing* **21**(1): 1.

Bialoskurski MM, Cox CL, Wiggins RD (2002) The relationship between maternal needs and priorities in a neonatal intensive care environment. *Journal of Advanced Nursing* **37**(1): 62–9.

Blencowe H, Cousens S, Oestergaard M, Chou S, Moller A, Narwal R, Adler A, et al. (2012) National, regional, and worldwide estimates of preterm birth rates in the year 2010 with time trends since 1990 for selected countries: a systematic analysis and implications. *Lancet* **379**: 2162–72.

Bliss (2010a) *Bliss baby report and manifesto: Wales 2010*. London: Bliss.

Bliss (2010b) *The chance of a lifetime? Bliss baby report 2010*. London: Bliss.

Bliss (2011) *The Bliss baby charter standards*, 2nd ed. London: Bliss.

Brennan C (1988) History of neonatology. Unpublished attachment prepared for presentation to the South West Thames Regional Health Authority Working Party on Neonatal Nursing and Education, London.

British Association of Perinatal Medicine (2001) *Categories of care*, 2nd ed. London: BAPM.

British Association of Perinatal Medicine (2010) *Service standards for hospitals providing neonatal care*, 3rd ed. London: BAPM.

British Association of Perinatal Medicine (2011) *Categories of care*, 3rd ed. London: BAPM.

British Association of Perinatal Medicine (2012) *Matching knowledge and skills for qualified in speciality (QIS) neonatal nurses: a core syllabus for clinical competency*. London: BAPM.

British Association of Perinatal Medicine (2016) Networks information. Available at www.bapm.org/networks_info.

Bromley P (2014) Clinical competence of neonatal intensive care nursing students: how do we evaluate the application of knowledge in students of postgraduate certificate in neonatal intensive care nursing? *Journal of Neonatal Nursing* **20**(4): 140–6.

Brown MS, Ohlinger J, Rusk C, Delmore P, Ittmann P (2003) Implementing potentially better practices for multidisciplinary team building: creating a neonatal intensive care unit culture of collaboration. *Pediatrics* **111**(4): e482–8.

Canadian Institute for Health Information (2006) *Giving birth in Canada: the costs.* Ottawa: CIHI. Available at www.cihi.ca.

Caplan G, Mason EA, Kaplan DM (1965) Four studies of crisis in parents of premature. *Community Mental Health Journal* **1**: 149–61.

Carter B, Bray L, Dickinson A, Edwards, Ford K (2014) *Child-centred nursing.* London: Sage.

Christie DA, Tansey EM (eds.) (2001) *Origins of neonatal intensive care. Wellcome witnesses to twentieth century medicine*, vol. 9. London: Wellcome Trust Centre for the History of Medicine at UCL.

Cockcroft S (2012) How can family centred care be improved to meet the needs of parents with a premature baby in neonatal intensive care? *Journal of Neonatal Nursing* **18**: 105–10.

Collard A (1986) Born early. One mother's account of giving birth 12 weeks too soon. London: Unpublished diary.

Department of Health (2004) *The NHS knowledge and skills framework (NHS KSF) and the development review process.* London: DH. Available at http://webarchive.nationalarchives.gov.uk/+/www.dh.gov.uk/en/publicationsandstatistics/publications/publicationspolicyandguidance/dh_4090843.

Department of Health (2009) *Toolkit for high quality neonatal services.* Available at www.dh.gov.uk/.

Department of Health (2012) *Compassion in practice: nursing, midwifery and care staff – our vision and strategy.* London: DH.

De Rouck S, Leys M (2009) Information needs of parents of children admitted to a neonatal intensive care unit: a review of the literature (1990–2008). *Patient Education and Counseling* **76**: 159–73.

Donn S, Boon W (2009) Mechanical ventilation of the neonate: should we target volume or pressure? *Respiratory Care* **54**(9): 1236–43.

Eklund W (2014) The challenge to identify the global neonatal workforce needed to meet the millennium developmental goals. *Journal of Neonatal Nursing* **20**(4): 165–70.

English National Board (1990) *Special and intensive nursing care of the newborn: course 405.* London: English National Board for Nursing, Midwifery and Health Visiting.

Ernst M, Messmer PR, Franco M, Gonzalez JL (2004) Nurses' job satisfaction, stress and recognition in a pediatric setting. *Pediatric Nursing* **30**(3): 219–27.

Federation of Nurses and Health Professionals (2001) *The nurse shortage: perspective from current direct care nurse and former direct care nurses.* Available at www.aft.org/pubs-reports/healthcare/Hart_Report.pdf.

Fegran L, Helseth S, Fagermoen MS (2008) A comparison of mothers' and fathers' experiences of the attachment process in a neonatal intensive care unit. *Journal of Clinical Nursing* **17**: 810–6.

Fenwick J, Barclay L, Schmied V (2000) Interaction in neonatal nurseries: women's perceptions of nurses and nursing. *Journal of Neonatal Nursing* **6**(6): 197–203.

Franck L, Cox S, Allen A, Winter I (2005) Measuring neonatal intensive care unit-related parental stress. *Journal of Advanced Nursing* **49**(6): 608–15.

Gale C, Santhakumaran S, Nagarajan S, Statnikov Y, Modi N (2012) Impact of managed clinical networks on NHS specialist neonatal services in England: population based study. *British Medical Journal* **344**: e2015.

Gallagher J, Botsko C, Schwalberg R (2004) *Influencing interventions to promote positive pregnancy outcomes and reduce the incidence of low birth weight and preterm infants, policies, programs and avenues for advocacy.* March of Dimes. Available at http://www.marchofdimes.org/materials/partner-positive-pregnancy-outcomes-reduce-low-birth-weight-preterm-infants.pdf.

Gavey J (2007) Parental perceptions of neonatal care. *Journal of Neonatal Nursing* **13**: 199–206.

Glasper A, Coad J, Richardson J (2015) *Children and young people's nursing at a glance.* Chichester: Wiley.

Gooding J, Cooper L, Blaine A, Franck L, Howse J, Berns S (2011) Family support and family-centred care in the neonatal intensive care unit: origins, advances, impact. *Seminars in Perinatology* **35**: 20–8.

Griffin T (2006) Family-centered care in the NICU. *Journal of Perinatal and Neonatal Nursing* **20**(1): 98–102.

Hack M, Flannery D, Schluchter M, Cartar M, Borawski E, Klein N (2002) Outcomes in young adulthood for very-low-birth-weight infants. *New England Journal of Medicine* **346**(3): 149–57.

Hack M, Taylor HG, Klein N, Eiben R, Schatschneider C, Mecuri-Minich N (1994) School-age outcomes in children with birth weights under 750 g. *New England Journal of Medicine* **331**(12): 753–9.

Hallsworth M, Farrands A, Oortwijn W, Hatziandreu E (2007) *The provision of neonatal services: data for international comparisons*. Cambridge: RAND Corporation.

Health Canada (2014) *About Health Canada*. Available at http://www.hc-sc.gc.ca/ahc-asc/index-eng.php.

Health Education England (2015) *About Health Education England*. Available at https://hee.nhs.uk/about/.

Hollywood M, Hollywood E (2011) The lived experiences of fathers of a premature baby on a neonatal intensive care unit. *Journal of Neonatal Nursing* **17**: 32–40.

Howell E, Graham C (2011) *Parents' experiences of neonatal care. A report on the findings from a national survey*. London: Picker Institute Europe.

Hummel P (2003) Parenting the high-risk infant. *Newborn and Infant Nursing Reviews* **3**(3): 88–92.

Jones L, Woodhouse D, Rowe J (2007) Effective nurse parent communication: a study of parent's perceptions in the NICU environment. *Patient Education and Counseling* **69**: 206–12.

Kaplan DM, Mason EA (1960) Maternal reactions to premature birth viewed as an acute emotional disorder. *American Journal of Orthopsychiatry* **30**: 539–47.

Kenner C, Boykova M, Eklund W (2011) Impact on neonatal nursing globally, exemplars of how US neonatal/perinatal nurses can get involved. *Journal of Perinatal and Neonatal Nursing* **25**(2): 119–22.

Klaus M, Kennel J (1976) *Maternal infant bonding*. St. Louis: Mosby.

Lindberg B, Axelsson K, Öhrling K (2007) The birth of premature infants: experiences from the fathers' perspective. *Journal of Neonatal Nursing* **13**: 142–9.

Liu L, Oza S, Hogan D, Perin J, Rudan I, Lawn JE, Cousens S, Mathers C, Black RE (2015)

Global, regional, and national causes of child mortality in 2000–13, with projections to inform post-2015 priorities: an updated systematic analysis. *Lancet* **385**: 430–40.

March of Dimes (2015) Born too soon – estimated rates of preterm birth in 2010. Available at http://www.marchofdimes.org/mission/global-preterm.aspx.

Marlow N, Gill AB (2007) Establishing neonatal networks: the reality. *Archives of Disease in Childhood, Fetal Neonatal Edition* **92**: F137–42.

Miles MS, Holditch-Davis D (1997) Parenting the prematurely born child: pathways of influence. *Seminars in Perinatology* **21**(3): 254–66.

Miljeteig I, Ali Sayeed S, Jesani A, Arne Johansson K, Frithjof Norheim O (2009) Impact of ethics and economics on end-of-life decisions in an Indian neonatal unit. *Pediatrics* **124**: e322–8.

Mills A, Blaesing S (2000) A lesson from the last nursing shortage. *Journal of Nursing Administration* **30**(6): 309–15.

Mulchay C, Betts L (2005) Transforming culture: an exploration of unit culture and nursing retention within a neonatal unit. *Journal of Nursing Management* **13**: 519–23.

Murray SF (1997) Neonatal care in developing countries. *Modern Midwife* **7**(10): 26–30.

National Audit Office (2007) *Caring for vulnerable babies: the reorganisation of neonatal services in England*. Available at www.nao.org.uk.

National Institute for Health and Clinical Excellence (2010) *Specialist neonatal care quality standards*. London: NICE.

Neonatal Expert Advisory Group (2013) *Neonatal care in Scotland: a quality framework*. Scottish government. Available at http://www.gov.scot/Resource/0041/00415230.pdf.

Neonatal Services Working Group Northern Ireland (2006) *Position paper on specialist neonatal services in Northern Ireland*. Northern Ireland: NSWG.

NHS England (2013) *Neonatal critical care retrieval (transport)*. Available at http://www.england.nhs.uk/commissioning/wp-content/uploads/sites/12/2015/01/e08-serv-spec-neonatal-critical-transp.pdf.

Northern Ireland Executive (2013) *Neonatal care is crucial to improving the lives of babies born too soon, too small or too sick – Poots*. Available at http://www.northernireland.gov.uk/news-dhssps-060913-neonatal-care-is.

Northern Ireland Executive (2014) *Expansion of specialist transport service will benefit sick children – Poots*. Available at http://www.northernireland.gov.uk/news-dhssps-200314-expansion-of-specialist.

Oates RK, Oates P (1995) Stress and mental health in neonatal intensive care units. *Archives of Disease in Childhood* **72**: F107–10.

O'Shea J, Timmins F (2002) An overview of parents' experiences of neonatal intensive care: do we care for both parents? *Journal of Neonatal Nursing* **8**(6): 178–83.

Petty J (2014) A global view of competency in neonatal care. *Journal of Neonatal Nursing* **20**(1): 3–10.

Podsiadly E (2008) Portrayal of the premature baby in the *Times* newspaper from 1930–2008. MSc dissertation, University of Surrey, Guildford.

POPPY Steering Group (2009) *Family-centred care in neonatal units. A summary of research results and recommendations from the POPPY project.* London: NCT.

Redshaw M, Harris A, Ingram JC (1993) *Delivering neonatal care: the neonatal unit as a working environment: a survey of neonatal unit nursing.* London: HMSO.

Rijken M, Veen S, Walther FJ (2007) Ethics of maintaining extremely preterm infants. *Paediatrics and Child Health* **12**(2): 58–63.

Roberts BJ, Jones C, Lynn M (2004) Job satisfaction of new baccalaureate nurses. *Journal of Nursing Administration* **34**(9): 428–35.

Rogowski J (1999) Measuring the cost of neonatal and perinatal care. *Pediatrics* **103**(1): 329–35.

Royal College of Nursing (2015) *Career, education and competence framework for neonatal nursing in the UK, RCN guidance for nursing staff.* London: RCN.

Royal College of Paediatrics and Child Health (2013) *Invited review of the options for provision of neonatal care in north Wales.* London: RCPCH.

Scottish Neonatal Nurses' Group (2005) *The competency framework and core clinical skills for neonatal nurses.* Edinburgh: SNNG.

Swedish Institute (2013–2015) *Healthcare in Sweden.* Available at https://sweden.se/society/health-care-in-sweden/.

Shin H, White-Traut R (2007) The conceptual structure of transition to motherhood in the neonatal intensive care unit. *Journal of Advanced Nursing* **58**(1): 90–8.

Smith L (2005) The ethics of neonatal care for the extremely preterm infant. *Journal of Neonatal Nursing* **11**: 33–7.

South West Neonatal Network (2015) *Developmental care.* Available at http://www.swneonatalnetwork.co.uk/parents-families/developmental-care/.

Surman G, Newdick H, King A, Gallagher M, Kurinczuk JJ (2009) *4 Child: four counties database of cerebral palsy, vision loss and hearing loss in children. Annual report 2009, including data for births 1984 to 2003.* Oxford: National Perinatal Epidemiology Unit.

Regulation and Quality Improvement Authority (2012) *Independent review of incidents of Pseudomonas aeruginosa infections in neonatal units in Northern Ireland, final report.* Available at http://www.rqia.org.uk/cms_resources/Pseudomonas%20Review%20Phase%20II%20Final%20Report.pdf.

Tommy's (2015) *Preterm birth.* Available at http://www.tommys.org/.

Turrill S (2015) Shape of caring review: neonatal nurse QIS education and competency project – audit tool, consultation background paper and rationale. Email communication, 2 April.

United Nations (2006) *Demographic year book: table 3, population by sex, rate of increase, surface area and density.* Available at http://unstats.un.org/unsd/demographic/products/dyb/dyb2006/Table03.pdf.

United Nations (2015a) *We can end poverty, Millennium Development Goals and beyond 2015.* Available at http://www.un.org/millenniumgoals/mdgmomentum.shtml.

United Nations (2015b) *We can end poverty, Millennium Development Goals and beyond 2015.* Fact sheet. Goal 4: reduced child mortality. Available at http://www.un.org/millenniumgoals/pdf/Goal_4_fs.pdf.

USA.gov (2015) *Health insurance.* Available at http://www.usa.gov/Citizen/Topics/Health/HealthInsurance.shtml.

VandenBerg KA (2007) Individualized developmental care for high risk newborns in the NICU: a practice guideline. *Early Human Development* **83**: 433–42.

Wales Neonatal Network (n.d.) *Neonatal transport service.* Available at http://www.walesneonatalnetwork.wales.nhs.uk/transfer.

Welsh Assembly Government (2013) *All Wales Neonatal Standards*, 2nd ed. Welsh Assembly Government. Available at http://www.walesneonatalnetwork.wales.nhs.uk/sitesplus/documents/1034/All%20Wales%20Neonatal%20Standards%202nd%20Edition%20v2%2005.08.13.pdf.

WG (1987) Nursing notes. From the past. *Midwives Chronicles and Nursing Notes*, March.

Wigert H, Johansson R, Berg M, Hellström A (2006) Mothers' experiences of having their newborn child in a neonatal intensive care unit. *Scandinavian Journal of Caring Science* **20**: 3541.

Wild L (2014) Nursing: past, present and future. In Peate I, Wild K, Muralitharan N (eds.) *Nursing practice: knowledge and care*, pp. 2–24. Chichester: Wiley.

Wilson-Costello D, Friedman H, Minch N, Siner B, Taylor, G, Schluchter M, Hack M (2007) Improved neurodevelopmental outcomes for extremely low birth weight infants in 2000–2002. *Pediatrics* **119**(1): 37–45.

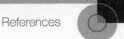

World Health Organization (2012a) *Born too soon. Global action on preterm birth*. Geneva: WHO.

World Health Organization (2012b) *Newborns: reducing mortality*. Fact Sheet No. 333. Available at http://www.who.int/mediacentre/factsheets/fs333/en/.

World Health Organization (2014) *Preterm birth*. Fact Sheet No. 363. Geneva: WHO. Available at http://www.who.int/mediacentre/factsheets/fs363/en/.

Yaktin U, Bou-Radd Azoury N, Doumit M (2003) Personal characteristics and job satisfaction among nurses in Lebanon. *Journal of Nursing Administration* **33**(7): 384–90.

Specialist community public health nursing: Health visiting and school nursing

CATHY TAYLOR AND SUSAN JONES

OVERVIEW

This chapter provides an overview of the history, development and current practice of health visitors (HVs) and school nurses (SNs) and shows how these have evolved in response to key health and social policy drivers and now come under the umbrella of specialist community public health nursing. Importantly, it shows how these disciplines complement each other by providing an integrated service which can ensure optimum health outcomes from the antenatal period and throughout a child and young person's school-aged years which can have lasting benefit in their adult years.

INTRODUCTION

Within the United Kingdom early intervention and prevention are high on the political and health agendas and are identified as key to improving outcomes for children, young people and families (Department of Health [DH] 2009a, Department of Health, Social Services and Public Safety [DHSSPSNI] 2010b; Welsh Government [WG] 2013). A public health approach may address inter-generational behaviours that negatively impact health and well-being. It will benefit society by reducing the financial burden of lifestyle-related chronic disease in adults such as obesity and will result in better outcomes for children and young people by empowering them to achieve their full potential throughout their childhood and adult life. This approach needs to begin pre-conceptually and be maintained throughout the early years and the school-aged years of a child's life. Health visitors and school nurses have a key role in ensuring universal provision in this vital area of public health.

HISTORY AND DEVELOPMENT OF HEALTH VISITING AND SCHOOL NURSING

Public health was initially influenced by poverty and environmental factors that were historically seen as the root causes of ill health, with food shortages and outbreaks of disease causing high levels of mortality and limiting population growth (Graham in Douglas et al. 2010). Public health development in the early nineteenth century created the foundation for 'sanitary reform' where public health programmes were built around environmental and engineering discoveries, the creation of vaccinations and preventative strategies for infectious disease. In 1848 the Public Health Act was introduced with the concept of cleanliness and personal hygiene viewed as critical to health and well-being, and in 1855 'sanitary inspectors' (the forerunners to health visitors) had been appointed by every local authority. Their role was to assist the poorer sections of the community, as they had the poorest health outcomes (identified in Edwin Chadwick's 1842 *Report on the Sanitary Condition of the Labouring Population*), often as a result of squalid and overcrowded living conditions.

REFLECTION POINT

Consider whether the causes attributed to poor health outcomes in the twenty-first century differ significantly from those identified in the nineteenth century.

The Ladies Sanitary Reform Association, established in Manchester and Salford in 1862, led to the employment of the first paid visitors, referred to as 'sanitary mission women'. Local women were paid to visit the homes of the poor and had a public health inspection remit. Infant mortality and poor health at this time were high, but interestingly the poor physical health of adult males only became apparent during recruitment for the Anglo-Boer War in 1899–1902 when men were enlisting to fight. A newspaper report suggested that 65% of those volunteering were rejected due to poor health and physique, which ultimately led to the government establishing the Inter-Departmental Committee on the Physical Deterioration of the Poor. The report from this committee in 1904 emphasized concerns over children's health, making the case that good health in children would lead to good health in adults. This resulted in a new national interest in maternal and child welfare.

KEY POINT

The Manchester and Salford Ladies Sanitary Reform Association is seen as the starting point of the health visiting profession.

The health visiting profession began to emerge, with the title *health visitor* accorded in 1891, and 11 years later, in 1902, the Midwives Act was passed. The aim of the act was to address infant and maternal mortality via provision of midwifery care from registered professionals. By 1917, health visitors were expected to visit all mothers, as soon after they had given birth as possible, to give direction and education regarding the care and health of the new baby. As it became recognized that knowledge of disease prevention, health and well-being was necessary for families, the expectation emerged that health visitors should be trained nurses. At this point the Ministry of Health took over training of health visitors, and in the 1920s the first university academic-level course was introduced.

Compulsory education for children in England and Wales began in 1870 with the introduction of the Elementary Education Act. This established schools where there had been no previous provision and enforced attendance for children from the age of 5 years. Northern Ireland and Scotland saw similar legislation such as the Scottish Education Act of 1872. This was followed in 1890 by the landmark Education Act that for the first time ensured free education for all children. Registers began to be recorded and absenteeism was noted to be mainly due to ill health, often related to poverty and resultant minor ailments, and in an effort to address the issues the school nurse role began to emerge.

In 1948 the National Health Service (NHS) was established resulting in healthcare reform with the move from a community perspective to a focus on hospital treatment. Concentrating on preventative work health visiting remained under the responsibility of local authority public health departments, but gradually the work of the health visitor expanded to include the health of the whole family and other groups, such as families with social problems and the recently bereaved. In the post-war years, as health visiting's association with general practice increased, there appeared to be a decline in public health work as health visitors tended to focus on a more individualistic approach.

The role of the health visitor expanded especially following the *Report of the Working Party on the Field, Training and Recruitment of Health Visitors* (Jameson 1956), which emphasized the importance of maternal mental health and care of the older person, offering a service from cradle to grave. However, this did lead to tension, as health visitors became increasingly 'attached' to general practices but were expected to maintain their responsibility for raising awareness of health needs and population-based work. Ambiguities with the role continued as health visitors became more involved in both health and social care and the protection of children. Health visitors were referred to by Jameson (1956) as generalist 'case finders' because of their access to all children and families and their ability to detect problems, whereas social workers differed, being described as 'case workers' and expected to use their skills to work with vulnerable at-risk families once identified.

Over a decade later, the 1959 School Health Regulations saw the move from universal to selective health inspections to cut costs and it also abolished the need for a health visitor qualification for schools. Subsequently the school nurse role was interpreted restrictively (Slack 1978), and the belief was that they were only capable of examining heads for lice and being known as the 'nit nurse' gave them little scope to fully utilize their skills. Health visitors and school nurses remained the responsibility of local education authorities under the supervision of the Medical Officer of Health until 1974 when the 1973 NHS Reorganisation Act was enforced, and the school health service became part of an integrated child health service in which school medical, dental and nursing services became the responsibility of the NHS. The court report (Court SMD 1976) identified that school nurses required specialist training for the role. At the same time the four principles of health visiting evolved: the search for health needs, the stimulation and awareness of health needs, the influencing policies affecting health and the facilitation of health-enhancing activities (Council for the Education and Training of Health Visitors [CETHV] 1977), later to be revised in 2006 by Cowley and Frost.

KEY POINT

The four principles of health visiting (CETHV 1977; Cowley and Frost 2006) continue to influence and guide health visiting and school nursing practice.

In 1996, the Patient's Charter established two rights for children and young people: the right of parents to know the name of their child's school nurse and how to contact them and their right to a health check during the first year of primary school (DH 1996). The development of the specialist practitioner qualification and educational changes required for community nursing in 1998 noted school nursing as one of the key roles that make up the community nursing family.

This was the beginning of a major shift in policy for school nurses as the profession had been in a decline owing to financial cutbacks. The Department of Health (1999a, 2000, 2003) cited the school nurse as a primary professional in the delivery of public health to the school-aged child representing a move from their involvement in screening programmes to a wider health promotion role. This new political climate enabled school nursing to develop professional leadership and contribute to the public health agenda for the school-aged child population. Although policy and education drivers were highlighting the importance of the public health role for school nurses, Clark et al. (2000) and others (Carlile 2002; DeBell and Tomkins 2006) all noted that they continued to be regarded as a 'Cinderella service' within the NHS despite being identified as the only NHS professional group whose focus is on meeting the health needs of the school-aged child. Alongside their health visiting colleagues, school nurses are now a distinct and specialist graduate profession registered on the Specialist Community Public Health Nursing, Part 3, of the Nursing and Midwifery Council (NMC).

Internationally, developments in Canada and the World Health Organization (WHO), specifically the Alma Ata Conference (WHO 1978) and the Ottawa Charter for Health Promotion (WHO 1986), were published as the biomedical model was being criticized for its narrow focus on disease and ignoring the effects of wider social, economic and environmental determinants. This, along with the notion of 'personal responsibility' for health becoming more prominent and the emergence of the concept of health promotion and empowerment, meant the 'new public health' movement had begun. The public health agenda was re-energized in the UK with publications of the Department of Health: *The New NHS* (DH 1997) and green paper *Our Healthier Nation* (DH 1998b). Emphasis was placed on the need for a multi-disciplinary public health workforce approach working with vulnerable families in communities where poor outcomes had been identified.

Working together to support families was acknowledged as vital and endorsed by UK government policy (DH 1991, 1998a). The need to tackle inequalities remained high on the political agenda and was identified in several documents of the twenty-first century, including the Wanless Report, *Securing Good Health for the Whole Population* (DH 2004b), and the Marmot Review (2010). Lord Laming's review (2009) following the death of Peter Connelly ('Baby P') highlighted a need to increase the numbers of qualified health visitors who had also been tasked with leading the development of the Healthy Child Programme (DH 2009a) in England.

> ### REFLECTION POINT
>
> In view of the current refocus on early intervention and prevention should health and social services be integrated?

HEALTH VISITING AND THE PRESENT-DAY SCOPE OF PRACTICE

There is no doubt that the historical background of health visiting has demonstrated its value as a worthwhile profession. Within the UK, it is known that the health of the nation has improved (more for some than others). Importantly, our population is ageing, with many causes of ill health in our communities being deep rooted and difficult to tackle (WG 2011b). Marmot (2010) in the *Independent Review of Health Inequalities in England Post-2010* report again highlighted the serious effects of health inequalities caused by social and economic differences, proposing that one significant way to help tackle issues would be to offer a strong commitment to the early years, focusing on giving children the best start in life. This once more put health visiting at the forefront of change to lead local child health initiatives providing vulnerable families the support they need.

A public health approach with a clear remit to positively influence the health of children in their early years (0–5 years) continues as the key focus of today's health visiting practice. The Health Visitor Implementation Plan 2011–2015, 'A Call to Action', (DH 2011) suggested that the health visiting profession should work on four different levels: community (community development work based on strategic needs assessment), universal (leadership on the Healthy Child Programme [HCP]), universal plus (provision of targeted services for those with additional needs) and universal partnership plus (additional specialist services for those with the highest need).

As specialist practitioners, health visitors understand what influences health and are aware of the effects of social determinants such as poverty, unemployment and poor housing. In order to work within communities, it is important that health visitors are able to understand what might influence health, having knowledge of the effects of the main social determinants. Gaining an understanding of a community is vital to assess current health need, so appropriate services can be designed and delivered. Searching for health needs can be challenging but provides the foundations for primary preventative work. Compiling a health needs assessment is a fundamental activity within health visiting so that an action plan to address the community's health needs can be formulated and acted upon. Early identification of need is paramount so that facilitation and stimulation of proactive interventions, working in partnership with communities and key partners within the multi-agency team and the voluntary sector, can be achieved. Building individual communities' capacity through health-enhancing activities is essential if the prevention of long-term chronic disease and protection against ill health is to be accomplished. This fits with the traditional work of the health visitor, acknowledged for their bottom-up community development work, in relation to leading groups and community initiatives. Various examples of this work can be seen at the local level and can range from traditional breastfeeding support groups to encouraging exercise and mental well-being by pram pushing, baby massage and the formation of local dads groups and community-wide activities.

Improving outcomes for children, families and communities through primary prevention and early intervention continues to be the key focus of the health visitor's role. It is well documented that having good social and emotional experiences in the early years can be critical in shaping an individual's health and well-being throughout life. Field's (2010) *Independent Review on Poverty and Life Chances* and Allen's (2011) independent report on early intervention offer significant evidence that children who grow up in dysfunctional families are more likely to create such families themselves, stating the importance of limiting the effects of negative experiences and influences so that children can obtain the best start in life. Many children find themselves having to live with the adverse effects of crime, unemployment, poverty and mental illness and are more likely to experience poorer outcomes in relation to developmental delay, behavioural problems, safeguarding concerns, low educational attainment and even offending behaviour (WG 2013). Even though it is parents and carers who are pivotal to providing these essential social and emotional foundations, it is the health visiting service that is crucial in providing a universal service to families regardless of where they live, their ethnic group, their language or their social circumstance (Welsh Assembly Government [WAG] 2005b; WG 2012).

Identifying and assessing need is a core skill of health visitors and a principle activity when working with families. Tickell (2011) stipulates that the early identification of need followed by appropriate support is essential if disadvantage is to be tackled within society. Assessing need can be complex, encompassing the collation of information over a period of time, requiring an ability to build relationships and work in partnership with families. There is a wealth of evidence stating that health visitors are well placed to undertake this role (DH 2009a; DHSSPSNI 2010b; Scottish Government 2012a) as they have a range of knowledge and skills to make judgements and prioritize those families which may need extra support or intervention (Appleton and Cowley 2008). Effective communication skills are vital to ensure families feel supported and empowered, and applied alongside structured assessment tools, such as the Common Assessment Framework (CAF) (DH 2000), they enable the health visitors to build a holistic assessment of families and identify the level of resilience and where support may be needed. Although they in no way replace professional judgement, expertise and intuition, accredited assessment tools in the UK (such as the CAF) (DfES 2003) help ensure a standardized approach and quality assurance that helps inform the health visitor's development of an action plan for individual families.

In line with this acknowledgement all families expecting new babies, and those who have preschool children, are allocated a health visitor who offers key contacts, advice and support in the family home and clinic settings. Described as the key professional working with the early years (0–5 years) age group and their families, they ensure universal application of the specific HCP in the four nations that comprise the UK (DH 2009a, 2009b; DHSSPSNI 2010a; Scottish Government 2012b).

REFLECTION POINT

Look at the CAF assessment tool and consider how this may be useful in aiding professional decision making.

HEALTH VISITORS AND THEIR SCOPE OF PRACTICE IN DELIVERING HEALTHY CHILD PROGRAMMES

The concept of child health promotion (CHP) has its roots in the last century, but it was the *Fit for the Future* report of the Committee on the Child Health Service (Court SMD 1976) which formally recommended a structured programme of health surveillance for all children. This was led by general practitioners in partnership with health visitors and proposed that the growth and developmental progress of all children should be monitored, together with provision of evidence-based immunization programmes and advice and support for parents. This concept went on to develop over time, but significantly it was Professor David Hall's review of these routine examinations for the British Paediatric Association that led to a review and the development of a new streamlined programme. Subsequent *Health for All Children* (HFAC) reports followed, but it was the final HFAC4 that provided the basis for the newly formed Healthy Child Programme (HCP) which was launched in England in the UK in 2009.

Acknowledged as the best placed and most appropriately qualified professional, health visitors were identified as the necessary lead in delivering the core elements of the HCP pregnancy and first 5 years (DH 2009a). A universal programme intended to improve the health and well-being of children, its goals are to help parents to care for their children, change health behaviours and therefore reduce inequalities. Through the provision of ongoing assessment, surveillance, reviews, health promotion, immunization programmes and parenting support, the programme is seen as essential especially for those families in need of additional support and advice.

Each of the four nations within the UK has a regional variation of an HCP, but all have the same core principles (DH 2009a, 2009b; DHSSPSNI 2010a; Scottish Government 2012b). They provide a standard approach to contacts, surveillance and public health approaches that inform and guide professional practice and decision making. The concept of the HCP begins in pregnancy and extends throughout childhood and school years with the health visitors remit being to focus on pregnancy and the first 5 years of a child's life.

The programmes (based on primary systematic evidence from Professor David Hall in 1989) emphasize the importance of regular surveillance of children's general health and development. They set key contact timings and suggest evidence-based interventions regarding pregnancy, mental health and the transition to parenting, neuroscience and early attachment, the promotion of health and well-being through infant feeding and nutrition, the promotion of the uptake of immunization, dental health and accident prevention. The goal of the programmes is to improve parenting, increase the rates of breastfeeding and physical activity, prevent communicable diseases and improve readiness for school.

Providing information to parents is a key component of the health visitor's role to help reduce infant mortality, improve routine screening and recognize early and minimize developmental delay. Essentially health visitors are skilled in evidence-based interventions such as behavioural management strategies, smoking cessation strategies and parenting programmes. Effectively, families are helped to manage and cope with problems as they arise (DH 2009a). There is necessarily an increased focus on families that may be viewed as 'vulnerable', in that specific aspects of the programme can be tailored to individual families depending on their level of need (for example parents with learning difficulties or teenage parents). This progressive universal approach to provision can be used to ensure that interventions are targeted where families are identified as having additional need in relation, for example, to parenting or access to support groups. Intensive support can be offered to families assessed as having high levels of risk or need; these may include children with complex needs or those in need of protection. Information sharing and effective team working with appropriate multi-agency partners is vital to achieving good outcomes. Examples of this work can be witnessed at the local level where health visitors in conjunction with the multi-agency team work closely with vulnerable groups such as teenage parents, travelling families or asylum seekers.

HEALTH VISITORS AND THEIR SCOPE OF PRACTICE IN SAFEGUARDING

Safeguarding continues to be everybody's responsibility and services should ensure a child-centred approach, based on a clear understanding of the rights and views of children. This is driven by the United Nations (UN) Convention on the Rights of the Child (UN 1989), which enshrines several rights and stipulates that all services should be child focused. Protecting and safeguarding children has always been a priority for the health visiting service and its contribution is well documented (Laming 2009; DH 2009c; HM Government 2013). Health visitors have always had a role in ensuring the safety and welfare of children; however, it is increasingly the protection of children which, despite being a key public health issue, can bring additional tension and challenges. Many children are being raised in a climate where several risk factors associated with poverty, mental illness, substance misuse, debt, poor housing and domestic violence (DH 2009c) are present, and the health visitor needs to be vigilant in being able to identify children who may be vulnerable or at risk of significant harm. Working with vulnerable children and families is demanding and often difficult as identification and assessment of neglect and abuse can be ambiguous, hard to detect and is often disguised or hidden (Munro 2011) (see Chapter 2).

Surveillance in this respect is challenging and can cause conflict, but agencies acknowledge the inability of a single profession to have the full picture or a complete overview of a child's needs. Lessons must continue to be learnt from historic serious case reviews (SCRs) and new child practice reviews, processes and lines of accountability need to be unambiguous and transparent and all lessons learnt must be embedded into practice to inform future approaches. It is recognized that recommendations from such reviews rarely refer or apply to a single agency and the impetus via recent policy direction (HM Government 2013) is on working together. This requires co-ordination between agencies including health, education, housing, police and the voluntary sector, and crucially effective sharing of information. It is essential for health visitors to be involved in early detection and intervention, making referrals to social services where appropriate, and attending and contributing to core groups, case conferences and legal proceedings as required. One of the key strengths of the Flying Start service in Wales has been the creation of local 'hubs' where many key agencies are located together, enabling communication and referral to become a much easier process.

To enable health visitors to meet these responsibilities, it is essential that they are able to maintain and update their knowledge and skills and are supported in accessing continuous professional development, shared training and child protection supervision with experienced colleagues to ensure they continue to be effective advocates for children and families.

KEY POINT

One of the main roles of the health visitor is to safeguard children.

REFLECTION POINT

How might this impact on their public health role?

HEALTH VISITORS' SCOPE OF PRACTICE IN DELIVERING ENHANCED MODEL PROGRAMMES

The Millennium Cohort Study (MCS) began in 2000 and aims to track social, economic and health circumstances of children born at the start of the twenty-first century (Bradshaw and Holmes 2010). Evidence suggests that there continues to be a significant difference in the wealthiest and poorest families, comparing factors including employment and income status, quality of housing, education, ethnicity and disability – all of which can influence a child's health, well-being and life in general. It has long been identified and documented (Department of Health and Human Services 1980; Acheson 1988; Marmot 2010) that poverty and social disadvantage can lead to continual inequality and social exclusion.

Breaking the cycle of deprivation is critical to improving health outcomes and reducing the pull on finite resources that are consumed when dealing with the expensive outcomes of providing health and social care services for the future. The four nations within the UK continue to produce policies that attempt to respond to identified health needs and significantly there has been increased emphasis on the importance of support in the early years. Giving every child the best start in life is acknowledged to be essential if long-term outcomes for children are to improve (DHSSPSNI 2010b; DH 2013a; Scottish Government 2014; WG 2013).

Children grow and develop rapidly within the first 5 years of their lives, with pregnancy and the early years being the most important time for physical, language, cognitive, social and emotional development, shaping health and well-being for the rest of a child's life. The UK government supports the fact that it is essential that children have a good start in life, having provided an increase in funding for early years investment. From this investment, both the Sure Start and Flying Start services were developed in England and Wales, respectively. This has supported additional training places for health visitors seen as key professionals to provide effective early intervention and support to families with the greatest need. The Flying Start Welsh government–funded programme provides additional resources in specifically identified areas of deprivation (http://gov.wales/topics/people-and-communities/people/children-and-young-people/parenting-support-guidance/help/flyingstart). The health visitor element of the programme is delivered by professionals who have smaller caseload allocations than their generic counterparts. This enables them to provide an enhanced programme in partnership with local authority and 'early years' settings colleagues to children of families in the most disadvantaged communities in Wales. Every child under 4 years of age living within these areas is offered an enhanced health visiting service providing additional home visits. Where a high level of need has been identified via professional judgement supported by assessment, additional input is offered along with referral to other appropriate services.

Contact with the service usually begins during the antenatal period following a referral from the midwifery service. This initial contact is critical to assess the needs of the family and the unborn child. Using a public health approach, health promotion and advice can be given related to preparation for parenthood, emotional health and well-being, importance of diet, promotion of breastfeeding and reducing risk around smoking, alcohol or substance misuse. Building a relationship with the family at this stage is paramount to encourage engagement so that a high-quality service can be delivered with the best interests of the child at the heart. A primary birth visit is planned for 10–14 days after the birth of the child, followed by further minimum contacts in line with the Flying Start Health Visiting Core Programme (WG 2012). Every contact is designed to promote health and assess the child's growth and development so that health interventions and health promotion activity can be planned and delivered to meet the individual family's needs.

The following scenario gives an example of how health visitors within the Flying Start service can help families optimize their health and well-being.

CASE STUDY

Sam and Emily have five children, three of whom are school aged and two are under 4 years. They live in council accommodation within a designated Flying Start area. Sam has recently become unemployed and has accrued gambling debts. Emily has been finding it hard to cope and the home has become unkempt. Some concerns had been raised with social services and Flying Start services were offered to provide additional support for the family.

Upon receiving information about the Flying Start programme all family members were keen to engage. Both parents attended a parenting group while the two younger children attended the Flying Start preschool nursery. Through their involvement in this group, Emily grew in confidence, discovering an artistic flair she never knew she had. She was receptive to constructive family planning advice and the group helped her to develop her parenting skills. Through the service, the school-aged children were also supported being encouraged to make greater use of the library and local leisure services.

Feedback from the family showed that the Flying Start service had made a small but significant difference to their lives.

REFLECTION POINT

Should the enhanced health visitor (HV) service model be available to all families assessed to be in need by the HV and not just those in designated areas?

Establishing effective relationships with parents is crucial in developing confidence and ability in parenting skills, and to meet the wide-ranging needs that may be identified Sure Start and Flying Start teams consist of myriad multi-disciplinary professional and skill mix colleagues. These include health visitors, family health workers, early years support officers, nursery nurses, dieticians, therapists, educationalists and voluntary sector and social workers. The specific health-related programmes and interventions that are delivered include topics such as healthy eating, smoking cessation, oral health, accident prevention and exercise. Additional support from partner agencies and the voluntary sector is available to help parents engage in their child's learning and develop skills with reading, singing and playing, helping to support early language development and numerical abilities.

In addition free, part-time quality child care is offered for all 2- to 3-year-olds within Flying Start areas which supports parents to access work or training and facilitates them making a contribution to the economy, which in turn enhances their self-esteem and well-being. This is reinforced by the provision of grants for targeted wrap-around and holiday child care to improve the quality of early education and child care provision. The health visitor also assesses the child's growth and social, emotional, behavioural and language development prior to them commencing school to enable effective transition to the foundation phase of formal education.

SCPHN (HV) HANDOVER OF CARE TO SCPHN (SN) COLLEAGUES

All four nation's versions of the Healthy Child Programme (HCP) identify explicit respective roles and clearly define health visiting involvement as being in the early years, pre-birth to 5 years, with a handover to school nursing services at 5 years of age (DH 2009a, 2009b, 2012; DHSSPSNI 2010a; Scottish Government 2012a, 2012b). The title of health visitor (HV) or school nurse (SN) is also standard with Scotland recently reverting from the public health nurse (PHN) title which had caused confusion (Chief Nursing Officer [Scotland] 2013).

SCHOOL NURSING AND THE PRESENT-DAY SCOPE OF PRACTICE

School nurses (SNs) are clearly identified as having a crucial leadership, co-ordination and delivery role within Healthy Child Programmes (DH 2012, 2014). In Northern Ireland and Scotland, the SN role is spilt into two distinct age groups: 5–11 years and 11–19 years. In England and Wales, the SN remit is described as being 5–19 years with no distinction between the primary and secondary school-aged years.

Actively engaged in what has been described as a complex field of practice that has developed into a well-defined specialty (Gleeson 2004), SNs are now far removed from the 'panadol and plaster' image of the nurse sited in an obscure area of a secondary school, providing a bolt hole from unpopular lessons in the curriculum, or the caricature 'nit nurse' figure from the primary school days memories of many adults.

Most SNs are Specialist Community Public Health Nurse (SCPHN) qualified and based in the community, work full-time as opposed to term-time and have a caseload of named schools. However, many remain contracted to local authority and individual schools, particularly in the independent sector, but there is a policy push, both professionally and politically, to bring all SNs into NHS employment (WAG 2009; DH 2009b). This will ensure they are afforded access to continual professional development, update and support, and the terms and conditions that many do not currently benefit from. This will be more essential as the new NMC revalidation process is rolled out in 2016 (NMC 2015a).

KEY POINT

Most SNs are public health qualified SCPHN (SN) graduates employed by the NHS.

From their young clients' perspective full-time availability of an NHS employed SN facilitates provision of a service that is available outside of school premises, can be accessed confidentially and is available outside of school hours and during school holidays. This is essential if SNs are to meet their young clients' rights and address their needs as they are not merely school children, but school-aged children who spend the majority of their time in their home and neighbourhood communities rather than their school community setting.

REFLECTION POINT

Consider how such provision would benefit the young people and what needs to be available to make it a reality.

In many areas, SNs provide drop-in sessions outside of school hours and terms in venues that include youth clubs and community schools where young people feel safe to attend as they are advised that within safeguarding parameters the service is confidential. Often the 'C Card' condom distribution scheme is provided by the SN, and as necessary and appropriate signposting to sexual health and contraception services is provided.

The SN service continues to be underresourced and has not benefited from the equivalent investment accorded to the health visitor (HV) service. This means they are unable to deliver enhanced services in the most deprived areas or give the same level of support offered by HVs once handover commences from the HV service to the SN service when the child starts full-time school. This is despite their documented role in building on the early years support and the identified need to ensure synergy between HV and SN services (DH 2012, 2014). Currently school-aged children in the UK equal a total of 11.184 million children and young people, and account for 17.7% of the population (Office for National Statistics [ONS] 2011). These statistics indicate that school-aged children represent a significant group of the population and, as such, deserve not just professional but also political commitment to providing them with long-term, sustainable and robust services that meet their documented rights (UN 1989; DH 2004c; Scottish Government 2014b). Present staffing levels therefore hamper the role of the SN as a public health specialist practitioner in meeting the public health agenda for children and young people at a population-level approach. In this connection, if SNs are to have a realistic chance of successfully addressing the identified public health priorities such as obesity, smoking, substance abuse, self-harm and unplanned teen pregnancy rates, it is essential that they utilize accredited tools (NHS Health Scotland 2004; Royal College Nursing 2014) to profile their named school communities and the neighbourhoods in which they are situated.

In times of austerity, when additional resources are unlikely to be available, this will inform the local priorities which can differ greatly in different localities and enable SNs to accurately target support for their young clients. It is worth noting the Welsh Government's 'prudent healthcare' approach which advocates 'only do what only you can do' (WG 2015). Embracing a skill mix service approach ensures appropriate delegation of elements of the SN role that maximize the effectiveness of the resources that are available. It is also essential that SNs remain up to date with the services available locally and signpost or refer to more appropriate multi-agency colleagues whose expertise may more effectively address children and young people's needs in specific areas.

KEY POINTS

School-aged children in the UK account for almost 18% of the population but SHNs are in short supply despite the following recommendations dating back 40 years:

- 1 SN to every 2500 children (Court SMD 1976)
- 1 SN to every 1500 children (Polnay 1995)
- 1 SN to every secondary school and related cluster of primary schools by 2010 (DH 2004a)
- 1 SN to every secondary school by 2011 (WAG 2007)

ENSURING A CLIENT-FOCUSED SCHOOL NURSING SERVICE

Children and young people are entitled to a school nursing service that they can identify with and which is relevant and appropriate to them. It is not acceptable ethically or professionally to merely provide a service that is informed according to what professionals, politicians and the adult society feel they should be given.

All children's nurses have a duty of advocacy on behalf of their young clients (DH 2012, 2014; NMC 2015b), and SNs must apply this documented responsibility to both lobby and advocate on behalf of their young clients who have the right to information, education and involvement in all issues that affect them (UN 1989; DH 2004; WG 2014). The ethos of such involvement is reaffirmed in the National Service Frameworks (NSFs) relevant to children and young people (Department for Education and Skills [DfES] 2004; National Assembly for Wales [NAW] 2005b). Of particular significance to all children and young people's nurses are the core aims which state that they should enjoy the best possible health, be listened to and have their views respected and be provided with a range of learning opportunities and education (see Chapter 1).

The following scenario gives an example of how the school nursing service can help children and young people optimize their health and well-being.

CASE STUDY

In one area, SNs aimed to provide confidential weekly drop-in sessions to pupils in school at lunchtime. They were poorly attended and the sessions were the first thing to be cancelled if priority issues, for example safeguarding, arose. The SNs presumed this may be the issue for the poor attendance.

Ensuring children's rights are met is central to their practice and in an effort to ensure the service was informed by them, the SNs engaged with pupils to confirm the reasons for poor attendance. Several reasons emerged including lunchtimes were too short to eat and attend the drop-in, the SN often cancelled so they weren't sure when they would be there and they didn't want to be seen attending by peers and certainly not by their teachers.

They advised they wanted a drop-in service but not in school hours and wanted it to be available during school holidays. The SN service used this information to negotiate with multi-agency partners' access to community facilities in the early evening in community schools and youth clubs. A pilot in a few venues on set evenings proved successful and attendance has evidenced the need for the change to meet young people's needs.

SNs AND THEIR SCOPE OF PRACTICE IN RELATION TO PUBLIC HEALTH PRACTICE

As defined by the WHO in 2013, public health refers to all organized measures to prevent disease, promote health and prolong life among the population as a whole. The population remit of the SN is the school aged, but they also have professional responsibility to address needs, particularly in relation to safeguarding, at an individual level for some of their young clients. As a result, to meet children and young people's needs within this contradictory stance, a multi-professional, multi-disciplinary and skill mix team approach is a prerequisite for SN practice (WAG 2009; DH 2009a, 2009b, 2012, 2014; DHSSPSNI 2010a, 2010b; Scottish Government 2012a, 2012b).

The SN's public health role is involved with statutory and non-statutory input. The statutory element includes as a minimum school entry screening for height, weight and vision, alongside the Child Measurement Programme in England and Wales and an ever-increasing vaccination programme, notably the new annual 'Fluenz Programme' (www.gov.uk/PHE-Childhoodinfluenza-programme-2015). Non-statutory input includes drop-in clinics for advice outside of school premises and school hours, and much of the health promotion and health education work in schools in support of their colleagues in education. Being aware of the plethora of policy and documentation that supports the role of the SN is essential to ensure that although much of their input is not presently considered to be of statutory nature, this fact does not render it dispensable. In particular issues related to safeguarding and specifically child sexual exploitation may be recognized via drop-in session attendance. It is therefore essential that SNs are in an informed position to lobby for appropriate interventions and activities to be included within their remit as statutory. There is also a need to produce evidence of effectiveness in improving children and young people's outcomes that is currently lacking, to argue the case for specific elements of the SN service to be sustainably resourced and to ensure they become embedded elements of their practice.

To meet their young clients' needs and documented rights (UN 1989; DfES 2003, 2004; DH 2004c, 2009a, 2009b; DHSSPSNI 2010a; Scottish Government 2012a) and professional standards (NMC 2015), SNs also need to be aware of the tools provided to assist them in implementing interventions that will enable them to achieve local and national targets for the future. Examples related to smoking cessation are available at www.ashwales. org.uk and www.nhsggcsmokefree.org.uk. SNs also need to develop tools to provide their own evidence base and sharing of best practice, networking at every opportunity via appropriate forums, and conference attendance can facilitate this aim being met. Reinventing the wheel is not necessary; learning what interventions have been successful for colleagues, developing, accessing and utilizing evidence-based tools will help ensure that school-aged children in all parts of the UK are receiving a robust, needs-led and constantly evolving service. This leads us naturally to the scope of practice SNs also have in relation to health promotion.

SNs AND THEIR SCOPE OF PRACTICE IN HEALTH PROMOTION

Long regarded as the 'bread and butter' of public health practice health education aims to empower people to take control of and responsibility for their own health (WHO 1986; DH 1999a; Wanless 2002). The public health agenda of current policy continues to highlight a lead role for SNs in promoting and maintaining the health of young people through education and health promotion (DH 2012, 2013a, 2014; DHSSPHNI 2010a, 2010b). Despite this SN involvement in health promotion is at the mercy of the resource constraints that have been identified previously in this chapter.

Equity of provision relates to providing input to meet identified needs, not providing the same to all regardless of whether there is an identified need, and the SN, like HV colleagues, can use accredited tools either to inform practice at the whole school population level or to assess an individual pupil's needs. Profiling of schools using evidence-based tools (NHS Health Scotland 2004; Scottish Government 2011; WAG 2009; DH 2009b; DHSSPSNI 2010b) will inform what issues exist and need to be prioritized as regards SN input in their named schools (Godson 2014). However, profiling is only useful if resources to address identified needs are available; this includes the availability of the SN.

Health promotion, particularly in primary schools, is largely, though not solely, related to the stated aims of the National Healthy Schools Programme (NHSP) (Department for Education and Employment [DfEE] 1999). All schools are encouraged to participate and achieve recognized standards leading to accreditation as a 'healthy school' in the Healthy Schools Scheme (HSS).

Each of the countries that constitute the UK has set targets for participation along with locally identified aims and priorities. The national and devolved government websites all have sections dedicated to news and updates on their area's achievements in regard to their specific programmes, and many schools also have dedicated web pages accessible via the individual school's web page. Although it was initially teacher led (DeBell et al. 2007) the programme is now a multi-disciplinary and multi-professional collaboration, of which the SN is an integral component (DH 2013a) as evidenced below.

Personal health and social education (PHSE) is a key component of the national curriculum throughout school-aged years and an area in which the SN's input is highly valued by teachers and pupils alike. While pupils report SNs as credible when delivering, for example, sessions in 'sex and relationships' education (SRE), it is important to keep in focus that although SNs lead and contribute to improving outcomes for children and young people it is not solely their responsibility (DH 2014). To achieve better outcomes for children and young people, a partnership approach with multi-agency and multi-disciplinary colleagues is necessary (WAG 2009; DH 2009a, 2009b, 2014; DHSSPSNI 2010b; Scottish Government 2011; Regulation Quality Improvement Authority [RQIA] 2011). The breadth of partners encompassed in work related to the SN role will be discussed later, but an example of effective working regarding SRE provision is where the local authority youth work service manager and the local education authority curriculum advisor worked with the HSS co-ordinator and the SN manager. Accredited training was delivered by the youth work service manager initially to the SNs, who then supported in-training teachers. A package of lesson plans was set and shared delivery of sessions to pupils was negotiated which included youth workers delivering some of the sessions in schools.

The dual role of the SN in relation to public health and health promotion has now been set out, and while it is outside the scope of this chapter to account for every aspect of their role, it would seem appropriate to discuss practice in relation to two important issues, namely immunization and vulnerable children and young people.

PRINCIPLES FOR PRACTICE

- SNs, as graduate specialist community public health practitioners, are aware of the political dimensions of practice.
- SNs have a dual role in relation to public health and health promotion.

IMMUNIZATION AND THE ROLE OF THE SN

Immunization programmes are one of the UK's most successful public health measures (Health Protection Agency [HPA] 2005). Historically SNs have delivered vaccination sessions for school-aged children and have been responsible for organizing, leading and conducting many successful mass vaccination campaigns as well as delivering the national vaccination programmes in school settings. Due to constant scientific advances, new vaccination programmes are regularly being introduced, as in the case of Fluenz currently being phased in for all pupils annually. Due to the continual introduction of new programmes this role is becoming untenable because it jeopardizes the wider public health role of the SN. As a result many areas are considering an alternative model of delivery (DH 2009a, 2014; DHSSPSNI 2010b) and it is essential, particularly in times of austerity, that SNs lobby to ensure that appropriate levels of new funding are secured. This will afford support for innovative approaches that utilize appropriately trained skill mix teams, to ensure that vaccination programmes are led but not fully delivered by SNs.

Minimum standards of training for all professionals who vaccinate were laid down by the HPA (2005) and anyone new to the role must undertake a minimum of 2 days training followed by a period of supervised practice and assessment of competency. There is ongoing discussion regarding healthcare support workers delivering vaccine to children and young people, but many contentious areas regarding the current legal definitions regarding application of patient group directives, delegation and professional accountability remain to be resolved. It is essential that SNs, in their advocacy role, actively engage in this debate to inform the outcomes to ensure they meet the rights and needs of children and young people. Linked to this SNs must also be aware of the issues with regard to information, input on decisions that affect them and the documented right to consent for themselves under Fraser guidelines, even if their parents disagree (*Gillick v West Norfolk and Wisbech AHA and DOHSS* [1985]; UN 1989; DH 2004c).

As this can only be achieved when both parties have had access to all the necessary information and an opportunity to ask questions about any areas of concern, SNs need to be confident, competent and able to explain to young people and their parents why vaccinations are still necessary (HPA 2005). As a result, the SN needs to be well versed on current advice and information on the immunizations that constitute the routine programme from birth to adolescence in the UK, all of which is provided in the *Green Book* (https://www.gov.uk/government/collections/immunisation-against-infectious-disease-the-green-book), which is now only available as an online resource.

The measles epidemic, centred in Swansea in South Wales in 2013–2014, was a result of undervaccination of children due to the now discredited research of Andrew Wakefield in 1998 and the controversy it fuelled regarding the safety of the MMR vaccination. The response was a true multi-agency public health approach which essentially involved SNs who both carried out vaccinations in schools and worked in the very successful mass vaccination clinics that were set up locally on weekends.

Eligible young people should be offered information and a chance to ask questions in sessions provided in their school and offered the opportunity to access individual advice as necessary. Local arrangements and provision for parents and carers to contact their child's named SN to discuss the issues also need to be in place. This will facilitate informed choice (see Chapter 1) and help ensure that local immunization rates are maintained at the level necessary to achieve 'herd immunity' and meet national public health targets. Collaborative working with the local education department and individual schools and staff is essential not least to facilitate provision of mutually agreed minimum requirements of the SN team for immunization sessions held on school premises. Negotiating requirements and working to a standard operating procedure ensures that sessions run smoothly and safely while causing the school as little disruption as possible.

PRINCIPLES FOR PRACTICE

- SNs need to be confident, knowledgeable and up to date when advising children and young people as well as their parents.
- Children, young people and their parents should be given the opportunity to ask questions to facilitate informed choice.

VULNERABLE CHILDREN AND YOUNG PEOPLE: THE ROLE OF THE SN

Vulnerability can result from myriad causes and is not always related to, but often co-exists with, safeguarding concerns. Some children will be identified to the SN by their HV colleague at handover as they are already receiving support, but problems can arise for a child or young person at any time. Issues from family problems and breakdown to poor health can result in increased vulnerability and vigilance to recognize the signs is essential. As already discussed profiling schools' needs informs the SN of issues specific to the particular locality and applying evidence-based tools to assess resilience at an individual level will inform and guide the SN regarding what support needs to be in place to protect some pupils.

When assessing risk and health needs of vulnerable children inter-agency collaboration and effective communication have been evidenced (DfEE 1999, 2006; DH 1999; HO 1999; HM Gov. 2006, 2010; All Wales Child Protection Procedures 2008; Laming 2009) to have positive outcomes for children. Safeguarding the welfare of children and young people is everyone's business and covers promoting children's welfare through to protection of children from maltreatment (DfEE 2006). As public health practitioners SNs are at the forefront of the preventative focus in working with vulnerable children to optimize their chances of health and well-being (WAG 2009; DH 2009b, 2014; DHSSPSNI 2010a, 2010b; Scottish Government 2010; RQIA 2011). It is essential in this regard that SNs access training to raise their awareness and develop their competence to deal with signs of possible child sexual exploitation. Young people may present in drop-in sessions or come to the SN's attention via behaviours in school, and the warning signs must be recognized to help ensure cases such as Rotherham are not repeated and vulnerable young people are protected. As an advocate, in line with (NMC 2015b) professional responsibilities, the SN can negotiate locally to ensure such issues are included for discussion in SRE sessions in school.

Although the vast majority of school-aged children enjoy good health and never require hospital admission or even outpatient attendance, it is not the case for all. Children and young people with special needs ranging from mild to complex medical conditions receive their education in appropriate settings. In 'special schools' for children with profound and complex needs, a children's community nurse is usually based in the school on a permanent basis. As registered children's nurses they have the training and expertise to meet the school-aged child's needs regarding clinical issues including ventilation, medication and enteral feeding.

In mainstream school, children with less complex but specific needs are supported to lead as normal a life as possible by clinical nurse specialists for conditions including asthma, epilepsy, diabetes and dermatological conditions, and Child and Adolescent Mental Health Services (CAMHS) nurses (Neill et al. 2009). Although mental and emotional health is a specialized area SNs are identified as being involved at tier 1 (WAG 2009; RQIA 2011) and their effectiveness in meeting children and young people's needs in this area is reliant on the support and expertise of colleagues in CAMHS and working in close partnership with school-based counsellors. Fostering strong links and excellent communication with colleagues whose expertise provides essential support to pupils with chronic health and mental and emotional health conditions will help to ensure that these young people achieve their full potential during their school years and maximize their health potential for adulthood.

The school-aged child with special needs may also receive input from a variety of medical disciplines and professionals, including speech and language therapists, physiotherapists, occupational therapists and paediatricians. Colleagues in education, including class teachers, classroom assistants, one-to-one support workers, education welfare officers, educational psychologists and peripatetic teachers, are often involved with the school-aged child whether or not they have identified special needs.

It is a prerequisite that SNs acknowledge their competency limits and are aware of colleagues' areas of expertise. They must be aware of the plethora of multi-disciplinary and multi-agency colleagues and professionals and their skills to ensure appropriate and effective support and signposting for their young clients. By forging and maintaining robust links they will, by working in partnership, achieve better outcomes for children and young people.

A discussion to cover the detail regarding the statutory duty and responsibility related to safeguarding requires a chapter to itself. As a result it will not be dealt with in any detail apart from reiterating that safeguarding professional responsibilities take precedence over all other areas of statutory and non-statutory SN practice.

REFLECTION POINT

Consider where and how SNs target and work with vulnerable children and their families.

PRINCIPLES FOR PRACTICE

- SNs can help support vulnerable children and young people and their parents and carers.
- Multi-disciplinary and multi-professional working is essential to meet the needs of vulnerable groups.
- The child or young person with special needs may receive input from a variety of disciplines and professionals.
- It is a statutory duty to be aware of and meet all safeguarding responsibilities.

REFLECTION POINT

Before reading the next section consider which professions or disciplines may be linked with the HV and SN.

MULTI-DISCIPLINARY AND MULTI-PROFESSIONAL WORKING: ROLE OF THE HV AND SN

Essential requirements for team working, if a collective goal is to be achieved, include shared vision, effective inter-agency communication and understanding and valuing each other's roles, particularly the recognition of individuals' responsibilities within roles (Freeman et al. 2000; Bryar and Griffiths 2003). It is important to recognize that some elements of HV and SN practice, particularly related to delivery of Healthy Child Programmes, require clinical and specialist public health nursing skills. It is equally important to be aware that some elements should and can be more effectively delivered by partners or by utilizing a skill mix approach with qualified HVs and SNs taking a leadership role (DH 2009a, 2009b, 2014; DHSSPSNI 2010a; WG 2012; Scottish Government 2012a).

To be effective in a leadership role ensuring that children, young people and their families' needs are addressed by appropriate multi-disciplinary and multi-professional colleagues, HVs and SNs need to be well informed regarding provision in their locality. They need to hone excellent communication skills to facilitate a mutually supportive climate with a collaborative teamwork ethos that essentially keeps the child as the central focus.

Having robust communication and appropriate information sharing, an understanding of each other's role, a willingness to share responsibility and mutual respect will ensure that multi-disciplinary and multi-professional teams collaborate effectively and serve the best interests of the child (Kenney 2002).

The identified role in safeguarding places a responsibility to work in partnership with all agencies involved and particularly social services. As identified earlier, many multi-disciplinary professionals and agencies are involved in providing input with children and families at home, in groups and in schools. The police and fire services often have strong links with the local community and schools, and HVs and SNs should be aware of what they can offer both at the individual and group level as well as on and off school premises and during school holidays.

Voluntary agencies, with a wealth of expertise working with groups and communities, play an essential role in many areas of individual family, community and school-based support and education. The voluntary sector is often the most appropriate people to provide everything from parenting programmes to up-to-date information to young people with regard to alcohol and drug abuse. Youth workers, who are also available outside school in youth clubs, are usually well accepted as relevant by young people and as a result can be invaluable in helping to engage school-aged children in health promotion activities outside school hours and in their local communities.

In fact HVs and SNs should always be mindful that, as specialist practitioners, they should act as the link professional to other professional or voluntary sector colleagues who have more specialized knowledge in specific areas of health promotion which fall outside their area of expertise (Scottish Government 2003; DH 2004a, 2009a, 2009b; NAW 2004; WAG 2009). There will be colleagues locally with far more in-depth and up-to-date knowledge on several subjects, including, for example, drugs and alcohol or dental health, who would be more appropriate and effective in offering input regarding such issues.

The HV and SN responsibility to advocate on behalf of their clients (NMC 2015b) can be effectively applied when engaging with multi-disciplinary colleagues to ensure that the family and essentially the child's voice (UN 1989; DH 2004c) is heard and listened to, especially with regard to service provision (Neill et al. 2009). Information sharing between agencies and partners can be contentious, but information-sharing agreements that meet all partners' governance needs can be negotiated. For example sharing the outcomes of school profiles with local authority education colleagues and ensuring that young people are appropriately represented on all relevant groups will mean that all their previously highlighted rights to involvement are met.

PRINCIPLE FOR PRACTICE

True collaboration with all relevant partners can ensure that the most appropriate support is provided to ensure better outcomes for the children, young people and families that HVs and SNs work with.

ISSUES FOR SCPHN HV AND SN PRACTICE

It has been well documented throughout this chapter that graduate specialist community public health practitioners are well versed in identifying and addressing the needs of children, young people and their families, but HVs and SNs need to keep in sharp focus that public health practice has a political dimension.

HVs and SNs need to work at a political and strategic level to improve services, and in this connection it is imperative that they are aware of and respond to all relevant consultations. Responding enables the process to be utilized as an opportunity to lobby for and advocate on behalf of their young clients' needs in line with their professional responsibilities (NMC 2015a, 2015b). The constant change endured by HVs and SNs in common with fellow practitioners can result in them failing to engage in policy debate, not least because they feel policymakers have no conception of the reality of the service they are attempting to deliver.

There is an identified need for a skill mix approach to delivering services within a finite resource, particularly in times of austerity. As a result it is essential that professionally SCPHNs recognize what can be safely delegated and do not fail to do so due to historic practice or professional protectionism. Delegation will allow them to focus their specialist skills on a leadership role with an overview that will enable them to ensure all necessary and appropriate interventions and support are afforded to meet needs in an equitable fashion.

Changes in policy in England have resulted in SNs, although employed by the NHS, being commissioned by local authorities, and this approach has been extended to HV services since October 2015 (DH 2014). Strong leadership for SCPHN practitioners will be paramount in ensuring they are both involved in and inform progress with this process including those countries where this approach has not been currently adopted.

PRINCIPLES FOR PRACTICE

- SCPHNs need to work at a political and strategic level to improve services.
- SCPHNs must be aware of and respond to all relevant consultations regarding the future of their service.
- Raising the profile of the HV and SN roles at the local and national level is essential to maintain, strengthen and improve services for children, young people and their families.
- The SCPHN is reliant on the collaboration, expertise and support of all who are involved in the life of their young clients and their families.
- Children and young people's nurses may consider a career as a HV or SN.

CONCLUSION

As identified throughout this chapter, the commitment to meeting the needs of children's early and school-aged years in regard to improving outcomes is well documented and evidenced in all four nations that comprise the UK. Notably the move to provision of a standardized child health programme clearly identifies the SCPHN qualified HVs and SNs as having a leadership role in ensuring the programmes are delivered and that appropriate support is offered to meet the needs particularly of the most deprived.

Accessing appropriate government, devolved government and local government websites and professional journals will facilitate maintenance of an informed stance. The profile of SCPHNs needs to be raised at the national level via devolved and central government, and at the local level within the employing NHS organization, local authority and local community level to ensure that their expertise and remit are fully understood and as a result valued. This can lead to much needed support when lobbying locally and nationally for resources to maintain, strengthen and improve services for the children and young people. Lastly, it must be emphasized that both health visiting and school nursing may offer another valuable career opportunity for those who have graduated as a children and young people's nurse.

REFERENCES

Acheson D (1998) *Independent inquiry into inequalities in health report.* London: HMSO.

All Wales Child Protection Procedures (2008) *Local safeguarding boards.* Available at http://www.childreninwales.org.uk/wp-content/uploads/2015/09/All-Wales-Child-Protection-Procedures-2008.pdf.

Allen G (2011) *Early intervention: the next steps.* London: Department for Work and Pensions and Cabinet Office.

Appleton JV, Cowley S (2008) Health visiting assessment processes under scrutiny: a case study of knowledge use during family health needs assessments. *International Journal of Nursing Studies* **45**(5): 682–696.

Bradshaw JR, Holmes J (2010) Child poverty in the first five years of life. In Hansen K, Joshi H, Dex S (eds.) *Children of the 21st century: the first five years.* Vol. 2. UK Millennium Cohort Study Series. Bristol: Policy Press, pp. 13–31.

Bryar RM, Griffiths JM (2003) *Practice development in community nursing. Principles and processes.* London: Arnold Publishers.

Carlile, Lord. (2002) *Too serious a thing. The review of safeguards for children and young people treated and cared for by the NHS in Wales.* Cardiff: National Assembly of Wales.

Chadwick E (1842) Report to Her Majesty's Principal Secretary of State for the Home Department, from the Poor Law Commissioners, on an enquiry into the Sanitary Condition of the Labouring Population of Great Britain. London: Clowes.

Chief Nursing Officer (Scotland) (2013) *CEL 13 2013.* Edinburgh: Scottish Government.

Clark J, Buttigieg M, Bodycombe-James M, et al. (2000) *A review of health visiting and school nursing in Wales.* Swansea: University of Swansea.

Council for the Education and Training of Health Visitors (1977) *An investigation into the principles of health visiting.* London: CETHV.

Council for the Education and Training of Health Visitors (1982) *Principles in practice.* London: CETHV.

Court SMD (1976) *Fit for the future. Report on the Committee on the Child Health Service.* London: HMSO.

Cowley S, Frost M (2006) *The principles of health visiting: opening the door to public health practice in the 21st century.* London: CPHVA.

DeBell D, Buttigieg M, Sherwin S, Lowe K (2007) The school as location for health promotion. In DeBell D (ed.) *Public health practice & the school age population.* London: Hodder Arnold, pp. 93–130.

DeBell D, Tomkins AS (2006) *Discovering the future of school nursing: the evidence base.* London: Amicus/CPHVA.

Department for Education and Employment (1999) *National healthy school standard.* Nottingham: DfEE.

Department for Education and Employment (2006) *Working together to safeguard children. A guide to inter-agency working to safeguard and promote the welfare of children.* London: TSO.

Department for Education and Skills (2003) *Every child matters.* London: Stationery Office.

Department for Education and Skills (2004) *Every child matters: change for children.* London: DfES.

Department of Health (1991) *Working together under the Children Act 1989: a guide to arrangements for inter-agency co-operation for the protection of children from abuse.* London: HMSO.

Department of Health (1996) *The patient's charter: services for children and young people.* London: HMSO.

Department of Health (1997) *The new NHS.* London: HMSO.

Department of Health (1998a) *A first class service: quality in the new NHS.* London: DH.

Department of Health (1998b) *Our healthier nation.* Green paper. London: HMSO.

Department of Health (1999a) *Making a difference.* London: TSO.

Department of Health (1999b) *Framework for the assessment of children in need and their families.* Consultation draft. London: DH.

Department of Health (2000) *Framework for the assessment of children in need and their families.* London: HMSO. Available at http://webarchive.nationalarchives.gov.uk/20130401151715/https:/www.education.gov.uk/publications/eOrderingDownload/Framework%20for%20the%20assessment%20of%20children%20in%20need%20and%20their%20families.pdf (accessed on 25 September 2015).

Department of Health (2003) *Tackling health inequalities — a programme for action.* London: DH.

Department of Health (2004a) *Choosing health.* London: DH.

Department of Health (DH) (2004b) *Securing good health for the whole population* (Wanless Report). London: HMSO.

Department of Health (2004c) *Children Act.* London: DH.

Department of Health (2009a) *Healthy Child Programme pregnancy and the first five years of life.* London: DH.

Department of Health (2009b) *Healthy Child Programme from 5–19 years old.* London: DH.

Department of Health (2009c) *Transforming community services: ambition, action, achievement. Transforming services for health, wellbeing and reducing inequalities.* London: DH.

Department of Health (2011) *Health visitor implementation plan 2011 to 2015: a call to action.* London: HMSO.

Department of Health (2012) *Getting in right for children, young people and families – maximising the contribution of the school nursing team: vision and call to action.* London: DH.

Department of Health (2013a) *Giving all children a healthy start in life.* London: HMSO.

Department of Health (2013b) *Our children deserve better: protection pays – annual report of the chief medical officer (2012).* London: DH.

Department of Health (2014) *Maximising the school nursing team contribution to the public health of school-aged children guidance to support the commissioning of public health provision for school-aged children 5–19.* London: DH.

Department of Health, Home Office, Department for Education and Employment (1999) *Working together to safeguard children: a guide to inter-agency working to safeguard and promote the welfare of children.* London: DH.

Department of Health and Human Services (1980) *Inequalities in health: a report of a research working group* (Black Report). London: HMSO.

Department of Health, Social Services and Public Safety (2010a) *Healthy futures: the contribution of health visitors and school nurses in Northern Ireland.* Belfast: DHSSPSNI.

Department of Health, Social Services and Public Safety (2010b) *Healthy child, healthy future: a framework for the universal Child Health Promotion Programme in Northern Ireland, pregnancy – 19 years.* Belfast: DHSSPSNI.

Douglas J, Earle S, Handsley S, Jones L, Lloyd CE, Spurr S (2010) *A reader in promoting public health challenge and controversy.* 2nd ed. London: Open University Press.

Field F (2010) *The foundation years: preventing poor children becoming poor adults. The report of the Independent Review on Poverty and Life Chances.* London: HMSO.

Freeman M, Miller C, Ross N (2000) The impact of individual philosophies of teamwork on multi-professional practice and the implications for education. *Journal of Interprofessional Care* **14**(3): 237–247.

Gillick v West Norfolk and Wisbech AHA and DOHSS [1985]. London: House of Lords.

Gleeson C (2004) School health nursing – evidence-based practice. *Primary Health Care* **14**(3): 38–41.

Godson R (2014) School nurse 121 campaign. *Community Practitioner* **87**(2): 15.

Hall DMB (1989) *Health for all children: a programme for child health surveillance; the report of the joint Working Party on Child Health Surveillance.* 1st ed. Oxford: Oxford University Press.

Health Protection Agency (2005) *National minimum standards for immunisation training.* London: HPA.

HM Government (2006) *Working together to safeguard children: a guide to inter-agency working to safeguard and promote the welfare of children.* London: HMSO.

HM Government (2010) *Working together to safeguard children: a guide to inter-agency working to safeguard and promote the welfare of children.* London: Department for Children, Schools and Families.

HM Government (2013) *Working together to safeguard children: a guide to inter-agency working to safeguard and promote the welfare of children.* London: Department for Education.

Jameson Report (1956) *Report of the Working Party on the field, training and recruitment of health visitors.* London: DH.

Kenney G (2002) Children's nursing and interprofessional collaboration: challenges and opportunities. *Journal of Clinical Nursing* **11**: 306–313.

Laming, Lord (2009) *The protection of children in England: a progress report.* London: TSO.

Marmot M (2010) *Fairer society, healthy lives: strategic review of health inequalities in England post 2010.* London: Marmot Review.

Munro E (2011) *The Munro review of child protection: final report.* London: Department for Education.

National Assembly for Wales (2004) *National service framework for children, young people and maternity services in Wales.* Full version. Cardiff: NAW.

Neill C, McPake K, Jones SA, Lewis N, Moyse K (2009) National perspectives. In Moyse K (ed.) *Promoting health in children and young people. The role of the nurse.* Chichester: Wiley-Blackwell, pp. 381–397.

NHS Health Scotland (2004) *School health profiling tool.* Available at www.healthscotland.com/documents/2239.aspx (accessed 29 May 2015).

Nursing and Midwifery Council (2015a) *How to revalidate with the NMC. Requirement for renewing your registration and demonstrating your continuing fitness for practice.* Provisional version. London: NMC.

Nursing and Midwifery Council (2015b) *The code.* London: NMC.

Office for National Statistics (2011) *Census.* Available at http://www.ons.gov.uk/ons/rel/census/2011-census/key-statistics-for-local-authorities-in-england-and-wales/index.html (accessed 24 September 2015).

Polnay L (ed.) (1995) *Health needs of the school age child: report of a joint Working Party of the British Paediatric Association.* London: BPA.

Royal College Nursing (2014) *An RCN toolkit for school nurses. Developing your practice to support children and young people in educational settings.* London: RCN.

Regulation Quality Improvement Authority (2011) *Independent review of Child and Adolescent Mental Health Services (CAMHS) in Northern Ireland.* Belfast: RQIA.

Scottish Government (2003) *A Scottish framework for nursing in schools.* Edinburgh: Scottish Government.

Scottish Government (2011) *Health and well-being in schools project final report.* Edinburgh: Scottish Government.

Scottish Government (2012a) *A guide to getting it right for every child.* Edinburgh: Scottish Government.

Scottish Government (2012b) *Getting it right for every child.* Edinburgh: Scottish Government.

Scottish Government (2014) *Children and Young People (Scotland) Act.* London: TSO.

Slack PA (1978) *School nursing.* London: Baillière Tindall.

Tickell C (2011) *The early years: foundations for life, health and learning. An independent report on the early years foundation stage to Her Majesty's Government.* London: Department for Education.

United Nations (1989) *Convention on the Rights of the Child.* Geneva: UN.

Wanless D (2002) *Securing our future health: taking a long term view.* Final report. London: Department of Health.

Welsh Assembly Government (2005a) *Designed for life: creating world class health and social care for Wales in the 21st century.* Cardiff: WAG.

Welsh Assembly Government (2005b) *National service framework for children, young people and maternity services.* Cardiff: WAG.

Welsh Assembly Government (2007) *One Wales. A progressive agenda for the government of Wales.* Cardiff: WAG.

Welsh Assembly Government (2009) *A framework for a school nursing service for Wales.* Cardiff: WAG.

Welsh Government (2011a) *The child poverty strategy for Wales.* Cardiff: WG.

Welsh Government (2011b) Together for health: a five year vision for the NHS in Wales. Cardiff: WG.

Welsh Government (2012) *A vision for health visiting in Wales.* Cardiff: WG.

Welsh Government (2013) *Building a brighter future. Early years and childcare plan.* Cardiff: WG.

Welsh Government (2014) *Children's rights scheme: arrangements of having due regard to the United Nations Convention on the Rights of the Child (UNCRC) when Welsh ministers exercise any of their functions.* Cardiff: WG.

Welsh Government (2015) *Prudent healthcare.* Available at http://gov.wales/topics/health/nhswales/prudent-healthcare/?lang=en (accessed 24 September 2015).

World Health Organization (1978) *Declaration of Alma Ata.* International Conference on Primary Health Care, Alma Ata, USSR, 6–12 September.

World Health Organization (1986) *Ottawa charter for health promotion.* Geneva: WHO.

Community children's nursing

9

RUTH DAVIES AND MARIE BODYCOMBE-JAMES

OVERVIEW

The increasing life expectancy of children with a chronic illness together with legislation that promotes the rights of the child means that the voice of the child must be listened to when decisions are made regarding their health care. Children with a chronic illness are more likely to be hospitalized due to complications or exacerbations of their condition. Research shows that children with a chronic illness do not want to be cared for in hospital but prefer to be cared for at home by a community children's nurse. Repeated hospital admissions for children have been shown to be detrimental to their psychological and physical well-being. However, being cared for at home by a community children's nursing service has been shown to be less stressful, and facilitative of normal family life. This chapter demonstrates the need to increase the availability of community children's nursing teams across the United Kingdom and also how the community children's nurse empowers children with a chronic illness to enable them to develop the knowledge and skills they require to manage their chronic illness at home. To set the scene the chapter begins with a historical overview of the care of sick children to show that care outside of the home is a relatively new development. In doing so it traces the early beginnings of community children's nursing and its continuing development. Present-day scope of practice, using real-life exemplars from research with children themselves, demonstrates that they want to be cared for at home by professionals who provide individualized holistic care.

CARE OF SICK CHILDREN AT HOME

People have always cared for sick children at home. Prior to the early beginnings of children's nursing in the nineteenth century, they would have been cared for by their mothers, female relatives or, as Versluysen (1980) has persuasively argued, 'women healers'. Caring has been seen as a 'virtue' since pre-Christian times, for, as Baly (1987) reminds us, Thucydides writing about the plague that visited Athens in 429 BC refers to the fact that people visited and cared for the sick in their own homes and in doing so lost their own lives.

Likewise, Judaism asserted that it was the responsibility of every Jew to visit the sick, while the prophet Mohammed required his followers to visit sick Muslims as well as non-Muslims. The rise of Christianity across the Mediterranean and Europe and eventual dominance within the Western world saw Christ's teachings on caring for the sick become an accepted Christian duty. Phoebe, commended by St Paul for her visits to the sick and poor, may be regarded as the first Christian role model of a community nurse and one that was emulated by many devout individuals and organizations in the centuries that followed. St Vincent de Paul, in the seventeenth century, with Louise de Marillac set up the Daughters of Charity, an order of French Catholic sisters, who worked outside of the convent caring for abandoned street children as well as the sick poor in their own homes (Purcell 1989). In contrast, in Great Britain no institutionalized discipline focused its work exclusively on the needs of sick children either in hospital or in the community until the nineteenth century (Jolley 2008). By then a small number of religious charities had been set up to care for the sick poor in their own homes. These included the Society of Protestant Sisters set up in 1840 by Elizabeth Fry and her sister, as well as the Sisters of Mercy, a Roman Catholic order, and the Sellonites, an Anglo-Catholic order (Dossey 1999), all of which would have had mixed caseloads of children and adults. Aside from these organizations, a system of outdoor relief was provided for the sick poor under the Old Poor Law, which derived from the time of Queen Elizabeth I. This included nursing care in the home, albeit by untrained nurses. The need to reform this antiquated system became apparent as the century progressed and, as will be shown, both government and individual reformers began to take a keen interest in the welfare of the sick poor on utilitarian as well as humanitarian grounds.

KEY POINT

Throughout history sick children have been cared for at home.

DEVELOPMENT OF DISTRICT NURSING AND HOME CARE FOR THE SICK POOR

By the nineteenth century Britain had evolved from an agrarian society to an industrial one, with a rapidly expanding population which had migrated from the countryside to work in the new industrial cities, towns and conurbations such as Belfast, Manchester, Glasgow, the South Wales Valleys and 'The Potteries'. Between 1751 and 1821 the population of Great Britain had doubled and there were real concerns about overpopulation and the high levels of mortality and morbidity which affected large swathes of the working classes because of overcrowded living conditions, poor sanitation and a general lack of public health. The provision of outdoor relief under the Old Poor Law to help people in times of need such as unemployment and sickness came to be regarded as encouraging a form of welfare dependency (Wilson 2005), and so was replaced by a chain of workhouses with their own purpose-built infirmaries across the country. The intention was to discourage entry by making admission a degrading and inhumane experience so only the most needy and desperate would apply. However, the sick poor denied any form of care within their own homes had no other option, and these infirmaries soon became overcrowded with the chronically ill or incurable cases that the voluntary hospitals rejected. This included large numbers of children who were either orphans or from families that were unable or unwilling to care for them. Many had conditions such as tuberculosis, epilepsy, learning disabilities or mental illness and once admitted were left in the 'care' of female able-bodied paupers under the supervision of paid but untrained nurses recruited from the ranks of maids or labourers (Dossey 1999). Workhouses and their infirmaries became places of dread to the working class, and national scandals reported in the public press that detailed the maltreatment of pauper patients probably prevented many a family from seeking admission for their sick child. This meant inevitably that the majority, apart from those able to gain access to a voluntary hospital, had no health care, with very few having the services of a trained nurse within their homes.

REFLECTION POINTS

- Why were the sick children of the poor treated so harshly in Victorian times?
- Are there any parallels with today's health service? For example, are services still focused on acute and curable conditions rather than chronic and incurable ones?

The precursor to today's community nursing service owes much to the work and vision of two Victorian luminaries, namely Florence Nightingale, who needs no introduction, and William Rathbone, a philanthropist and a member of a wealthy Liverpool shipping dynasty. Rathbone's desire to help the sick poor was based on personal experience when his first wife had been ably nursed at home in her final illness by Mrs Mary Robinson. After his wife's death in 1859, he engaged Mrs Robinson to nurse the sick in some of the poorest areas of Liverpool and it quickly became apparent that more nurses were needed. In 1860, Rathbone wrote to and visited Nightingale to seek her advice on this and sent Elizabeth and Mary Merryweather as observers to the Nightingale School, St Thomas's, London. Four Nightingale nurses returned to Liverpool with the Merryweathers and set up what was in effect the first district nursing service (Stocks 1960).

This system spread to other cities, towns and villages so that by the end of the nineteenth century there was a network of district nursing associations supported by various charities across Great Britain. Many of the great and good supported these, including Queen Victoria, and money raised by the women of Great Britain to commemorate her Jubilee in 1887 was used to set up the Queen's Nursing Institute. Admittance to the ranks of a queen's nurse was stringent, with applicants having to show they had undergone general hospital training and 3 months of training in a maternity hospital or lying-in hospital plus 6 months of training in the practice of district nursing under the tutelage of a trained district superintendent (Craven 1890; Baly 1987). District nurses, regardless of which association they belonged to or whether they were based in cities, towns or villages, had caseloads which included sick children and adults. Given the high childhood morbidity and mortality during this time their workload would have been considerable. Florence Lees, the first superintendent of district nursing, wrote the first handbook for practitioners under her married name of Mrs Dacre Craven, in which she gave practical advice, based on her own extensive experience as a district nurse. In discussing the care of babies and children with diphtheria, croup and bronchitis, she advised a warm and moist atmosphere and suggested that the child's cradle be brought as near to the side of the fire as possible. Recognizing that many of the children visited lacked even the most basic necessities such as a cradle or individual sick bed, she advised, 'An extemporary cradle for a sick child can be made out of clothes-basket or a large drawer, and an extemporary bedstead by arranging chairs back and front alternatively tied together by the legs' (Craven 1890, p. 48).

Mrs Craven also gave advice on caring for cases of scarlet fever, typhoid and smallpox, which were endemic at this time. The many pages devoted by her on the best position for the dying patient as well as 'last offices' highlight the fact that the majority of deaths, including those of babies and children, took place in the family home. Thoughtfulness and compassion toward the patient were evident throughout her book and, as she observed, 'A district nurse must have real love for the poor, and a real desire to lessen the misery she may see' (Craven 1890, p. 13). Their work must have lessened this misery not only through their skilled care of the sick and dying but also in their role as health advisors. This was an important aspect of their role in the days before a health visiting or school nursing service, and it is notable that district nursing associations expected them to teach families not only how to care for their sick relative but also how to provide a clean and well-ventilated environment as well as nutritious meals (Craven 1890; Stocks 1960; Baly 1987).

SURGERY AT HOME AND DAY SURGERY FOR CHILDREN

District nurses were also involved at all stages of the many surgical cases that took place at home on the kitchen or dining room table, including procedures such as tonsillectomies, adenoidectomies and circumcision as well as emergency operations for appendectomies and tracheostomies. There were many cases that voluntary hospitals would not or could not accept, but the positive aspects of surgery at home were not lost on the Victorians or Edwardians, who noted that it caused less family disruption and was often safer (Baly 1987). That children fared better at home cared for by their own mothers was also recognized by James Nicholl, a surgeon at the Glasgow Hospital for Sick Children (1894–1920), who pioneered the use of day surgery for procedures such as pyloric stenosis, hernia and cleft palate to avoid the hospitalization of young children which he not only considered unnecessary but also harmful, involving as it did separation of the child from his mother (Nicholl 1909). In this he was supported by a 'domiciliary nursing service', which enabled children to be discharged home immediately post-surgery where their progress was monitored by daily visits from a team of nurses. Nicholl not only believed that children fared better at home but cannily identified that the cost of day surgery was one-tenth of inpatient care. Sadly, his innovative scheme was not adopted elsewhere and it was to take nearly another 100 years before this was put into practice again.

> **KEY POINT**
>
> Early district nursing teams, funded by charities, had mixed caseloads of children and adults and cared for the sick poor children. Some children's nurses operated outside of children's hospitals but for a fee.

Middle- and upper-class children had access to trained nurses within the home as many voluntary hospitals, including children's hospitals, had a system of providing trained hospital nurses in the home but for a fee. Great Ormond Street Hospital for Sick Children, for example, set up a private domiciliary nursing service to supplement its income that ran successfully from 1888 to 1948 (Hunt and Whiting 1999). Throughout the nineteenth century, with the exception of Wales, voluntary children's hospitals had been built in most of the major cities across Great Britain (Lomax 1996). However, these catered to only a minority of sick children while the majority continued to be housed in workhouse infirmaries. During the 1850s and 1860s Charles Dickens, Florence Nightingale and Louisa Twining campaigned with other reformers against the harsh conditions that prevailed within these, which eventually led to the passing of the Metropolitan Poor Act 1867. This was an important landmark, which, as Abel-Smith (1964, p. 82) noted, acknowledged for the first time 'that it is the duty of the state to provide hospitals for the poor' and effectively paved the way for the National Health Service (NHS) that was to follow 80 years later.

SICK CHILDREN'S CARE DURING THE FIRST HALF OF THE TWENTIETH CENTURY

By the twentieth century improvements had been made in workhouse infirmaries, including the employment of trained nurses. Finally, in 1929, responsibility for these was transferred from the Poor Law Board of Guardians to county and county borough councils. Enlightened councils such as London, Manchester and Birmingham invested in these 'municipal infirmaries' by developing nursing staff and ensuring full-time, salaried medical staff so that, by 1939, these rivalled the elite voluntary hospitals. In the meantime, the majority of children requiring nursing care at home continued to receive this from district nursing teams funded by charitable nursing associations. By the 1930s voluntary hospitals were in serious financial trouble and became fee-charging institutions. The setting up of the Emergency Medical Service for civilians during the Second World War provided a blueprint of what a comprehensive state-funded service could provide. Most nurses, as Baly (1988, p. 44) observed, 'were all too aware of the inequalities of health before the war, particularly the hardship of mothers and children and the everlasting dread of the doctors' bill'. Inevitably, the publication of the Beveridge Report (1942), which outlined a comprehensive NHS, combined with the post-war consensus for a more just and fair society ushered in a Labour government committed to an NHS funded by general taxation, which was duly set up in 1948. This took over responsibility for the care of children in hospital and the community and in the words of Nye Bevan, first Minister of Health, finally put in place an ethos which recognized that 'rich and poor are treated alike … poverty is not a disability and wealth is not advantaged' (Bevan 1953, p. 77).

FIRST STATE-FUNDED 'DOMICILIARY' OR COMMUNITY CHILDREN'S NURSING TEAMS

In 1949, the first publicly funded community-based nursing service for children was set up in Rotherham in an attempt to reduce high infant mortality caused by cross-infection in hospital (Gillett 1954). A more ambitious home care programme operated out of St Mary's Hospital, Paddington, and cared for nearly 3000 children, aged 0–10 years, at home during 1954–1964. This multidisciplinary team comprised a paediatrician, two children's nurses, a student nurse, a medical student, a part-time secretary, a social worker and a physiotherapist. Between them they carried out what, even today, may be described as fairly sophisticated procedures, including lumbar punctures, subdural taps, duodenal intubations, electrocardiography and intravenous infusions. The caseload included newborns with pyloric stenosis, jaundice and prematurity. They also cared for children with acute conditions such as upper respiratory tract infections and gastroenteritis as well as chronic conditions such as cystic fibrosis, asthma and children with cancers. It was concluded that the 'use of the nurse to *support* mothering, rather than take it over, has appeared to have gratifying results in some families' and that the cost of care was roughly one-third the average cost per case of several London children's hospitals (Bergman et al. 1965).

Community children's nursing, or 'domiciliary care' as it was referred to in a paper by Professor Smellie in the *British Medical Journal* of 1956, was now perceived as a means of children avoiding hospitals or having earlier discharge. Reporting on the success of the Birmingham Children's Home Nursing Unit, set up in 1954, he noted that over a 1-year period 454 children were cared for at home, totalling 3295 visits. Only 26 of these required hospital admission, and in some of these cases mothers were unwilling to have their child nursed at home, particularly if, as he noted, they had to go out to work, had large families or lived in overcrowded or inadequate housing. The caseload included conditions such as respiratory infections, tonsillitis, otitis media, abscesses and gastroenteritis. Reflecting their role as health educators as well as 'hands-on nurses', he reported:

> Often the nurses have been called in initially to give an injection of penicillin etc., but they have always seized this opportunity to teach the mother general nursing care and to advise on diet, clothing, general hygiene, and the like.… In particular, evening visits have been found to be the most important in allaying the fears and worries and anxieties of mothers, so that there have been very few emergency calls during the night.

Smellie 1956, p. 256

The publication of the Platt Report (Ministry of Health 1959; Davies 2010a) raised awareness of the adverse emotional effects of hospitalization on children and recommended that they should not be admitted if it could possibly be avoided. Home care was put forward as a better alternative, with both the St Mary's, Paddington, and Birmingham schemes identified as exemplars of good practice (Ministry of Health 1959). Whether children should be cared for at home or in hospital (Essex-Cater 1962) was the subject of much debate within the professions, especially in the light of Illingworth and Knowelden's (1961) study of 22 provincial English hospitals, which showed that paediatric hospital admissions had actually risen from 65,385 in 1950 to 83,184 by 1959. However, despite Platt's recommendation for an increase in home care, which was also reiterated in the court report (Court 1976), this did not happen, and by 1985 there were still only 17 community children's nursing teams in existence across the whole of the UK (Whiting 1985).

EXPANSION OF COMMUNITY CHILDREN'S NURSING TEAMS FROM THE 1980s ONWARD

The number of community children's nursing teams provided across the UK accelerated during the 1980s. Research by Whiting (1985) showed that 22 districts in England provided these, although, as he noted, only two provided a 24-hour, 7-days-a-week (24/7) service. A decade later, Tatman and Woodruffe (1993), in their postal survey across the UK, identified 62 general and 124 specialist paediatric home care services. However, reflecting Whiting's (1985) findings, they found only a few provided a 24/7 service. For the purposes of their study, a general home care service was defined as that provided by paediatric community nurses based in the community, whereas specialist home care was defined as that provided by hospital-based clinical nurses, e.g. paediatric oncology outreach nurses or specialist nurses for conditions such as diabetes. They found that most services lacked a budget within that of the hospital or community where they were based and identified that the boundary between hospital and community created a barrier to an efficient and effective system of care. In 1997, a House of Commons select committee report (House of Commons 1997) expressed concern that less than 50% of children in the UK had access to community children's nursing services, with less than 10% having access to a 24/7 service. This report was strongly in favour of increasing provision, recommending that all children should have access to a 24/7 community children's nursing service and that every GP should have access to a named community children's nurse. However, as Whiting (1998) noted, it did not make any clear recommendations of how these services might be formulated. This has since resulted in services being developed in an ad hoc fashion with a wide range of service models, variation in funding (i.e. through hospital, community or combined hospital–community trusts) as well as management and location of services.

Nevertheless, expansion continued and a factor, as Bradley (1997) has argued, must have been the realization by child care professionals that parents were just as capable of meeting their sick child's needs at home as they were in hospital. The end of this decade and century saw the setting up of 10 Diana Community Children's Nursing Teams to commemorate the life and work of the late Princess of Wales (Davies 1999). These, as well as providing palliative care to children with life-limiting conditions, raised public and political awareness of the need to have dedicated services for children in their homes and communities.

KEY POINT

Community children's nursing teams started to expand rapidly from the mid-1980s onward as successive governments aimed to reduce the hospitalization of children on humanitarian and cost grounds.

By 2000, While and Dyson's (2000) postal survey across the UK found that more than half of the current community children's nursing teams had been founded after 1990, and that there were two dominant models of paediatric home care: the community model with strong links to primary care and the hospital outreach model with strong links to the hospital. Again, reflecting previous findings, few provided a 24/7 service. Furthermore, Eaton (2000), in her review of the literature on community children's nursing services, found six models of paediatric home care delivery: (1) hospital outreach generalists, (2) hospital outreach specialists, (3) community-based teams, (4) hospitals-at-home, (5) district nursing services and (6) ambulatory assessment units. These, as Eaton concluded, had been set up in response to local needs or as a result of hero-innovators and so had not been developed strategically, which may, as noted previously, be traced back to the consistent failure at the government level to make recommendations on how a comprehensive community children's nursing service may be formulated.

It should be noted that until fairly recently health services have been based on professionals' understandings of what children and young people need and meant they were rarely consulted about the services or care they received. Recent research with children and young people by children and young people's (CYP) nurses who are also leading researchers in the field (Pontin and Lewis 2008; Carter and Coad 2009; Bodycombe-James 2012) has done much to inform us about what children and young people really want from the children's community nursing service as well as the children's community nurse (CCN) or CYP nurse who cares for them. As the following section of this chapter will demonstrate, it is vital that CYP nurses continue to research their own practice and undertake research with children and young people for this not only respects their right to be consulted but also takes account of children's agency.

CHILDREN'S AGENCY

Historically children's lives have been described and evaluated almost exclusively by adults. However, the sociology of childhood questions whether children are passive, incomplete and incompetent and instead promotes the view that children are agents in their own right who can shape their own experiences and take control over their own lives (James and Prout 1997; Balen and Blyth 2006; Clark 2010). Legislation such as the Children Act (Department of Health [DH] 1989; DfES 2004) and the United Nations Convention on the Rights of the Child 1989 also promote the importance of ascertaining the wishes and feelings of children regarding decisions that are made about their welfare.

As consumers of health care, children with a chronic or life-threatening illness must therefore be consulted regarding the care they receive as they are no longer the passive outputs of child-rearing practices, but social agents who take part in moulding their childhood experiences (James and James 2004; Jones and

Welch 2010). The Royal College of Nursing guidance *Children and Young People's Nursing: A Philosophy of Care* (RCN 2014a, p. 3) states that all nurses should 'listen to children and young people, providing them with a means for them to convey their opinions and feelings and using these to guide decisions about the way health care is delivered'.

Children are able to determine where they wish to receive care and provide valid reasons as to why this care should be provided at home (Bodycombe-James 2012). Children rate their quality of life as better when cared for at home as opposed to being looked after in hospital (Speyer et al. 2009). This is because children who are cared for in hospital often suffer from home sickness, boredom and loss of control. Being cared for at home by a community children's nurse, however, is more conducive to family life as children are able to eat family meals, have their own possessions around them and spend time with family members. Children with a chronic illness need and want to maintain normality in their lives; to facilitate this they require a flexible CCN service that ensures the continuation of family routines (Bodycombe-James 2012).

Enabling families to maintain their usual life patterns is a significant aspect of the role of the CCN as it leads to less disruption, isolation and conflict for the child and family (Carter 2000). The RCN position paper (2009b) maintains that 'every child and young person has the right to expect care to be provided at home unless they need to be admitted to a hospital environment' (p. 1). However, in the United Kingdom the availability of the CCN service remains limited to a 9:00 a.m. to 5:00 p.m. service from Monday to Friday, which does not reflect a service that is responsive to the needs of sick children and their families (Carter and Coad 2009). Indeed the RCN (2014b) confirms that many locations within the UK still have no CCN service provision and that very few are able to provide a 24/7 service.

> **KEY POINT**
>
> Children have their own opinions about the environment in which they are cared for and are able to provide valid reasons for preferring home care to hospital care.

The following extracts are based on findings from a qualitative study of children's stories of managing their chronic condition at home (Bodycombe-James 2012) and demonstrate the importance of consulting children.

If the nurses did not come I would have to go to hospital for a finger prick. Yes I think that is what I would have to do it would be a bit of a pain every week as it's an hour, it's better that they [CCN] come here it would be a pain to go to hospital once a week. It's better if the nurse comes so I don't miss out on school. When it's a school day she comes to school and takes it. When I am home I have got different places to go after school and do stuff and that's what I like about being home and staying with my pets a fish and cat.

Ellie, age 7, leukaemia

She [CCN] rings my Mum and says I am coming or I am going to be five minutes it [going to hospital] would tire us out a lot we would not have time to do anything we would have to go in the car to hospital a lot more now we can stay at home and the nurse can come and take bloods and then you can go back to doing what you were doing before the nurse came.

Blue, age 9, leukaemia

Providing care at home for children with life-threatening conditions such as cancer means that treatment can be fitted into the family's normal day. This is important as children with cancer do not want the treatment to interfere with the ordinariness of their lives (Stewart 2003). Soanes et al. (2009) conducted a longitudinal exploratory study which aimed to understand the health care experiences of children with a brain tumor and found a preference to home care as opposed to hospitalization.

Children who are cared for at home want more than just clinical care; they want the CCN be interested in their everyday lives, to be cheerful, kind and happy (Bodycombe-James 2012). In order to deliver effective care that is acceptable to the child, it is vital that the CCN develop a relationship with the child and family. It is important that children are valued for who they are, are seen as individuals in their own right and are respected by the professionals who care for them. Carter (2005) in her study also found that children want competent nurses who when caring for them are funny and nice.

Here, three children talk about how they perceive their CCN.

I like her [CCN] she is kind and happy.

Ruby, age 9, cystic fibrosis

She [CCN] is happy when she comes she asks me how my Gran is and how is Tiny [dog].

Alesha, age 11, epilepsy and precocious puberty

She talks to me like what am I doing this week and stuff.

Holly, age 8, growth concern

The provision of care to children in their own homes requires special and comprehensive nursing skills; the role of the CCN is complex and multifaceted and includes facilitating independence in children, building a trusting relationship and the maintenance of continuity of care (Bodycombe-James 2012). Carter (2000) in her qualitative study examined the role and skills of the CCN; results showed that skills such as empathy, compassion, facilitation and listening were thought to be as essential to CCN practice as technical expertise. These skills are the hallmark of an expert practitioner who has a deep understanding of complex situations and knows more than they can say. The work of the CCN is often invisible, and the intricacy and depth of knowledge used when caring for children with complex needs in the community is often not captured. Pontin and Lewis (2008) in a qualitative action research study describe the CCN as a proactive practitioner who aims to promote family independence and maximize continuity of care for the child and family.

Below two children talk about the importance of continuity of care.

I have been looked after at home I see Y [CCN] she comes every few months I was in hospital with food poisoning last year and she was there too.

Jake, age 10, diabetes

My nurse taught her [Mum] in the hospital the same one that comes to the house.

Ruby, age 9, cystic fibrosis

Families who are visited consistently by the same CCN are more likely to develop a trusting relationship which is an essential element of partnership working. Partnership working is one of the key concepts of family-centred care (FCC) which has become the foundation for children's nursing practice. FCC recognizes the central role of the family in the child's life and actively encourages parents to be involved in the care process.

Caring places a heavy responsibility on parents, who run the risk of becoming physically and emotionally exhausted. Community children's nurses can support families by providing practical 'hands-on' care and respite in the home and liaising with health and social services as well as voluntary agencies such as children's hospices. They can also provide an FCC approach to care and, in doing so, support not only the affected child but also their parents, siblings and grandparents. They may take on the role of an 'informed friend' to the whole family, often over many years (Davies 1999); this is a relationship which, while rightly acknowledging parents as the experts in the care of their child, also respects their right to be first and foremost parents rather than just carers. This is a point worth making and is expressed by Blue, a 9-year-old girl with leukaemia, as she describes how the community children's nurse supports her mother.

Because she has taken a bit off Mum as well because my Mum does not have to worry about taking my bloods and she does not have to worry about asking me these questions. Yes well my Mum would have to take all my bloods and things she would have to know well she does know but without the nurse Mum would have to know all my medicines my Mum would have to come to school to take my bloods.

Children with a chronic illness need to go through a transition period where the responsibility for their care moves from the parent to the child. Enabling children with a chronic illness to develop agency in relation to their own health care needs is a significant role of the CCN. The process to successful self-management occurs gradually and the development of autonomy requires the support, encouragement and guidance of the CCN and the child's family. In order to gain independence children with a chronic illness require education about their condition, and to learn the skills necessary to maintain their health. However, children need to do more than master clinical skills to ensure independence; they need to assimilate knowledge and understanding about their condition to ensure they make autonomous informed decisions about their health care needs.

The following extract is from Rhiannon, an 11-year-old girl with diabetes. She describes her CCN as a problem solver and someone who would find her solutions to her problems.

V [CCN] is always there if I need her I can give her a ring. I know she is there whenever I need her I can give her a ring and I can tell her anything and she will give me the solutions of how I can get around doing the solution like when I go out in public. I am having the shakes in the middle of the street or something I feels shy and I was having a 'hypo' in the middle of the street I was shy to do a BM because everyone was watching me but now I am not as shy because I have had help. Yes I do feel if I did not have V I probably would be in a coma now because I would not have had anyone to help me or adjust me because at first me and my Mam when it was new we was a bit unsure what to do and its frightening.

This story shows that the work of the CCN should not be underestimated as they play a vital role in educating and enabling children to manage their chronic illness and develop agency in their lives (Bodycombe-James 2012). Children need to be seen as partners in care if they are going to successfully manage their illness and make autonomous decisions about their health care needs. Being cared for by a CCN empowers children to become self-caring individuals who can manage their condition themselves with the support of the CCN and their family.

KEY POINTS

- The CCN teaches and supports children and parents to manage chronic illness.
- Transition of responsibility from parent to child facilitates independence; facilitating this process is a major role for the community children's nurse.

PROVIDING A COMMUNITY CHILDREN'S NURSING SERVICE THAT MEETS THE NEEDS OF CHILDREN IN THE TWENTY-FIRST CENTURY

The *Future for Community Children's Nursing: Challenges and Opportunities* (RCN 2014b) recommends that a CCN service needs to be provided for four groups of ill and disabled children:

1. Children with acute and short-term conditions
2. Children with long-term conditions
3. Children with disabilities and complex conditions, including those requiring continuing care and neonates
4. Children with life-limiting and life-threatening illnesses, including those requiring palliative and end of life care.

Currently there are too few community children's nursing teams available that can meet the needs of these four groups of children (Carter and Coad 2009; RCN 2009, 2014b; DH 2011) even though there is clear evidence that children prefer to be cared for at home as they find hospitals frightening and boring, have less opportunities for normal development and suffer from homesickness (Bodycombe-James 2012). The Royal College of Nursing (2014b) advocates for a community children's nursing service that is safe, comprehensive and sustainable. The report also recommends that 'for an average sized district, with a child population of 50,000, a minimum of 20 whole time equivalent (WTE) community children's nurses are required to provide a holistic CCN service in addition to any individual child specific continuing care investment' (RCN 2014b, p. 10).

The provision of a comprehensive community children's nursing service can prove to be cost-effective as shown by the *NHS at Home: Community Children's Nursing Services* (DH 2011) report which found that a CCN service in Lambeth, Lewisham and Southwark was able to provide home care at a cost that was between 30% and 50% cheaper than that of hospital care. The report also found that a children's community nursing team in Newcastle provided care for 274 patients in 2008–2009 which resulted in 1996 potential hospital bed/cubicle days saved and the equivalent of £1.1 million in hospital costs. After accounting for staffing and equipment for the community children's nursing team, the potential savings for the NHS was £923,768.

However, some words of caution would seem necessary. Parker et al. (2002), in their systematic review of the costs and effectiveness of different models of home care, question whether it should always be assumed that families necessarily want to provide care at home, especially if it involves 'high technology'. They argue, quite rightly, that just because it may be cheaper for the health service, this is not reason in itself for 'pushing as much care as possible into the home, particularly if it imposes both short and longer-term costs on parents and other children in the family' (Parker et al. 2002, p. 78). Similarly, Noyes (2006), in a helpful and detailed case study of a 12-year-old child with quadriplegia cared for at home on 24/7 ventilation, found the burden of care may well be pushed onto the family, or, in this particular case, a single mother. As Noyes reported, the child in question, Nathan, accessed or used 11 different services and was cared for by 5 different doctors (GP, community paediatrician attached to the special school and consultants in cardiac, orthopaedic and respiratory care). This, in itself, must have involved many separate appointments for there was no single shared health care plan or lead paediatrician. Although Nathan was supposed to receive 24/7 care at home, major problems had been experienced by his mother at weekends and on nights because of staff sickness. Understandably, she had been prescribed antidepressants as she found it difficult to cope with all these demands. Nathan was also affected and felt that he spent too much time with adults rather than with friends his own age. This case study, which probably reflects many others, shows all too well how an inadequate care package benefits neither the child nor the mother, although it may benefit the NHS by savings on expensive hospital care.

In the final analysis, increasing community children's nursing provision is not just about cost savings but also about giving children and their families choice about place of care; as research findings show, most would prefer to be cared for in their own homes and communities. It is also about giving them choice with regard to end of life care at home too, if that is their wish. Research across the developed world has shown that most children and young people prefer to die at home and that most parents also prefer this option (Davies 2009). However, despite this, most children continue to die in hospital because of a lack of CCN provision.

REFLECTION POINTS

- In your present clinical hospital placement or ward, how many children could possibly be cared for at home instead?
- Does your present clinical hospital placement or ward have access to a local community children's nursing team?

CONTRIBUTION TO CARE BY COMMUNITY CHILDREN'S NURSES AND THE CASE FOR EXPANDING PROVISION

Although it is outside the scope of this chapter to describe every role played by community children's nurses, it is clear that their contribution is an increasingly important one in the care of sick children, as reflected by their continuing expansion. A major reason for this has, of course, been the desire by successive governments to reduce the number of children admitted to hospital on both humanitarian and cost grounds. Fewer children are now admitted to hospital and those who are will potentially experience early discharge, with day surgery (Calder et al. 2001) and ambulatory care (Ogilvie 2005) also reducing the number of hospital admissions and length of stay. Hospital-based children's and young people nurses, including specialist nurses, play a crucial role in transferring care to home by liaising and working closely with community children's nurse teams and individual community children's nurses.

PRINCIPLES FOR PRACTICE

Currently all children, regardless of where they live, have access to a hospital. The ideal would be for all children to also have access to a community children's nursing team and only be hospitalized if absolutely necessary.

However, demand for this service continues to exceed supply with Wales, our own country, providing a typical example of the situation that exists in parts of the other three countries that make up the UK.

COMMUNITY CHILDREN'S NURSING PROVISION IN WALES: NOTES FROM A SMALL COUNTRY

Wales has its own government elected by the people of Wales and is responsible for deciding on issues in relation to health, education, language, culture and public services. Wales has its own particular problems with a gross domestic product well below the European average, and parts of west Wales and former mining communities experiencing high levels of deprivation, social exclusion and health inequalities (Osmond 2004). Welsh government policy is refocusing on community-based care with an emphasis on placing the patient at the heart of services (WG 2014, 2015). The Welsh government health care policy is based on the principles of prudent health care which aims to create a patient-centred system ensuring patients receive the most appropriate agreed treatments while recognizing the fact that individuals can make a contribution to their own health and well-being. The Welsh government states that it is committed to providing consistent quality care and services across all geographical areas of Wales (WG 2014).

Wales has a child population (0–15 years) mid-year estimate for 2014 of 554,841 representing 17.9% of the population (Stats Wales 2014), and the Welsh Health Survey 2014 reported that 21% of children in Wales have a long-standing illness, including 6% who have a limiting long-standing illness. The National Service Framework for Children, Young People and Maternity Services in Wales (Welsh Assembly Government 2005) identified the need to develop community children's nursing to provide 'a children's community service available to meet the local needs in every local area of Wales' (Welsh Assembly Government 2005). This also identified the need to provide 'an appropriate range of outreach services as close to home as possible particularly to meet the need of families living in rural Wales' (Welsh Assembly Government 2005). The ideals expressed with these child-specific policy documents are clearly reflected in the more contemporary policies discussed earlier (WG 2014, 2015). In 2010, in response to the Welsh government consultation on community nursing in Wales, the All Wales Community Children's Nursing Forum conducted a scoping exercise to identify the number of qualified community children's nurses who currently practice in Wales (Davies 2009). This found that, although the number of community children's nursing teams had increased over the last 10 years, there were still only 12 working across the whole of Wales, and these teams varied considerably in size. While older and well-established teams such as Gwent (South Wales) have an effective number of community children's nurses, others are small, with some comprising less than one or two WTEs covering vast rural areas in north and mid-Wales. Small teams of one or two community children's nurses are a concern, for, as the Royal College of Nursing (2009a) warns, these are vulnerable in times of staff sickness and may lead to 'burn-out' among staff.

In all, outcomes from the scoping exercise found less than 60 qualified community children's nurses (WTEs) working across Wales, providing hospital-at-home and continuing care to children and young people within their own homes. It highlighted that provision was 'patchy' across Wales with rural areas, in particular, being poorly served. Unsurprisingly, no team was able to provide a 24/7 service, although, anecdotally, some did work outside their contracted hours to meet the wishes of the child and family and provide end of life care at home. The Royal College of Nursing (2009b) has recommended that for a child population of 50,000 a minimum of 20 WTE community children's nurses are required to provide a holistic service. Using this formula, the number in Wales would have to increase, i.e. more than quadruple to 280, based on the current child population of 700,000 to provide such a service. In addition, each community children's nursing team would have to consist of six WTEs to provide a 24-hour service (Forys 2001). It should be emphasized that this 'snapshot' of Wales only reflects what is happening elsewhere and, as identified throughout this chapter, there is an urgent need to increase community children's nursing provision to meet the needs of children, young people and their families across all four countries that make up the UK.

ROLE OF COMMUNITY CHILDREN'S NURSES IN EXPANDING PROVISION: EDUCATIONAL PRIORITIES AND PROFESSIONAL DEVELOPMENT

The Royal College of Nursing (2014b) describes a good community children's nursing service as a safe service with consistency of care, and a comprehensive service that meets local need 7 days a week with 24-hour provision through an on-call service. It also must be sustainable with clear workforce planning and the use of individuals with the right skills available in the locality. For community children's nursing teams and qualified community children's nurses to deliver a service based on these principles, those currently in post must work together to make this happen. This calls upon leaders within the profession to demonstrate and, in doing so, publicize the contribution they make already as well as identifying how further expansion will benefit children and their families. This may be difficult for a profession that is perhaps overmodest and more used to getting on with the job rather than self-promotion, but work at a strategic and political level is vital if children and families are to receive the services they so clearly desire and need. The Royal College of Nursing/ WellChild (2009) initiative has shown that politically there is cross-party support in England for increasing provision, and the same probably holds true for other countries in the UK, which brings us naturally on to the thorny question of funding. Although there may be some savings in transferring care from hospital to home, it will still require a substantial investment and rebalancing of services to provide a 24/7 service across the whole of the UK. In Scotland (RCN 2009c), it was proposed that the £28 million set aside for consultants' merit awards should be used to fund a Scottish community children's nursing service instead, but such a redistribution of wealth is unlikely. In the midst of a worldwide recession, seeking funding on the scale put forward may seem overambitious, but we should recall that the setting up of the NHS in 1948 was also at a time when the nation was experiencing economic difficulties but took place because of the post-war desire for a better society. Investment in a nationwide community children's nursing service may strike a similar chord in the nation's collective conscience given that children are usually perceived as the most deserving of causes and how we care for and treat them as the yardstick upon which any civilized country is measured.

Expansion of services on any scale will mean looking not only at future workforce planning but also at how educational places may be increased at the pre-registration level, this being the pool from which future community children's nurses are recruited. There are a range of community children's nursing programmes across the UK offering post-registration study at the diploma, bachelor and master levels, but an increase in capacity is also dependent on sufficient clinical placements and clinical practice teachers as well as mentors. In parallel with these programmes there must be professional development to support community children's nurses in practice who wish to progress horizontally or vertically. A comprehensive and high-quality community children's nursing service is dependent on a range of roles from staff nurse to advanced practitioner through to consultant. The few consultant community children's nurses who presently practice in the UK have already made a contribution, taking on leadership at a strategic level as well as combining excellence in clinical practice with strong links to education and research, but more are needed if community children's nurses are to develop their own evidence base upon which to continuously improve practice. Those who aspire to become a consultant may be well advised to study at the doctoral level, for possession of a doctorate is likely to be seen as 'essential' rather than 'desirable' for this role in the future (Rolfe and Davies 2009). To this end, educational and career development opportunities need to be made explicit to those considering a career as a children's nurse and as a future community children's nurse if we are to recruit and retain the 'brightest and best'. In Wales, the predominant programme in preparing community children's nurses is the Specialist Practice Qualification (SPQ) Programme, which is based on an amalgam of work by the Scottish government and the Welsh Assembly Government (2009). This clearly sets out the career pathways available to nurses and the levels of education required for practice without losing sight of the fact that caring for children and their families in their own homes and communities is reward in itself.

This chapter has shown how the provision of community children's nurses can prevent hospital admissions and enable earlier discharge. Importantly, this can give children and young people as well as their parents/carers a choice between hospital and home care.

PRINCIPLES FOR PRACTICE

- Community children's nurses must demonstrate their contribution to care at a strategic and political level, and any expansion of service must take into account future educational and professional needs to ensure a comprehensive service that combines practice, education and research.
- Community children's nursing offers another rewarding career opportunity for CYP nurses.
- Continuing research with children and young people by CYP nurses about CCN provision is vital if care and services are to be evidence based.

CONCLUSION

This chapter began by showing that throughout most of history the place of care for a sick child was the family home, and that their removal to other institutions, namely hospitals, only began in the nineteenth century und continued unabated until the Platt Report (Ministry of Health 1959) began to question this practice and advocated home care. Also, while a few community children's nursing teams resulted following the setting up of the NHS in 1948, these did not catch on immediately, and their expansion only started in earnest in the late 1980s owing to changes in professional attitudes toward parental involvement in their sick child's care as well as the desire by successive governments to shift hospital to home on humanitarian as well as cost grounds.

The chapter identified how community children's nurses and their teams make a substantial contribution to the care of children in their own homes in a number of roles. It has also shown that community children's nursing teams have not, in the main, been developed strategically and as a consequence, although every child has access to a hospital, not every child has access to such a nurse or team. This has led to inequity of provision across the UK, with Wales being a prime example. This is regrettable, for, as research and exemplars from practice highlight, this service can make a real difference in terms of choice between hospital and home for the child and family and can provide a family-centred and holistic approach to care. This is reflected in calls from within and outside the profession to increase provision, with the Royal College of Nursing (2009, 2014b) reports still demanding a 24/7 community children's nursing service.

The case for shifting hospital to home has been discussed in relation to children with complex needs with a strong plea being made for this to be for the benefit of the individual child and their family rather than merely a cost-saving exercise for the NHS. The argument put forward throughout this chapter is that children are capable of providing evidence to support their choices with respect to health care, and that research has shown that children with a chronic illness do not wish to be cared for in hospital but prefer to be cared for at home by a community children's nurse. Providing a 24/7 service that is properly funded and underpinned by educational programmes and continuing professional development has also been put forward as a means of ensuring high-quality, evidence-based care. Lastly, in researching this chapter, it is clear that community children's nurses not only have increased in number over the last 10 years but also have made great strides in their practice, education and particularly research, all of which bodes well for their future development and aspiration to provide a comprehensive 24/7 service across the length and breadth of the UK to ensure 'more hands and hearts in the home'.

SUMMARY OF PRINCIPLES FOR PRACTICE

- Children and young people should only be admitted to hospital if absolutely necessary. Both they and their parents/carers must have access to community children's nurses to enable choice between hospital or home care.
- Children should be consulted about their health care preferences.
- Children and young people's nurses, whether based in hospital or in community settings, must work together at a political and strategic level to increase community children's nursing provision.
- Any increase in community children's nursing provision must be matched by an increase in educational provision to ensure a safe, effective and high-quality community children's nursing service.
- Children and young people's nurses must continue to research with children and young people to ensure CCN provision and care is evidence based.

ACKNOWLEDGEMENTS

Marie Bodycombe-James would like to thank all the children from Wales who took part in her research study and who contributed to this chapter.

REFERENCES

Abel-Smith B (1964) *The hospitals 1800–1948: a study in social administration in England and Wales.* London: Heinemann.

Baly ME (1987) *A history of the Queen's Nursing Institute: 100 years 1887–1987.* London: Croom Helm.

Balen R, Blyth E, Calbretto H, Fraser C, Horrocks C, Manby M (2006) Involving Children in Health and Social Research 'Human becomings' or 'active beings'? *Childhood* 13(1): 29–42.

Baly ME (1988) NHS thoughts from home and abroad. *International History of Nursing Journal* **3**(3): 44–6.

Bergman AB, Shand MDH, Oppe TE (1965) A pediatric home care program in London: ten years experience. *Pediatrics* **36**(3): 314–21.

Bevan A (1953) *In place of fear*. London: Heinemann.

Beveridge W (1942) *Report on social insurance and allied services*. London: HMSO.

Bodycombe-James (2012) Children's stories on managing their chronic illness at home. Unpublished doctorate in nursing science thesis, Swansea University, Wales.

Bradley SF (1997) Better late than never? An evaluation of community nursing service for children in the UK. *Journal of Community Nursing* **6**: 411–18.

Calder F, Hurley P, Fernandez C (2001) Paediatric day-case surgery in a district general hospital: a safe option in a dedicated unit. *Annals of the Royal College of Surgeons, England* **83**: 54–7.

Carter, B (2000) Ways of working: CCNs and chronic illness. *Journal of Child Health Care* 4(2): 66–72.

Carter B (2005) They've got to be as good as man and dad: Children with complex health care needs and siblings' perceptions of a Diana community nursing service. *Clinical Effectiveness in Nursing* **9**: 49–61.

Carter B, and Coad J (2009) Community Children's Nursing in England. An appreciative review of CCNs in England.

Clark A (2010) Young children as protagonists and role of participatory, visual methods in engaging multiple perspectives. *American Journal of Community Psychology* **46**(1–2): 115–23.

Court S (1976) *The report of the Committee on Child Health Services: fit for the future*. London: HMSO.

Craven D (1890) *A guide to district nurses and home nursing*. London: Macmillan and Co.

Davies R (2009) Caring for the child at end of life. In Price J, McNeilly P (eds.) *Palliative care for children and families: an interdisciplinary approach*. Basingstoke: Palgrave MacMillan.

Davies R (2010a) Marking the fiftieth anniversary of the Platt Report: from exclusion, to toleration and parental participation in the care of the hospitalised child. *Journal of Child Health Care* **14**(1): 6–23.

Davies R (2010b) Community Children's Nursing Provision 2010: Position paper and scoping exercise. *Nursing Praxis International* (ISBN 1-903625-20-3).

Davies RE (1999) The Diana community nursing team and paediatric palliative care. *British Journal of Nursing* **8**: 506–11.

Department for Education and Skills (2004) *Children Act*. London: Stationary Office.

Department of Health (1989) *Children Act*. London: Stationary Office.

Department of Health (2011) *NHS at home: community children's nursing services*. London: DH.

Dossey BM (1999) *Florence Nightingale: mystic, visionary, healer*. Springhouse, PA: Springhouse Corporation.

Eaton N (2000) Children's community nursing services: models of care delivery. A review of the United Kingdom literature. *Journal of Advanced Nursing* **32**(1): 49–56.

Essex-Cater AJ (1962) The sick child: home or hospital care. *Public Health* March: 157–66.

Forys J (2001) Do children's nurses offer 24 hour care? *Primary Health Care* **11**(6): 31–6.

Gillett J (1954) Domiciliary treatment for sick children. *Practitioner* **172**: 281–3.

House of Commons (1997) *Health Committee Session 1996–7: third report. Health services for children and young people in the community: home and school*. London: HMSO.

Hunt J, Whiting M (1999) A re-examination of the history of children's community nursing. *Paediatric Nursing* **11**(4): 33–6.

Illingworth RS, Knowelden J (1961) The demand on provincial children's hospitals. *Lancet* **1**(7182): 877–9.

James A, James A (2004) *Constructing childhood. Theory, policy and social practice*. Hampshire: Palgrave Macmillan.

James A, Prout A (eds.) (1997) *Constructing and reconstructing childhood: contemporary issues in the sociological study of childhood*. 2nd ed. London: Falmer Press.

Jolley J (2008) The emergence of the 21st century children's nurse. In Hughes J, Lyte G (eds.) *Developing nursing practice with children and young people*. London: Wiley-Blackwell.

Jones P, Welch S (2010) *Rethinking children's rights*. London: Continuum International Publishing Group.

Lewis M, Noyes J (2008) The children's community nurse. *Paediatrics and Child Health* **18**(5): 227–32.

Lomax EMR (1996) *Small and special: the development of hospitals for children in Victorian Britain*. London: Wellcome Institute for the History of Medicine.

Maunder EZ (2004) The challenge of transitional care for young people with life-limiting illness. *British Journal of Nursing* **13**(10): 594.

Ministry of Health (1959) *The welfare of children in hospital*. Platt Report. London: HMSO.

Nicholl JH (1909) The surgery of infancy. *British Medical Journal* 753–4.

Noyes J (2006) The key to success: managing children's complex packages of community support. *Archives of Disease in Childhood* **91**: 106–10.

Ogilvie D (2005) Hospital based alternatives to acute paediatric admission: a systematic review. *Archives of Disease in Childhood* **90**: 138–42.

Osmond J (ed.) (2004) *End of the corporate body: monitoring the National Assembly December 2003–2004.* Cardiff: Institute for Welsh Affairs.

Palliative Care Planning Group (2008) *Report to the Minister for Health and Social Services.* Cardiff: Palliative Care Planning Group.

Parker B, Lovett P, Paisley CA, et al. (2002) A systematic review of the costs and effectiveness of different models of paediatric home care. *Health Technology Assessment* **6**(35): iii–108.

Pontin D, Lewis M (2008) Managing the caseload: a qualitative action research study exploring how community children's nurses deliver services to children living with life-limiting, life-threatening, and chronic conditions. *Journal for Specialists in Pediatric Nursing* **13**(1): 26–34.

Purcell M (1989) *Politics, philosophy and religion: the work of Monsieur Vincent, Life of St Vincent de Paul.* Dublin: Veritas Publications.

Rolfe G, Davies R (2009) Second generation professional doctorates in nursing. *International Journal of Nursing Studies* **46**: 1265–73.

Royal College of Nursing (2009a) *Preparing nurses to care for children at home and community settings.* London: RCN. Available at http://rcn.org.uk.

Royal College of Nursing (2009b) *A child's right to care at home.* London: RCN. Available at http://rcn.org.uk.

Royal College of Nursing (2009c) Spend on services – not consultant awards. *RCN Bulletin*, 17 June.

Royal College of Nursing (2014a) *Children and young people's nursing: a philosophy of care.* London: RCN.

Royal College of Nursing (2014b) *The future for community children's nursing: challenges and opportunities.* London: RCN.

Royal College of Nursing/WellChild (2009) Better at home campaign. Interim report for MP reception, 10 March 2009 House of Commons, hosted by Tom Clarke MP. Available at http://wellchild.org.uk.

Sartain SA, Maxwell MJ, Todd PJ, et al. (2002) Randomised controlled trial comparing an acute paediatric hospital at home service with conventional hospital care. *Archives of Disease in Childhood* **87**: 371–5.

Smellie JM (1956) Domiciliary nursing service for infants and children. *British Medical Journal* **1**(Suppl. 2676): 256.

Soanes L, Hargrave D, Smith L, Gibsin F (2009) What are the experiences of the child with a brain tumour and their parents? *European Journal of Oncology Nursing* **13**: 255–61.

Speyer E, Herbinet A, Vuillemin A, Chastagner P, Briancon S (2009) *Child: Care, Health and Development* **35**(4): 489–95.

Stats Wales (2014) Available at https://statswales.gov.uk/catalogue/population (accessed 18 October 2015).

Stewart JL (2003) 'Getting used to it': children finding the ordinary and routine in the uncertain context of cancer. *Qualitative Health Research* **13**(3): 394–407.

Stocks M (1960) *A hundred years of district nursing.* London: George Allen and Unwin.

Tatman MA, Woodruffe C (1993) Paediatric home care in the UK. *Archives of Disease in Childhood* **69**: 677–80.

Versluysen MC (1980) Old wives' tales: women healers in English history. In Davies C (ed.) *Rewriting nursing history.* London: Croom Helm.

Welsh Assembly Government (2005) *National service framework for children, young people and maternity services in Wales.* Cardiff: WAG.

Welsh Assembly Government (2009) *A community nursing strategy for Wales: consultation document.* Cardiff: WAG.

Welsh Health Survey (2014) Available at http://www.Gov.wales/statistics-and-research/Welsh Health Survey. Accessed on 26 April 2016.

Welsh Government (2014) *Our plan for primary care services in Wales up to March 2018.* Cardiff: WG.

Welsh Government (2015) *Programme for government summary report.* Cardiff: WG.

While AE, Dyson L (2000) Characteristics of paediatric home care provision: the two dominant models in England. *Child: Care, Health and Development* **26**(4): 263–76.

Whiting M (1985) Building a nationwide community paediatric nursing service. *Nursing Standard* **17**: 5.

Whiting M (1998) Expanding community children's nursing services. *British Journal of Nursing* **3**(4): 183–90.

Wilson AN (2005) *The Victorians.* London: Hutchinson.

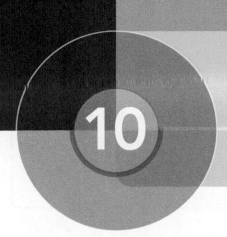

Children and young people's mental health

JULIA TERRY AND ALYSON DAVIES

OVERVIEW

Children and young people's nurses provide a wide range of interventions to children, young people and their families, which include addressing issues pertaining to mental health. Emotional health is part of a child or young person's overall well-being, as neither physical nor mental health exists separately. As most children and young people with mental health problems are managed outside specialized mental health services, all staff who work with them need an understanding of how to assess and address their emotional well-being, identify problems at an early stage and liaise with appropriate services. This chapter is intended as an introduction to the topic of children and young people's mental health issues and begins with a discussion of the role of the children and young people's nurses in relation to mental health. It is widely accepted that a comprehensive, multidisciplinary approach is needed to care for children and young people when they may be at their most vulnerable. While it is recognized that children and young people's nurses often feel they have had little or inadequate training on mental health issues, with support and advice from partner agencies they are often well placed to contribute significantly to the plan of care. It is acknowledged that specialist child and adolescent mental health services teams have limited resources, and therefore focus on serving those with the most severe mental illness. Therefore children and young people's nurses are key players in assessing, planning, implementing and evaluating the mental health of children and young people in their care.

INTRODUCTION

This chapter sets out the risks and protective factors that impact the mental health of children and young people. The provision of child and adolescent mental health services (CAMHS) is also discussed, including the roles that are available to support and advise children and young people's nurses in any mental health work they undertake. Emotional literacy and its context is alluded to as well as the importance of identifying how children and young people learn to understand and manage their feelings, and when a problem may require intervention. This is followed by a brief discussion of three common mental health problems that they may experience – anxiety, trauma and depression – together with some case study examples. There follows a section addressing the importance of communication, boundaries, managing risk and engaging with them in a therapeutic relationship. The chapter concludes by highlighting the need for increased training and education in children and young people's mental health issues for children and young people's nurses and all fields of the nursing profession.

ISSUES FOR CHILDREN AND YOUNG PEOPLE'S NURSES

The foundations for good mental health are laid down in childhood, ensuring that children and young people have the potential to lead positive fulfilling lives and develop resilience and the ability to cope with stressful life events. Their mental health and psychological health are fundamental to their broader health and well-being, as mental health problems significantly compromise the ability to cope, leading to low self-esteem, poor body image, social isolation or exclusion and dysfunctional relationships with the potential for long-term consequences lasting into adulthood (Department for Children, Schools and Families and Department of Health 2008; Parry-Langdon 2008; Department of Health 2009; Patton et al. 2014).

The incidence of mental health problems among young people, especially those who are looked after, is rising (National Institute of Health and Care Excellence [NICE] 2010). Patton et al. (2014) suggest that adolescence is a high-risk phase for the onset of common mental disorders due to complex neurological, psychological and physical developmental changes taking place. Emotional and behavioural disorders are the most frequently occurring problems, with boys and children who experience a serious or chronic condition being significantly more at risk (Bone and Knight 2009; Department for Children, Schools and Families and Department of Health 2009). One in ten children aged between 5 and 16 years has a mental health problem and many continue to have mental health problems into adulthood (Department of Health 2011; Welsh Government 2012). It is suggested that one in five young people suffer with clinical depression and that the rate of self-harm and suicide among them is still alarmingly high with 10%–13% of 15- and 16-year-olds having self-harmed (Department of Health 2011), despite initiatives to reduce the incidence (Green et al. 2005; World Health Organization 2005). Half of those with lifetime mental health problems first experience symptoms by the age of 14 and three-quarters before their mid-20s (Department of Health 2011; Welsh Government 2012; Patton et al. 2014). The increase is multifactorial and symptomatic of the increasingly complex society in which children and young people live and to which they are expected to contribute (Parry-Langdon 2008; Department for Children, Schools and Families and Department of Health 2009; Claveirole 2011).

Mental health issues are key targets on the health and social agenda and require serious attention by all parties involved in caring for children and young people with mental health problems, including children and young people's nurses. Children and young people with mental health problems may be encountered via routes and settings not traditionally associated with mental healthcare, and it is essential to recognize that those admitted to the acute care setting may also have underlying or accompanying mental health issues (Department for Children, Schools and Families and Department of Health 2008, 2009; Royal College of Nursing (RCN) 2014a, 2014b). Physical ill health has been strongly linked to the onset of emotional disorders, with children who experience a serious or chronic condition being twice as likely to develop an emotional disorder. Such children are a visible group for targeted mental health interventions (Valentine and McNee 2007; Lowes 2007; Fuhr and De Silva 2008; Parry-Langdon 2008; RCN 2014a, 2014b). Thus it is vital that children and young people's nurses have knowledge and insight into mental health issues in order to meet the care needs of this vulnerable group.

Perceptions of mental health, publicly and professionally, are important as they influence the care delivered. Mental health problems still carry a stigma which can isolate the child and young person, excluding them from their peer group and mainstream society, thus compromising their self-esteem and social competence (Department for Children, Schools and Families and Department of Health 2008, 2009; Jorm and Wright 2008). In recent years UK mental health charities have recognized that children and young people can suffer greatly from the effects of mental health stigma and have prioritized combating it, e.g. Young Minds – Children and Young People's Manifesto, Mind, Rethink leading Time to Change Campaign, Comic Relief and the Big Lottery Funding (Department of Health 2011). In comparison the response from some health professionals has been less positive and many children and young people who seek their help feel belittled and denigrated by them at a time when they are most vulnerable and already feel stigmatized. Sadly, they may be seen by a professional who has had little experience or training in the care of those with mental health problems (Jorm and Wright 2008; Department for Children, Schools and Families and Department of Health 2009). This is regrettable for it is imperative that the child or young person and their family are treated with dignity and respect by a competent, experienced children and young people's nurse whose professional interests encompass mental health issues (Department for Children, Schools and Families and Department of Health 2008, 2009; RCN 2014a, 2014b).

However, it has been recorded that children and young people's nurses have had strong reservations about caring for children or young people with mental health problems and have a perception that this is best left to the mental health professionals (Watson 2006; Buckley 2010). Some children and young people's nurses feel that they are only trained to care for those with physical healthcare needs and that their knowledge and experience in mental health issues is limited and beyond their professional remit (Watson 2006; Wilson et al. 2007; Buckley 2010). Children and young people's nurses cite lack of experience, confidence and evidence-based knowledge in the care of this client group, and for these reasons feel emotionally challenged, inadequate and vulnerable and are sometimes judgmental of their patients. As a result, they are often uncertain of what is required of them and are overwhelmed by the number and complexity of the cases they face, finding it difficult to transfer knowledge into practice (Watson 2006; Wilson et al. 2007; Buckley 2010). This situation is compounded by the slow rate of recovery in that the outcome of care may never be witnessed by the staff and the client never appears to 'get better' (Buckley 2010; RCN 2014b). This deficit in knowledge, skills and experience only becomes apparent when children and young people's nurses begin to work with an emotionally distressed child or young person and their families (Jones 2004; Watson 2006; Wilson et al. 2007; RCN 2014a, 2014b). Thus it may be argued that mental health nurses should be a part of the nursing team so that the professionals and children and young people benefit from their knowledge and expertise (Department for Children, Schools and Families and Department of Health 2010). However, on a cautionary note it should not be assumed that only mental health nurses should have sole responsibility for the care of those with mental health problems.

At this point we need to ask, 'Whose job it is to care for the mental health of the child or young person?' The response must be that this is not just a mental health or children and young people's nursing issue but a need that can only be met through a wide range of services and professionals. It has to be stated that mental health is everybody's business wherever and whenever children and young people present with needs and is not just the domain of mental health professionals. No one professional has the remit for mental health and it is incumbent upon everyone to meet the needs of the child or young person presenting with mental health problems (Department for Children, Schools and Families and Department of Health 2008, 2010; RCN 2014a). All professionals throughout the children and young people's workforce have an invaluable role to play in identifying mental health issues, promoting and maintaining positive mental health as well as providing help or access to support services (Department for Children, Schools and Families and Department of Health 2008, 2009, 2010). If children and young people's nurses are to care holistically for their patients, then mental health issues must be addressed with as much care and attention as physical health needs and without discrimination. Children and young people's nurses are in a prime position to model positive attitudes toward mental health issues; to promote the psychological and emotional well-being of children, young people and their families; to identify mental health problems; and to lead by example in coordinating and planning compassionate and non-discriminatory care (Wilson et al. 2007; RCN 2014a, 2014b).

PRINCIPLE FOR PRACTICE

The mental health of children and young people is everybody's business.

MENTAL HEALTH PROBLEMS IN CHILDREN AND YOUNG PEOPLE

It is recognized that a comprehensive approach is required across and between agencies, in order to deliver effective mental health interventions to all young people (Department of Health 2011, 2014; Welsh Government 2012). The demand on specialist CAMHS is exceeding capacity, which has had a reputation for lengthy waiting lists (House of Commons Health Committee 2014). It is therefore essential that children's nurses, and other primary care staff, are able to identify less severe mental health issues (Gale and Vostanis 2003). There is a desperate need for early intervention and recognition of these young people's needs (Lowenhoff 2004), so difficulties do not become more complex. It may be seen that such an approach results in a reduction in the financial cost of services, as early intervention by one provider may eliminate later intervention by another, with enormous benefits for the mental health of the child or young person (Department of Health 2011, 2014).

Concerns have been raised about young people exposed to a range of risk factors, including socioeconomic disadvantage, family breakdown, abuse and neglect, which may predict later mental health problems (Hawkins et al. 2000; Callaghan et al. 2003; World Health Organization 2012) (Box 10.1). Traumatic experiences in childhood affect individuals' core beliefs and are likely to compromise future chances of developing healthy and trusting relationships (Gumley and Schwannauer 2006). Findings from three national studies of the lives of people born in 1946, 1958 and 1970 highlight that mental health problems in children and young people have a significant impact on their chances of success in employment and family life, as well as contact with the criminal justice system (Sainsbury Centre for Mental Health 2009). For example, a 'looked after' young person is by definition somewhat separated from his or her family and far more likely to experience a mental disorder, teenage pregnancy and involvement in crime (McAuley and Day 2009). One of the principal aims of the youth justice system is to provide intervention that tackles family, social, educational and health factors which put the young person at risk of offending, and that helps them to develop a sense of personal responsibility (Department for Children, Schools and Families and Department of Health 2009).

Young people are particularly at risk between the ages of 16 and 18 years, so it is vital that health strategies address their needs particularly in relation to sexual health, substance misuse and accident prevention, which directly relate to their mental health (Royal College of Paediatrics and Child Health 2003; Patton et al. 2014). There are particular concerns about young people with mental health problems who require inpatient care and those who make the transition to adult services. In recent years media reports have highlighted concerns over the inappropriate use of adult inpatient beds for young people (Townley and Williams 2009), as well as young people being taken overnight to police cells as an intended place of safety when there has been a lack of appropriate facilities (Department of Health 2014). Likewise, it has been identified that there is frequently a lack of information around transition and that young people have found that adult mental health services may not see them as eligible for a service (Clutton and Thomas 2008). This is sometimes referred to as the cliff edge of lost support (Department of Health 2014) and the scale of the problem is significant for it is estimated that more than 40% of young people have recognizable risk factors (Green et al. 2005), which only serves to identify the need for greater and improved inter-agency working as well as greater clarity of each other's roles in supporting these young and vulnerable young people.

There may be issues within the family setting or context which means that a child is more likely to develop mental health problems (Box 10.2). Additionally, parents who require support may have a sense of guilt and so

---

BOX 10.1: Child risk factors

- Poverty
- Family breakdown
- Single-parent family
- Parent mental ill health
- Parent criminality, alcoholism or substance abuse
- Overt parental conflict
- Lack of boundaries
- Frequent family moves/being homeless
- Overprotection
- Hostile and rejecting relationships
- Parental failure to adapt to the child's development needs
- Death and loss, including loss of friendships
- Caring for a disabled parent
- School non-attendance

Source: Royal College of Nursing, *Children and young people's mental health – every nurse's business*, 2014a, available at http://www.rcn.org.uk/professional-development/publications/pub-004587; Royal College of Nursing, *Mental Health in Children and Young People: An RCN Toolkit for Nurses Who Are Not Mental Health Specialists*, RCN, London, 2014.

BOX 10.2: Family risk factors

- Learning disability
- Abuse
- Domestic violence
- Prematurity or low birthweight
- Difficult temperament
- Physical illness
- Lack of boundaries
- Looked after children
- Lack of attachment to carer
- Academic failure
- Low self-esteem
- Shy, anxious or difficult temperament
- Young offenders
- Chronic illness

Source: Department of Health, *The National Service Framework For Children, Young People and Maternity Services: The Mental Health and Psychological Well Being of Children and Young People*, Standard 9, DH, London, 2004.

refrain from seeking help, meaning that their child's mental health problems often increase in severity until crisis point is reached. This frequently leads to further problems, including increased rates of self-harm, alcohol and substance misuse and the long-term risk of developing adult mental health difficulties (Walker 2008). Therefore early identification of mental health problems is essential.

We have already highlighted in Boxes 10.1 and 10.2 the risk factors pertaining to the child and his or her environment and how this may affect their mental health, so at this point it is also worth considering the part that brain development plays. If there is a history of mental illness within the family, the likelihood of a child developing a mental health problem is greatly increased (Maybery et al. 2009). The experiences a child has during his or her early years can affect brain development, and therefore a child's mental health. From birth, children develop their abilities to express and experience emotions, as well as the capacity to manage a variety of feelings. Traditionally, motor control, cognition and communication receive a lot of attention, while emotional development may have less focus for health professionals. Certainly, families themselves may be less aware of emotional difficulties initially.

The human brain, formed before birth, continues to develop for another 20 years, constantly receiving information from the sensory nervous system to shape its connections and neuronal pathways (Coyne et al. 2010), or, to put it another way, environmental experiences mould the mind. A serious loss of any sensory system or the exposure to severe adverse stimuli can have profound and often permanent effects on the way the brain functions and perceives the world. Sensory deprivation and environmental factors, such as drugs or alcohol at key stages of development, can have a permanent detrimental influence on brain function. Child abuse, be it physical or psychological, has severe implications for brain development, usually with lifelong consequences, and may well threaten the mental capabilities of future generations (Coyne et al. 2010) – hence the importance of parental bonding, play and positive communication in the early years.

PRINCIPLE FOR PRACTICE

Child mental health problems are more likely to develop when a range of social, economic, environmental and familial risk factors are present.

Other external risk factors may impact children and young people's mental health, such as bullying and peer rejection or peer pressure, or situations where discipline is unclear and they are not recognized as individuals (RCN 2014a, 2014b). It is important for staff working with them to have knowledge about the factors that increase the likelihood of mental health problems developing, in order to increase awareness, especially identification of children most at risk. On a more optimistic note, there are also protective factors that enable children to be more resilient and less likely to develop mental health problems (Box 10.3).

> ## BOX 10.3: Protective factors
>
> - Intelligence
> - Being loved and feeling secure
> - Living in a stable home environment
> - Parental employment
> - Good parenting
> - Good parental mental health
> - Activities and interests
> - Positive peer relationships
> - Emotional resilience and positive thinking
> - Sense of humour
> - Full engagement with education
>
> *Source:* Royal College of Nursing, *Children and young people's mental health – every nurse's business*, 2014a, available at http://www.rcn.org.uk/professional-development/publications/pub-004587; Royal College of Nursing, *Mental Health in Children and Young People: An RCN Toolkit for Nurses Who Are Not Mental Health Specialists*, RCN, London, 2014.

PROVISION OF CHILD AND ADOLESCENT MENTAL HEALTH SERVICES

Mental health services for children and young people first emerged in the UK in the 1920s in the form of the child guidance clinic model, with most health authorities providing a basic service by the 1940s. After the birth of the NHS, inpatient and outpatient services began to develop, with medical models of care dominating. It is within the last 20 years that the role of nurses across CAMHS has begun to develop more rapidly, mainly because of changes in roles for social workers and educational psychologists, whose professional time working directly with them has been reduced (Townley and Williams 2009). This has resulted in increased opportunities for nurses, who are now the largest discipline in CAMHS, with many working across the full range of CAMHS. Anywhere that children are, whether this is school, hospital, playgroup or voluntary sector club, children's workers have a responsibility for children's well-being, which includes mental health.

Only 10% of children with emotional and behavioural issues are seen at any one time in specialist CAMHS, with many children's mental health problems managed in primary care or remaining undetected (RCN 2014a, 2014b). National frameworks have been instrumental in setting out a tiered approach illustrating how and where children's mental health needs can best be met (Health Advisory Service 1995; National Assembly for Wales 2001; Welsh Assembly Government 2008). The CAMHS tiered model outlines the different levels at which services working with children and young people operate and contribute toward the promotion of mental health and the care and treatment of this client group (RCN 2014a, 2014b). This four-tiered approach proposed to unite service provision according to the complexity of children's mental health needs, also highlighting the importance of links between the tiers of service (Townley and Williams 2009). The tiered approach is now rooted in the philosophy of service delivery in CAMHS throughout England and Wales (Department for Children, Schools and Families and Department of Health 2008) and has been instrumental in promoting the development of a wide range of services for children and young people. Scotland has implemented the 'Getting It Right for Every Child' (GIRFEC) model (Scottish Government 2004), which emphasizes the responsibility of services to work together to ensure appropriate support, and uses 10 core components and a set of principles based on the Children's Charter for Scotland (2004).

Access to CAMHS should be available to all children and young people, regardless of age, gender, race, religion, sexuality, class, culture or ability (United Nations 1990, 2013; UNICEF 2014). The universal children's workforce includes education, health, social, family and community support; youth justice and crime prevention; sports and culture; and early years, and is sometimes referred to as 'comprehensive CAMHS' (National CAMHS Support Service 2007). Indeed, all staff who work with children and young people work under the CAMHS umbrella. In order to plan care effectively, service delivery and commissioning activity need to be informed by regular audit and multiagency assessment of groups of children and young people with their views sought as well as those of families and stakeholders (Department of Health 2007). This will help meet the mental health needs of children and young people in the most appropriate way.

It is worth recognizing that children and young people's mental health problems can change over time, requiring different help from different levels of service. Notably, teams have sometimes differentiated which service they provide to reflect the educational and training background of those involved. However, what is fundamental is that children and young people receive the most appropriate, and responsive, care for them as individuals, in the most convenient setting for them and their families. In this connection reports have highlighted the worrying state of CAMHS regarding cuts to staff and budgets (Young Minds 2012), and the problems with the commissioning and provision of CAMHS services (House of Commons Health Committee 2014). Sufficient funding across all tiers of CAMHS services is long overdue. Children's services have experienced a 'double whammy' with cuts to CAMHS services and voluntary sector cuts. It is important that future CAMHS service commissioners focus on cost-effective services that are offered as locally as possible, and need to include:

- Universal services, e.g. schools, children's centres and GPs, which will play a pivotal role in promotion, prevention and early detection of emotional well-being and mental health issues, bringing in other professionals as appropriate
- Targeted services, which will provide additional help to particular groups such as children in care or those with learning difficulties or disabilities
- Specialist services, which will meet the needs of children and young people with complex, severe or persistent problems

Each of these elements is essential to effective local provision (Department for Children, Schools and Families and Department of Health 2010).

In terms of referring children and young people to the most appropriate service, it is essential to know the remit of specialist CAMHS at tiers 2–4 (Boxes 10.4 and 10.5).

The delivery of CAMHS is fraught with a number of challenges, including the increasing demand on services and prioritizing who receives a service with limited available resources (Williams et al. 2005). In addition, there have been frequent reconfigurations of service structures, and the commissioning of CAMHS has been slow to develop.

KEY POINT

Child and adolescent mental health services are delivered by a range of different services and are aimed at universal, targeted and specific groups of children.

BOX 10.4: Framework for child and adolescent mental health services

Tier 1: Universal services provided by professionals whose main role and training is not in mental health. This may be in primary care, education and the voluntary sector, who see children with less severe mental health issues, identifying problems early and providing short-term interventions in a variety of settings (e.g. school health nurses, health visitors, children's nurses, GPs, support workers and voluntary sector staff).

Tier 2: Specialist trained mental health professionals, usually working in a uni-disciplinary way (although many also work in Tier 3 services too), with children who have more pronounced mental health problems and may not have responded to intervention at Tier 1. Staff working in Tier 2 may provide training, consultation and advice to Tier 1 (e.g. school counsellors, community mental health nurses and primary mental health workers).

Tier 3: Usually a multidisciplinary team working in a community mental health clinic or outpatient service providing specialized CAMHS service to children who have more severe, complex and persistent mental health problems and disorders, which may be more complex and who need to be seen by members of a multidisciplinary team (e.g. community mental health nurses, psychologists and psychiatrists).

Tier 4: Tertiary-level services for children and young people with the most serious problems, highly specialized teams and inpatient units – children who have very severe mental disorders and require intervention from a specialist, intensive service, which may include forensic units and eating disorder services.

Source: Department for Children, Schools and Families and Department of Health, *Keeping Children and Young People in Mind: Full Government Response to the CAMHS Review*, DCSF/DH, London, 2010.

> ## BOX 10.5: Remit of specialist child and adolescent mental health services
>
> - Psychosis
> - Depressive disorders
> - Attention deficit hyperactivity disorder (ADHD)
> - Autistic spectrum disorders (ASDs)
> - Tourette's syndrome and complex tic disorders
> - Self-harm and suicide attempts
> - Eating disorders
> - Obsessive–compulsive disorder (OCD)
> - Phobias and anxiety disorders
> - Post-traumatic stress disorder (PTSD)
> - Mental health problems secondary to abusive experiences
> - Mental health problems associated with physical health problems and somatoform disorders
> - Behavioural challenges associated with a learning disability
>
> *Source:* Reproduced from Royal College of Psychiatrists, *Building and Sustaining Specialist Child and Adolescent Mental Health Services*, Council report CR137, RCP, London, 2006. With permission.

A helpful role in guiding staff and families around the provision of CAMHS has been that of the primary mental health worker (PMHW). Staff in this role operate at the crucial interface between primary care and Specialist CAMHS (Health Advisory Service 1995), to strengthen and enhance mental health service provision in schools and primary care (Gale and Vostanis 2003). The majority of child mental health problems may be dealt with in primary care with specialist support from PMHWs, through consultation and liaison with Tier 1 workers or direct work with children and their families, or a combination of both (Atkinson et al. 2010) (see case study below).

Early identification of mental health problems and intervention may prevent deterioration and referral onto SCAMHS (Health Advisory Service 1995). The PMHW is well placed to bring both agencies, information and specialist mental health knowledge, together (Dogra et al. 2002) to enable primary care staff to engage in more efficient assessments and to ensure that the needs of children and young people at risk of mental health problems are fully recognized (Department for Education and Skills 2003; Department of Health 2004).

> ## CASE STUDY
>
> Ben is a 12-year-old boy who has been recently diagnosed with diabetes. He recently attended the young person's diabetic clinic and has been referred to Gemma, a local community children's nurse. She is worried about Ben as he has said he feels different to his friends now, and is angry that he has to 'mess about before rugby or going out because of this stupid diabetes'. Ben's mother says he seems embarrassed about the diabetes and does not want to talk about it. Gemma is worried by Ben's lack of self-esteem, that his mood is low and that he will be at risk if he does not learn to look after his diabetes.
>
> On return to the office, she decides to telephone Max, the PMHW, for advice. Gemma discusses Ben with Max, who says Gemma is right to be concerned, and that it would be a good idea to:
>
> - Monitor Ben's mood over the next few weeks
> - Suggest to Ben that he writes down a list of activities he enjoys and, in discussion with his family, starts to think how he can manage his diabetes so he can participate
> - Ben needs to engage in one-to-one time with each parent, to allow time to talk and share his worries
> - Suggest to Ben that he may like to keep a diary of how he is feeling and what he has been doing; this would give Ben and Gemma something to focus on when she visits
> - Contact him again if she is concerned that Ben's emotional health is not improving.
>
> Gemma puts this plan into place when she next visits. After 3 weeks, Ben has learned more about his diabetes, and is more comfortable talking about it. Mum says he has been smiling and talking more, and is more engaged in his usual activities. Gemma, although very familiar with diabetes and some of the emotional effects on children, was glad to ask a colleague for advice and suggestions regarding interventions to improve Ben's emotional health.
>
> Although a simple example, this serves to illustrate the importance of early intervention. The community children's nurse was assessing and monitoring Ben's mental health and providing early intervention, which in this case prevented the situation worsening.

EMOTIONAL LITERACY

Emotional literacy is best defined as the ability to understand, express and manage our own emotions, and respond to the emotions of others in ways that are helpful (Weare 2004). Emotional literacy originates from Goleman's (1995) concept of emotional intelligence. This can be broken down into a combination of five characteristics: self-awareness, managing one's emotions (e.g. handling fear and anxiety), self-motivation, empathy and handling relationships (e.g. conflict) (Osborne 2004). It has been said that emotional literacy defines emotional development in educational terms (Hoyos 2005), recognizing that emotions are an integral part of cognitive development. As the importance of emotional development of children has been recognized (Liau et al. 2003), there has been an increase in emotional literacy programmes, particularly within school settings. Circle time and anger management groups have become common practice in many schools (Hoyos 2005), with a focus on children interpreting emotions in themselves (see the example below).

EXAMPLE OF GOOD PRACTICE

The Student Assistance Programme (SAP) is an early intervention and prevention model through school-based support groups, facilitated by staff over an 8-week period (Watkins 2009). Each course can be tailored to need, e.g. exploring bereavement, divorce and parents with substance misuse issues. The SAP is designed to have a proactive impact on the entire school community, helping with problems that include physical, drug/alcohol and emotional health issues, and has shown evidence of improved grades, decreased illegal drug use, positive peer relationships and improved attendance. In Caerphilly, South Wales, the SAP is supported through consultation and training by the local primary mental health team. This model was developed in the US and has now been rolled out in 30 countries worldwide.

Another initiative, the Emotional Literacy Support Assistants (ELSA) Network, is prominent in England and Wales. Its role is to support children and young people to regulate their own emotions (ELSA Network 2015), with ELSAs usually located in schools.

KEY POINT

Emotional literacy programmes can improve children's mental health, as they learn to understand and recognize their feelings and emotions, and how this affects their relationships with other people.

Children's emotional literacy can be improved by encouraging listening, talking and discussing feelings, using books, stories and pictures. Bibliotherapy is the guided use of reading with a therapeutic outcome in mind (Katz and Watt 1992), and can be as simple as reading, looking through or discussing a book with a child. There are many books available that address the issues that children encounter, including death, divorce, siblings who are ill and moving house. Promoting early discussion of these feelings can prevent problems arising later. Further training on emotional development and emotional literacy for people who work with children and young people in all sectors would increase the likelihood of early identification of mental health problems.

EMOTIONAL AND BEHAVIOURAL PROBLEMS IN CHILDREN AND YOUNG PEOPLE

Although emotional and behavioural problems in young children can be common, it is important to consider the severity and impact of these. Problems such as anxiety, tantrums and poor sleeping patterns may emerge for many reasons, including difficulties with development as well as the parenting the child or young person receives (Thompson 2005). Emotional and behavioural problems may sometimes be mild and short-lived, with no lasting impact, and can be identified by a change in their mood, such as sadness or anger, whereas behavioural problems are usually noticed by a difference in actions, such as sleeping or eating problems. Some problems can be identified by a trigger or precipitant, such as a change or an adjustment reaction (Dogra and Leighton 2009). A child or young person may show a difference in their mood or behaviour after moving school or house, experiencing the death of a family member or pet, experiencing bullying or knowing a family member or friend is ill. Although, as set out in Box 10.6, it is possible to indicate at what point the situation may become a problem, it is not always possible to identify why this occurs at a particular time.

Parents may have difficulties with children who continually cry, have eating problems, have difficulty sleeping, have wetting or soiling problems or have temper tantrums. In the main, these are not considered mental health problems, unless they persist over time, in which case parents and carers are best advised to seek help through primary care or paediatric referral.

The following sections cover three common mental health problems: anxiety, trauma and depression, which may exist on their own or be the basis of a more complex mental disorder (more severe mental health issues, such as eating disorders, self-harm and suicide, are discussed in Chapter 11).

ANXIETY

Anxiety and fear are powerful emotions that have a strong effect on our minds and bodies (Mental Health Foundation 2009). This can be useful in emergency situations and is often called the 'fight or flight' response, as the increase in adrenaline helps us to run away or stay and deal with the situation at hand. It is a natural response to a perceived threat, and in small doses can be useful when we are faced with non-dangerous situations, such as examinations, dates or meeting new people. Indeed, children and young people's nurses would expect a child or young person to experience some level of anxiety before an appointment or coming into hospital. Box 10.7 lists common symptoms of anxiety that children may experience.

However, feelings of anxiety can last much longer, and commonly occur in school-aged children (see the case study below), sometimes resulting in social isolation, interpersonal difficulties and impaired school adjustment (Rubin et al. 2009). This can lead to children becoming overwhelmed by fear and wanting to avoid situations that might make them frightened or anxious. Anxiety is at the root of a number of mental health problems, including phobias, panic attacks, generalized anxiety disorder, separation anxiety, social anxiety and obsessive–compulsive disorder. The main aim is for the child or young person to learn to cope with the anxiety so it no longer affects them and prevents them enjoying life. In terms of co-morbidity, depression is eight times more likely to be present in young people who have an anxiety disorder (Costello et al. 2004).

CASE STUDY

Chelsea is 9 years old; she has told her school teacher that she feels worried every morning because she does not like to leave her mother at home on her own. Chelsea's attendance has been poor this term, and she has missed many school days. Chelsea says when she thinks about leaving the house she feels hot and shaky and sick. She has been referred to the school health nurse.

BOX 10.7: Symptoms of anxiety in children and young people

- Physical signs: Headache, nausea, raised blood pressure, increased heart rate, vomiting, pain, diarrhoea, needing to urinate more often, poor sleep, feeling faint or dizzy, changes to breathing, sweating
- Psychological signs: Feeling nervous or afraid, sense of apprehension or distress, having difficulty concentrating, hard to make decisions, feeling tired and irritable
- Behavioural signs: Avoiding people or situations, isolating self or becoming more clingy, constantly seeking reassurance, pacing around, not being able to settle to an activity

REFLECTION POINTS

- What could be the cause of Chelsea's worried feelings before school?
- How would you approach this with Chelsea and her mother?

Parents may be unsure whether their child's behaviour is something to be concerned about or whether it is typical behaviour for a child of that age. For many years it was believed that children did not experience anxiety or depression, and that those who appeared to were just malingering or attention seeking. This has changed and it is now widely accepted that as many as one in six children and adolescents suffer from anxiety that affects their ability to get on with their lives (Young Minds 2015).

A child's world can be a frightening and unpredictable place, and the same holds for young people, who experience a time of rapid physical and emotional change. Feelings of anxiety, misery and worry are common, and they can be particularly sensitive to what happens around them, sometimes feeling things that happen are their fault (such as rows or parents becoming ill). These feelings can lead to further anxiety and guilt, as not all children's emotions are logical. It is usual for small children to have fears about the dark, insects, ghosts, kidnappers and getting lost; usually children grow out of these, but they can persist as the child gets older (Mental Health Foundation 1997).

Anxious children can be irritable and demanding, and a real worry for parents. In addition to this, it often takes a lot of patience for parents to see that behind the difficult behaviour there is anxiety and uncertainty. It is common for parents to respond angrily to their children's behaviour, when what the children need is for their parents to be calm and to know exactly how they are feeling and why (Huberty 2009). If parents appear not to understand, children can feel ignored, which may exacerbate their difficult behaviour. During the period of adolescence there is much uncertainty, which can produce anxiety in both children and their families. Anxiety symptoms may include overeating or undereating, excessive sleepiness and overconcern with appearance, and some will experience phobias and panic attacks. Adolescents' anxieties often relate to relationships, financial concerns and educational performance (Rogers and Dunsmuir 2015). Although the majority will experience feelings of unhappiness at times that are all part of adolescence, there will be a minority who go on to develop more serious problems.

Panic can happen even when there is no immediate threat, and these are often called 'panic attacks' (Black et al. 2005). Panic attacks are one of the most common psychological problems in the Western world, affecting 2%–3% of the population in any one year. Many people get over this with no need for treatment; when treatment is required, it is usually short and often successful (Hands on Scotland 2009). A child or young person experiencing these distressing feelings and thoughts is often not really aware why they feel so frightened. If panic attacks happen regularly they can start to interfere with normal daily activities such as school and social life. This can add to distress and lead to the child avoiding things or places that they may associate with a time when they experienced panic. This avoidance might be called agoraphobia, school phobia or social phobia, depending on which area of the child's life is affected.

Agoraphobia, as with adults, is when a child or young person fears open space, queues and public places, which may affect their school attendance. Social phobia can mean that people fear talking or eating in public or just being looked at, which can result in the young person not being able to face other people at all. School phobia is when the individual develops a powerful fear of attending school and finds themselves unable to leave home and go to school, which highlights the question of whether the child or young person is refusing to attend school as opposed to refusing to leave home, or whether both these factors are interacting (Rethink 2016). How this problem is resolved is significant, as to whether treatment should be directed primarily toward returning the individual to school or resolving parent–child relationships in the home. After a significant absence from school, e.g. after a lengthy illness, it is understandable that a child or young person may fear returning to school. However, they can also develop more irrational phobias which appear to have no trigger or source. Generalized anxiety disorder is present in about 3% of children (World Federation for Mental Health 2008), who experience persistent anxieties and worries that are unrelated to any particular event or situation.

A third of adults who have obsessive–compulsive disorder find that it started when they were in childhood (Basu and Padmore 2009). Obsessions are repetitive thoughts that crowd the mind and are difficult to get rid of (even though the person knows they may make no sense). These obsessions prompt compulsive rituals such as counting, handwashing or cleaning, which are intended to ward off such thoughts or deal with the anxieties (Krebs and Heyman 2010). For instance, children may feel they have to say goodnight to their toys nine times or they might die in their sleep. While child development and learning theory often encourages parents to develop routines with children, e.g. dinner time, followed by a bath, a story, then saying goodnight, these are simply patterns of living that promote safety and security. Obsessive rituals can be unpleasant and much more distressing.

> ### PRINCIPLE FOR PRACTICE
> Anxiety in children that is persistent can be debilitating and can have a profound effect on family and peer relationships, education and day-to-day functioning.

TREATMENT FOR CHILDREN AND YOUNG PEOPLE WITH ANXIETY PROBLEMS

The most important intervention when working with an anxious child or young person is to encourage them to be calm and to explain what is happening and why their body has 'gone into overdrive'. Simple explanations can help the child realize that things may feel overwhelming, but that they will soon feel better and are not alone in experiencing these symptoms. It is common for people with anxiety or panic to feel that they may faint or die, and simple deep-breathing techniques can help the child or young person regain control.

During the past two decades, much progress has been made in treating those experiencing anxiety; cognitive behaviour therapy (CBT) has emerged as the treatment of choice (Krebs and Heyman 2010), whether in individual or group format. During CBT children are taught to cope with anxious feelings and thoughts, and to learn increased positive self-talk and relaxation techniques (Muris et al. 2009).

TRAUMA

Children and young people experience events that are unplanned and significant, which may include traumatic experiences such as sexual, physical or emotional abuse; violent crime; suicide; assault; or even natural disasters such as floods or fires as well as medical procedures. Non-fatal injuries occur in 10 million to 30 million children each year (World Health Organization 2008), and research suggests that 14%–43% of these have experienced at least one traumatic event in their lifetime that can have lasting effects on their mental health. Indeed, children and young people's nurses will encounter children and young people all the time who have experienced trauma, in the form of illness or accident, and this will have a different impact on each individual, according to their own situation.

Some children and young people may experience short-term anxieties after a trauma that improve quickly, whereas others experience long-term problems such as depression, anger, haunting memories and regressive behaviour (Veenema et al. 2002). Reactions can occur immediately after the event or weeks later (International Society for Traumatic Stress Studies 2009) (Box 10.8). They may play in ways that repeat something from their traumatic experiences (e.g. hiding from an attacker or escaping from a threat) and recreate aspects of the traumatic experience in their behaviour, which can be important to help them process and think about what has happened. Children and young people may display sadness, have less emotion or feel guilty about things they did or did not do related to the traumatic experience. These thoughts may not be verbalized, and it is important that distress is identified by parents and carers.

The greater the severity of the trauma, the greater the likelihood of the child or young person developing problems. They may go on to develop post-traumatic stress disorder, and this can be screened for using

> ### BOX 10.8: How children and young people respond to trauma
>
> - Young children (age 5 years and younger): May experience new fears such as separation anxiety or fear of strangers or animals. They can become clingier or may act like a younger child.
> - School-aged children (6–11 years): May get parts of the traumatic experience confused or out of order when recalling the memory. They may complain of body symptoms that have no medical cause (e.g. stomach aches). They may stare into space or startle easily.
> - Adolescents (12–18 years): May experience visual, auditory or bodily flashbacks of the events, have unwanted distressing thoughts or images of the events, demonstrate impulsive and aggressive behaviours, or use alcohol or drugs to try to feel better. They may feel depressed or have suicidal thoughts.
>
> *Source:* International Society for Traumatic Stress Studies, *Children and trauma*, 2009, available at https://www.istss.org/

BOX 10.9: Coping with trauma in children and young people

- Create a safe environment
- Provide children with reassurance and extra emotional support
- Be honest with children about what happened
- Monitor exposure to the media (if the event was publicized)
- Try to put the event into perspective

Source: Cardiff Council, *Coping With Trauma in Children: Some Practical Advice,* Cardiff and Vale Traumatic Stress Initiative: Cardiff, 2009, available at https://www.cardiff.gov.uk/ENG/Your-Council/Strategies-plans-and-policies/Emergency-Planning-and-Resilience/Emergency-Planning-and-Resilience/Documents/Coping_with_trauma_in_children.pdf.

the Child Trauma Screening Questionnaire (Kenardy et al. 2006). If close family members were extremely distressed after the trauma, this may have an impact on them. Additionally, risk increases if the event is an interpersonal trauma (caused by another person), such as rape or assault, or if the child or young person has been exposed to numerous stressful life events in the past or has a pre-existing mental health problem. For all these reasons, it is crucial to support them at this time, as set out in Box 10.9.

Children and young people's nurses at some time in their career may care for a child or young person who has experienced trauma and can support both them and their family during this difficult time, as shown in the case study below.

CASE STUDY

Emily (aged 6) saw her mother hit by a car on a zebra crossing. Emily's mother was not badly hurt, and mostly had bruises and grazes from the accident. Emily talks about the accident at school, and the teacher suggests Emily see the school health nurse, as Emily has been drawing pictures of people being hit by cars in class.

Donna, the school health nurse, makes time to sit with Emily and her mother to make sense of what has happened and how children can react after a traumatic event.

Emily's mother was reassured to hear that experiencing nightmares, talking a lot about the incident and re-enacting the trauma were behaviours often necessary to help children start to come to terms with what had happened.

Donna encouraged Emily's mother to:

- Talk with Emily about what had happened in a way that Emily could understand
- Invite Emily to play or draw what had happened if Emily wanted to
- Seek support for herself as a parent, to ensure she had others to support her
- Notice any concerns or changes in Emily's behaviour that may be present after a few weeks, and to seek further advice if she was concerned

While it is often said that children are resilient and cope with change, traumas will occur in all families, and it can be hard to predict how children will respond to them. Children and young people's nurses need to consider the thoughts, feelings and potential anxieties of children at all times. How trauma is talked about and managed will affect the child's current and future mental health (Box 10.9). As nurses we are in a primary position to encourage family discussion, provide age-appropriate information and provide support to children and their families.

PRINCIPLE FOR PRACTICE

Children who have experienced trauma need to feel safe, supported and have age-appropriate information about their traumatic experience.

DEPRESSION

The majority of children and young people will feel 'low' or 'down' at times, as this is a normal reaction to stressful experiences. However, if these feelings continue or begin to interfere with the child's day-to-day activities this can deteriorate into depression. In the early 1980s, many psychiatrists believed children did not experience depression because they lacked the emotional maturity to feel hopeless. Depression probably affects 1 in every 200 children under 12 years old and 2 or 3 in every 100 teenagers (Royal College of Psychiatrists 2005). Although figures are variable for young people experiencing depression, with reports of between 4% and 20%, there is evidence that there is an increase in children and young people experiencing depression in the last three decades (Green et al. 2005).

A higher incidence of depression has been found in children and young people whose parents are not working or have no educational qualifications, or are in a lone-parent family (Green et al. 2005). While no direct causes have been found in children and young people who come from homes where families have separated, research has shown that there does appear to be a link, as the incidence of emotional problems in this group is significantly higher (Office for National Statistics 2016). This suggests that sociological as well as genetic and environmental factors are linked to depression (Walsh 2009). The concept of 'learned hopelessness' has been influential in childhood research, as a child may learn an expectation of hopelessness or helplessness within the family, leading to negative thinking and ultimately depression (Thompson and Nelson 2005). Signs and symptoms of depression are set out in Box 10.10.

Depression is still not understood clearly, but we do know that some children and young people are more at risk, particularly those who have a physical illness, have experienced abuse or come from a home where there is family breakdown or refugee status. Depression can lead to academic difficulties and social isolation, and can create relationship problems with family and friends. Depression in children is also associated with an increased risk of suicide. It has been estimated that more than 90% of children and young people who complete suicide had a depressive illness. The risk is greatest among young men if accompanied by alcohol or substance misuse (Rethink 2016). Suicide is discussed in greater detail in Chapter 11.

WHAT CAUSES DEPRESSION?

Depression can occur for many reasons, with events or personal experiences often acting as a trigger, such as bereavement or loss, bullying, neglect or a physical illness. Depression may also be triggered if too many changes happen in a child or young person's life too quickly. They are also more at risk if they have no one to share their worries with and lack practical support (see Box 10.11 for further risk factors). Depression seems to be linked with chemical changes in the part of the brain that controls mood. These changes prevent normal functioning of the brain and cause many of the symptoms of depression shown in Box 10.10.

TREATMENT FOR DEPRESSION

The National Institute of Health and Care Excellence Quality Standard for depression in children and young people is a useful template in identifying the steps in treating it (NICE 2013). The guidelines cover assessment and identifying risk, through to recognition and treating mild, moderate and severe depression.

BOX 10.10: What are the signs of depression?

- Having a depressed mood most of the day, nearly every day (children and young people are often irritable rather than sad)
- Having no interest in activities that used to be fun
- Losing weight, gaining weight or having a change in appetite
- Having problems sleeping or needing too much sleep
- Feeling restless or sluggish
- Being tired and having no energy
- Feeling worthless or guilty for no reason
- Having trouble concentrating or making decisions
- Thinking about death or suicide

BOX 10.11: Risk factors for children

- Past psychosocial risk factors, such as age, gender, family discord, bullying and physical, sexual or emotional abuse
- Co-morbid disorders, including drug and alcohol use
- A history of parental depression, significant loss and multiple risks, e.g. homelessness, refugee status and living in institutions

There is clear guidance as to when the child or young person should be referred on to specialist services for assessment (NICE 2013).

For those with moderate to severe depression, as a first-line treatment, a specific psychological therapy should be offered, such as individual CBT or family therapy, for at least 3 months. Antidepressant medication should only be offered in conjunction with current psychological therapy, and monitoring arrangements must be made to observe for adverse drug reactions and to review the child's mental state (NICE 2013) and progress.

> **PRINCIPLE FOR PRACTICE**
>
> Depression in children may arise from a number of risk factors or triggers, and requires prompt assessment and treatment.

COMMUNICATION, BOUNDARIES AND MANAGING RISK

COMMUNICATING WITH CHILDREN AND YOUNG PEOPLE

It is important that all children and young people's nurses have the ability to talk with and engage with children and young people, and although this may be something that you do on a daily basis, it needs careful thought and skill. Whether in a community or hospital environment, there may be certain staff who are employed to work with children and young people for a specific purpose with regard to mental health, such as play therapists or psychologists. However, we all have the ability to engage with them and need to build on these essential skills, while recognizing that there are times we need to engage with the services of other staff.

All children and young people's nurses engage in work with children and young people that has therapeutic value, which may be as simple as talking with them about favourite toys and hobbies, depending on their age and their health condition (Box 10.12). The ease with which we engage with each child or young person will vary enormously.

Using play media and art means the child and young person can explore their own thoughts and stories, which helps them understand their experiences and gain greater resilience. Play media with children may include sand tray work, water, puppets, clay, books and soft toys, which can help them learn about feelings and increase their emotional literacy. In addition to talking with children and spending time with them, using play therapeutically can be one of the most important interventions in preparing children for painful or invasive procedures, as demonstrated in the example of good practice below. Play therapy provides developmentally appropriate ways to facilitate children's coping strategies when faced with the stresses of being in hospital (Goymour et al. 2000). There are a number of useful activities that children and young people's nurses can use to get to know children and encourage them to help explore their feelings, such as 'the feelings pie' as described by Sori and Biank (2006). For this, a child is asked to draw a circle and make six or eight sections, and then label these happy, sad, angry, proud, worried, etc., thus leaving the child or yourself space to include other relevant feelings. The child can then name, write or draw in the sections in response to, for example, 'tell me a time when you feel happy'. This leads to the child discussing a wide variety of situations and relationships within their life, is of great therapeutic value and helps to identify areas where there may be problems.

> **BOX 10.12: Important points when engaging in therapeutic work with children and young people**
>
> - Know how to create appropriate boundaries
> - Consider different ways of working through the use of play and the creative arts
> - Remember that therapeutic work can help children and young people make sense of current and past experiences
> - Contemplate how therapeutic work can add to the actual assessment
> - Understand that this can be a valuable part of their care

IMPROVING COMMUNICATION BETWEEN CHILDREN AND YOUNG PEOPLE AND HOSPITAL STAFF: AN EXAMPLE OF GOOD PRACTICE

In Leicester, third-year medical students (the 'teddy doctors') work alongside children to 'look after' poorly or injured teddy bears. This play with a purpose provides a chance to reduce the fear and anxiety that children may feel on either being admitted to hospital themselves or visiting a sick relative. Each child has an appointment with the teddy doctor and, through role play, they have treatments for teddy and get a certificate and teddy gets a sticker. The doctors answer questions, as this is also a learning experience which has an impact on emotional development as fear is reduced. Familiarizing children with the hospital through fun helps them to clarify and demystify their worries, know what the instruments are and how they may be used, and know who the staff are and how they would help. Likewise, the scheme helps medical students to improve their communication skills with children. Such a scheme could be easily adapted across a range of settings where children and young people's nurses work including students.

BOUNDARIES AND MANAGING RISK

It is essential that all people working with children and young people do so in a way that is appropriate to the child or young person's age and ability as well as level of development and understanding. It should also be in a way that is consistent with organizational policies, practices and procedures, and within regulatory and legislative frameworks. The Nursing and Midwifery Council Code (Nursing and Midwifery Council 2015) states that nurses must make the care of people their first concern, treating them as individuals and respecting their dignity; this includes maintaining clear professional boundaries.

A child-centred approach is vital, and a values-based approach must be demonstrated in terms of equality of opportunity and inclusivity, which demonstrates respect for children, young people and their families. It is vital to acknowledge that children are often discriminated against, and their ideas, rights and experiences are often considered less important than those of adults (Pavord et al. 2014). Core nursing values include human dignity, integrity, autonomy, altruism and social justice (Fahrenwald et al. 2005). It is important for us as nurses to have an awareness of our own underlying values, beliefs and principles. This can help us to identify, reflect on, review and apply personal and professional boundaries in relation to our care of children and young people. At times you may need to set achievable goals and boundaries with or for children and young people, and it is important that they and their families understand them. For example, this may relate to behaviour that is challenging, where it is important that boundaries are consistently applied. You can act as a good role model by ensuring that your own actions and behaviour are appropriate. Children and young people need to know what behaviour is acceptable, and learn to recognize and understand their own behaviour and its consequences.

As nurses we too must know our limitations, and not overstretch ourselves. Engaging with a child or young person about emotional health can be challenging at times. However, if we keep in mind good safeguarding practices, we will serve to keep the child safe, observe confidentiality and liaise with other members of the multidisciplinary team, who are best placed to work with the child or young person and their family. It is vital that children and young people's nurses are aware of those who are most at risk of harm, and those who may develop mental health problems, in order to safeguard them and plan the most appropriate care. Agreed protocols are essential in order to effectively manage the interface between CAMHS and other agencies, which will clearly set out the respective roles and responsibilities of those involved in a child or young person's care (Department of Health, Social Services and Public Safety 2008), thus strengthening joint working. In order to protect and promote their health and well-being this must also include managing risk (Nursing and Midwifery Council 2015).

PRINCIPLES FOR PRACTICE

- Communicating and developing therapeutic relationships is the key to finding out more about children and young people's emotional well-being.
- Identifying and managing risk is fundamental for mental health practice.

NEED FOR INCREASED TRAINING AND EDUCATION ABOUT MENTAL HEALTH ISSUES IN CHILDREN AND YOUNG PEOPLE FOR ALL NURSES

The need for robust and rigorous education in children and young people's mental health is a recurrent theme addressed in a number of policy and research documents (Department for Children, Schools and Families and Department of Health 2008; Welsh Government 2012, 2013; RCN 2014a, 2014b). What emerges with distinct clarity is that children and young people's nurses perceive their training and education with regard to this as inadequate and preventing them from caring effectively for children and young people with mental health problems. This would appear to emanate from pre-registration nursing education, resulting in a lack of confidence, evidence-based knowledge, experience and the necessary skills and abilities to deal with complex issues in order to effectively support the children, young people and their families (Watson 2006; Wilson et al. 2007; Buckley 2010). Such research highlights the need for ongoing multidisciplinary education at all levels. This must be addressed in pre-registration nursing programmes and the curricula should address this highly pertinent issue throughout the course for all students and not just during specialized placements (Department for Children, Schools and Families and Department of Health 2008, 2010; Department of Health 2009; Welsh Government 2012, 2013; RCN 2014a, 2014b). Several educational initiatives have demonstrated the value of interdisciplinary teaching, illustrating that where students are exposed to intensive, interactive, experiential learning about mental health issues, they develop positive attitudes. Such an approach facilitates the sharing of evidence-based knowledge and experience which can be honed and developed (Curtis 2007; Happell et al. 2008; Happell 2009; Terry et al. 2009).

It is essential that the skills and competencies of the CAMHS workforce at all levels of service provision meet the mental health needs of children and young people. The children and young people's nurse has a vital role in ensuring a multidisciplinary approach to care is adopted so that professional boundaries are broken down, enabling practitioners to communicate effectively across all sectors (Mental Health Foundation 2006; Department for Children, Schools and Families and Department of Health 2008, 2009; Department of Health 2009; RCN 2014a, 2014b; Welsh Government 2012, 2013, 2015). Professional roles, responsibilities and access to services must be transparent to the child, young person and their families. Children and young people's mental healthcare is an integral part of the role of all children's nurses across the diverse settings in which they work; it is every nurse's business (Department for Children, Schools and Families and Department of Health 2008; Nursing and Midwifery Council 2015; Welsh Government 2012, 2013, 2015; RCN 2014a, 2014b). Lastly, in order to address the mental health needs of children and young people nurses need increased pre- and post-registration training opportunities to assist them to develop skills and expertise in this area and across all healthcare settings (Townley and Williams 2009).

PRINCIPLE FOR PRACTICE

It is essential that education about children and young people's mental health and well-being is provided at the pre-registration and post-registration level to ensure that children and young people's nurses can deliver competent and compassionate care.

Children and young people's nurses need to seek out training opportunities to better understand mental health issues.

CONCLUSION

This chapter began by highlighting that the mental health of children and young people is everybody's business, and it has been shown that even though children and young people's nurses may feel unprepared for this, they may, through a collaborative approach with other agencies, contribute positively toward it. This chapter has also drawn attention to the individual, familial and environmental risk factors that may be present in children's and young people's lives and the need to have an understanding of the way CAMHS are structured to ensure that the individual child or young person and their family can access the most appropriate help. A number of interventions, such as advice from the primary mental health worker, parent support groups and emotional literacy programmes, have demonstrated that these can make a real difference to a child's mental health and that it is essential to take opportunities to promote the resilience of vulnerable children and their families.

This chapter has also discussed how anxiety, trauma and depression are common mental health problems which may require short-term support or referral on to a more specialist service. In this respect, the importance of engaging and communicating with children and young people cannot be overstated, as this forms the basis of a therapeutic relationship, and is central to the work of the children and young people's nurse. Identifying problems at an early stage and managing risk may be viewed as safeguarding children and young people as this has the potential to prevent problems escalating. On reflection, it may be stated that all children and young people's nurses are engaged in supporting the mental health needs of children and young people in whatever setting they may practice, and how we engage with them has a great bearing on their overall emotional and mental well-being and is integral to our care and practice.

SUMMARY OF PRINCIPLES FOR PRACTICE

- Everyone who works with children and young people in whatever setting has a responsibility for their mental health. Child and adolescent mental health is everybody's business.
- Emotional literacy programmes offer a range of opportunities for children to recognize and understand their feelings and relationships, increase their self-esteem and reduce the stigma associated with mental health problems.
- Early identification of a child's or young person's mental health problem leads to early intervention and may prevent problems becoming worse for both them and their family at a later stage.
- Children and young people who experience mental health problems need to feel safe and supported and to have age-appropriate information which may help them and their families understand the situation. Professionals need to identify and manage risk effectively when working with the individual child or young person.
- The training and education of all nurses, particularly children and young people's nurses, in the mental health issues that affect children and young people is essential if the individual child or young person is to receive the compassionate and informed care they are entitled to.

REFERENCES

Basu R, Padmore J (2009) Mental health problems in childhood and adolescence. In Norman I, Ryrie I (eds.) *The art and science of mental health nursing*, 2nd ed. Milton Keynes: Open University Press.

Black S, Donald R, Henderson M (2005) What is a panic attack? Available at http://www.scotland.gov.uk/Resource/Doc/98780/0023930.pdf.

Bone D, Knight D (2009) The mental health of children and young people: the EMHA role. *Community Practitioner* **82**: 27–30.

Buckley S (2010) Caring for those with mental health conditions on a children's ward. *British Journal of Nursing* **19**(19): 226–30.

Callaghan J, Pace F, Young B, Vostanis P (2003) Primary mental health workers within youth offending teams: a new service model. *Journal of Adolescence* **26**: 185–99.

Cardiff Council (2009) Coping with trauma in children: some practical advice. Cardiff: Cardiff and Vale Traumatic Stress Initiative. Available at https://www.cardiff.gov.uk/ENG/Your-Council/Strategies-plans-and-policies/Emergency-Planning-and-Resilience/Emergency-Planning-and-Resilience/Documents/Coping_with_trauma_in_children.pdf.

Claveirole A (2011) Setting the scene. In Claveirole A, Gaughan (eds.) *Understanding children and young people's mental health*, Chapter 1, pp. 4–28. London: Blackwell Publishing.

Clutton S, Thomas M (2008) Mental health provision for 16 and 17 year olds in Wales: policy and practice briefing. Cardiff: Barnardo's Cymru.

Costello E, Egger H, Angold A (2004) Developmental epidemiology of anxiety disorders. In Ollendicdk T, March J (eds.) *Phobic and anxiety disorders in children and adolescents: a clinician's guide to effective psychosocial and pharmacological interventions*. New York: Oxford University Press.

Coyne I, Neill F, Timmins F (2010) Clinical skills in children's nursing. Oxford: Oxford University Press.

Curtis J (2007) Working together: a joint initiative between academics and clinicians to prepare undergraduate nursing students to work in mental health settings. *International Journal of Mental Health Nursing* **16**(4): 285–93.

Department for Children, Schools and Families and Department of Health (2008) *Children and young people in mind: the final report of the National CAMHS Review*. London: DCSF/DH.

Department for Children, Schools and Families and Department of Health (2009) *Healthy lives, brighter futures: the strategy for children and young people's health*. London: DCSF/DH.

Department for Children, Schools and Families and Department of Health (2010) *Keeping children and young people in mind: full government response to the CAMHS review*. London: DCSF/DH.

Department for Education and Skills (2003) *Every child matters*. Nottingham: DfES.

Department of Health (2004) *The national service framework for children, young people and maternity services: the mental health and psychological well being of children and young people*. Standard 9. London: DH.

Department of Health (2007) *The national service framework for children, young people and maternity services: the mental health and psychological wellbeing of children and young people*. Standard 9. London: DH.

Department of Health (2009) *New horizons: towards a shared vision for mental health – consultation*. London: DH.

Department of Health (2011) *No health without mental health: a cross-government mental health outcomes strategy for people of all ages*. London: DH. Available at https://www.gov.uk/government/uploads/system/uploads/attachment_data/file/213761/dh_124058.pdf.

Department of Health (2014) *Closing the gap: priorities for essential change in mental health*. Available at https://www.gov.uk/government/uploads/system/uploads/attachment_data/file/281250/Closing_the_gap_V2_-_17_Feb_2014.pdf.

Department of Health, Social Services and Public Safety (2008) *Standards for child protection services*. London: DHSSPSNI.

Dogra N, Leighton S (2009) *Nursing in child and adolescent mental health*. Milton Keynes: Open University Press.

Dogra N, Parkin A, Gale F, Frake C (2002) *A multidisciplinary handbook of child and adolescent mental health for front-line professionals*. London: Jessica Kingsley.

Egeland B, Kalkoseke M, Gottesman N (1990) Pre-school behaviour problem: stability and factors accounting for change. *Journal of Child Psychology and Psychiatry* **31**(6): 891–909.

Emotional Literacy Support Assistants Network (2015) *ELSA Network building for success*. Available at http://www.elsanetwork.org/.

Fahrenwald N, Bassett S, Tschetter L, et al. (2005) Teaching core nursing values. *Journal of Professional Nursing* **21**: 46–51.

Fuhr D, De Silva M (2008) Physical long-term health problems and mental comorbidity: evidence from Vietnam. *Archives of Diseases in Childhood* **93**: 686–9.

Gale F, Vostanis P (2003) The primary mental health worker within child and adolescent mental health services. *Clinical Child Psychology and Psychiatry* **8**(2): 227–40.

Goleman D (1995) *Emotional intelligence*. New York: Bantam Books.

Goymour K, Stephenson C, Goodenough B, Boulton C (2000) Evaluating the role of play therapy in the paediatric emergency department. *Australian Emergency Nursing Journal* **3**(2): 10–2.

Green H, McGinnity A, Meltzer H, et al. (2005) *Mental health of children and young people in Great Britain 2004*. London: Palgrave Macmillan.

Gumley A, Schwannauer M (2006) *Staying well after psychosis: a cognitive interpersonal approach to recovery and relapse prevention*. Chichester: John Wiley.

Hands on Scotland (2009) *Anxiety*. Available at http://www.handsonscotland.co.uk/topics/anxiety/panic.html.

Happell B (2009) Influencing undergraduate nursing students' attitudes towards mental health nursing: acknowledging a role for theory. *Issues in Mental Health Nursing* **30**: 39–46.

Happell B, Robins A, Gough K (2008) Developing more positive attitudes towards mental health nursing in undergraduate students, part 3: the impact of theory and clinical experience. *Journal of Psychiatric Mental Health Nursing* **15**(7): 527–36.

Hawkins JD, Herrenkohl TI, Farrington DP, et al. (2000) *Predictors of youth violence*. Washington, DC: Office of Justice Programs, Office of Juvenile Justice and Delinquency Prevention.

Health Advisory Service (1995) *Together we stand*. London: HMSO.

House of Commons Health Committee (2014) *Children's and adolescents' mental health and CAMHS*. Third report of session 2014–2015. Available at http://www.publications.parliament.uk/pa/cm201415/cmselect/cmhealth/342/342.pdf.

Hoyos C (2005) Emotional development and emotional literacy. In Cooper M, Hooper C, Thompson M (eds.) *Child and adolescent mental health: theory and practice*, pp. 21–7. London: Hodder Arnold.

Huberty T (2009) *Anxiety and anxiety disorders in children: information for parents*. Available at http://www.nasponline.org/resources/intonline/anxiety_huberty.pdf.

International Society for Traumatic Stress Studies (2009) *Children and trauma*. Available at https://www.istss.org/.

Jones J (2004) *The post registration education and training needs of nurses working with children and young people with mental health problems in the UK*. London: Royal College of Nursing.

Jorm AF, Wright A (2008) Influences on young people's stigmatising attitudes towards peers with mental disorders: national survey of young Australians and their parents. *British Journal of Psychiatry* **192**: 144–9.

Katz G, Watt J (1992) Bibliotherapy: the use of self help books in psychiatric treatment. *Canadian Journal of Psychiatry* **37**: 1730–8.

Kenardy JA, Spence SH, Macleod AC (2006) Screening for posttraumatic stress disorder in children after accidental injury. *Pediatrics* **118**: 1002–9.

Krebs G, Heyman, I (2010) Treatment resistant obsessive-compulsive disorder in young people: assessment and treatment strategies. *Child and Adolescent Mental Health* **15**(1): 2–11.

Liau A, Liau A, Teoh G, Liau M (2003) The case for emotional literacy: the influence of emotional intelligence on problem behaviours in Malaysian secondary school students. *Journal of Moral Education* **32**: 51–66.

Lowenhoff C (2004) Emotional and behavioural problems in children: the benefits of training professionals in primary care to identify relationships at risk. *Work Based Learning in Primary Care* **2**: 18–25.

Lowes L (2007) Impact upon the child and family. In Valerntine F, Lowes L (eds.) *Nursing care of children and young people with chronic illness*. London: Blackwell Publishing.

Maybery D, Reupert A, Patrick K (2009) Prevalence of parental mental illness in Australian families. *Psychiatric Bulletin* **33**(22): 26.

McAuley C, Day T (2009) Emotional well-being and mental health of looked after children in England. *Child and Family Social Work* **14**(2): 147–55.

Mental Health Foundation (1997) *The anxious child: a booklet for parents*. London: MHF.

Mental Health Foundation (2006) *Truth hurts*. London: MHF.

Mental Health Foundation (2009) *What is fear and anxiety*. London: MHF. Available at https://www.mentalhealth.org.uk/publications/overcome-fear-anxiety.

Muris P, Mayer B, den Adel M, et al. (2009) Predictors of change following cognitive-behavioural treatment of children with anxiety problems: a preliminary investigation on negative automatic thought and anxiety control. *Child Psychiatry Human Development* **40**: 139–51.

National Assembly for Wales (2001) *Child and Adolescent Mental Health Services: Everybody's Business*. Cardiff: National Assembly for Wales.

National CAMHS Support Service (2007) *Learning perspectives from the National Child and Adolescent Mental Health Service Improvement Programme*. Available at http://www.chimat.org.uk/resource/view.aspx?RID=58397

National Institute for Health and Care Excellence (2010) *Looked after children*. PH28. NICE: London.

National Institute for Health and Care Excellence (2013) Depression in children and young people. QS48. Available at https://www.nice.org.uk/guidance/qs48/chapter/list-of-quality-statements.

Nursing and Midwifery Council (2015) *The code: professional standards of practice and behaviour for nurses and midwives*. London: NMC.

Office for National Statistics (2016) *Measuring National Well-being: Life in the UK: 2016*. Available at https://www.ons.gov.uk/peoplepopulationandcommunity/wellbeing/articles/measuringnationalwellbeing/2016

Osborne S (2004) Can we teach emotional literacy? *Mental Health Nursing* **24**(2): 20.

Parry-Langdon N (2008) *Three years on: survey of the emotional development and well-being of children and young people*. Newport: Office for National Statistics.

Patton GC, Coffey C, Romaniuk H, MacKinnon A, Carlin JB, Degenhardt L, Olsson CA, Moran P (2014) The prognosis of common mental disorders in adolescents: a 14 year prospective study. *Lancet* **383**: 1404–11.

Pavord E, Williams B, Burton M (2014) Values, attitudes, beliefs and inequalities when working with children, young people and their families. In Burton M, Pavord E, Williams B, *An introduction to child and adolescent mental health*. London: Sage.

Rethink (2016) *Depression: factsheet*. Available at https://www.rethink.org/resources/d/depression-factsheet.

Rogers A, Dunsmuir S (2015) A controlled evaluation of the 'FRIENDS for life' emotional resiliency program on overall anxiety levels, anxiety sub-type levels and school adjustment. *Child and Adolescent Mental Health* 20(1): 13–19.

Royal College of Nursing (2014a) *Children and young people's mental health – every nurse's business*. Available at https://www2.rcn.org.uk/__data/assets/pdf_file/0005/587615/004_587_WEB.pdf.

Royal College of Nursing (2014b) *Mental health in children and young people: an RCN toolkit for nurses who are not mental health specialists*. London: RCN.

Royal College of Paediatrics and Child Health (2003) *Bridging the gaps: healthcare for adolescents*. Royal College of Psychiatrists Council Report CR114. London: RCPCH.

Royal College of Psychiatrists (2005) *Depression in children and young people*. Factsheet 34. London: RCP.

Royal College of Psychiatrists (2006) *Building and sustaining specialist child and adolescent mental health services*. Council report CR137. London: RCP.

Rubin KH, Coplan RJ, Bowker JC (2009) Social withdrawal in childhood. *Annual Review of Psychology* **60**: 141–71.

Rutter M (1986) Meyerian psychobiology, personality, development, and the role of life experiences. *American Journal of Psychiatry* **143**(9): 1077–87.

Sainsbury Centre for Mental Health (2009) *Childhood mental health and life chances in post-war Britain*. London: Sainsbury Centre for Mental Health.

Scottish Government (2004) *Protecting Children and Young People – The Charter*. Available at http://www.gov.scot/Publications/2004/04/19082/34410.

Smari J, Petursdottir G, Portsteindottir V (2001) Social anxiety and depression in adolescents in relation to perceived competence and situational appraisal: panic attacks, phobias, and obsessive compulsive disorder (OCD). *Journal of Adolescence* **24**: 199–207.

Sori C, Biank N (2006) Counselling children and families experiencing serious illness. In Sori C (ed.) *Engaging children in family therapy: creative approaches to integrating theory and research in clinical practice*. Abingdon: Routledge.

Terry J, Maunder EZ, Bowler N, Williams D (2009) Interbranch initiative to improve children's mental health. *British Journal of Nursing* **18**(5): 282–7.

Thompson M (2005) Problems in young children. In Cooper M, Hooper C, Thompson M (eds.) *Child and adolescent mental health: theory and practice*, pp. 73–109. London: Hodder Arnold.

Thompson M, Nelson R (2005) Mood disorders. In Cooper M, Hooper C, Thompson M (eds.) *Child and adolescent mental health: theory and practice*, pp. 120–5. London: Hodder Arnold.

Townley M, Williams R (2009) Developing mental health service for children and adolescents. In Dogra N, Leighton S (eds.) *Nursing in child and adolescent mental health*, pp. 181–92. Milton Keynes: Open University Press.

UNICEF (2014) *Advancing the CRC*. Available at http://www.unicef.org/crc/index_protocols.html.

United Nations (1990) *Convention on the Rights of the Child*. Available at https://treaties.un.org/Pages/ViewDetails.aspx?src=TREATY&mtdsg_no=IV-11&chapter=4&lang=en.

United Nations (2013) *Convention on the Rights of the Child in Wales*. Cardiff: University of Wales Press.

Valentine F, McNee P (2007) Context of care and service delivery. In Valentine F, Lowes L, *Nursing care of children and young people with chronic illness*. London: Blackwell Publishing.

Veenema TG, Schroeder-Bruce K (2002) The aftermath of violence: children, disaster, and posttraumatic stress disorder. *Journal of Pediatric Health Care* **16**(5): 235–44.

Walker S (2008) The challenge of child and adolescent mental health. *British Journal of School Nursing* **3**(7): 349–52.

Walsh L (2009) *Depression care across the lifespan*. Chichester: Wiley-Blackwell.

Watkins C (2009) *Student assistance program*. Available at http://www.cwsap.com/.

Watson E (2006) CAMHS liaison: supporting care in general paediatric settings. *Paediatric Nursing* **18**: 30–3.

Weare K (2004) *Developing the emotionally literate school*. London: Sage.

Welsh Assembly Government (2008) *Annual operating framework CAMHS targets 2008–2009:* Cardiff: WAG.

Welsh Government (2012) *Together for mental health: a strategy for mental health and well-being in Wales*. Cardiff: Welsh Government. Available at http://gov.wales/docs/dhss/publications/121031tmhfinalen.pdf.

Welsh Government (2013) *Breaking the barriers: Final report*. Cardiff: Welsh Government. Available at http://www.cmryu.org.uk.

Welsh Government (2015) *Talk to me 2: suicide and self harm prevention strategy for Wales 2015–2020*. Cardiff: Welsh Government. Available at http://gov.wales/topics/health/publications/health/reports/talk2/?lang=en.

Williams R, Rawlinson S, Davies O, Barber W (2005) Demand for and use of public sector child and adolescent mental health services. In Williams R, Kerfoot M (eds.) *Child and adolescent mental health services: strategy, planning, delivery and evaluation*, pp. 445–70. Oxford: Oxford University Press.

Wilson P, Furnivall J, Barbour RS, et al. (2007) The work of the health visitor and school nurse with children with psychological and behavioural problems. *Journal of Advanced Nursing* **61**(4): 445–55.

World Federation for Mental Health (2008) *Understanding generalised anxiety disorder. An international mental health awareness packet.* Available at http://wfmh.com/wp-content/uploads/2013/11/WFMH_GIAS_ UnderstandingGeneralizedAnxiety.pdf.

World Health Organization (2005) *Child and adolescent injury prevention: a global call to action.* Geneva: WHO.

World Health Organization (2008) *Preventable injuries kill 2000 children every day.* Available at http://www. who.int/mediacentre/news/releases/2008/pr46/en/index.html.

World Health Organization (2012) *Adolescent Mental Health.* Available at http://apps.who.int/iris/bitstream/ 10665/44875/1/9789241503648_eng.pdf.

Young Minds (2012) *Survey reveals worrying state of CAMHS.* Available at http://www.youngminds.org.uk/ news/news/1182_survey_reveals_worrying_state_of_camhs.

Young Minds (2015) *Anxiety and phobias.* Available at http://www.youngminds.org.uk/for_children_ young_people/whats_worrying_you/anxiety.

Caring for children and young people with complex mental health problems

ALYSON DAVIES AND JULIA TERRY

OVERVIEW

This chapter discusses from a national and international perspective a number of complex mental health problems which the children and young people's nurse may encounter among the children and young people who attend healthcare settings. The topics include suicide, self-harm, anorexia nervosa, autistic spectrum disorders and attention deficit hyperactivity disorder. The incidence and causative and contributory factors will be discussed, highlighting the role of the children and young people's nurse within the therapeutic relationship that should occur between the nurse and patient. The discussion draws on the relevant research and policy to inform the debate and provide further reading material for practice. This chapter should be read in conjunction with 'Children and Young People's Mental Health' (Chapter 10) as complex mental health problems are influenced significantly by the issues raised in this chapter. Depression, anxiety and emotional disorders are contributory factors in more complex problems. Also, the role of the children and young people's nurse and his or her knowledge and expertise are interwoven with the issues raised in this chapter, as it is often the quality of their education and skills concerning mental health issues which influences the care delivered to the patient with complex mental health problems.

INTRODUCTION

It is widely recognized that the incidence of complex mental health problems is increasing among children and young people (Department for Children, Schools and Families and Department of Health 2008, 2009, 2010; Department of Health 2011; Patton et al. 2014; Welsh Government 2012). It can be argued that psychological pressures on young people have increased, with high value being placed on academic achievement, personal success and material acquisition; all of these can oppress children and young people, affecting their mental health as they strive to cope with their development and fit into a modern society which can appear toxic to their well-being. Health professionals have a heightened awareness and knowledge of such issues and so diagnosis, support and interventions can be offered at an earlier stage than was done so previously. This is pertinent to the diagnosis of neurodevelopmental disorders such as autistic spectrum disorders (ASDs) and attention deficit hyperactivity disorder (ADHD), in which early diagnosis and intervention ensure that timely support is offered to the child, young person and their family. It is this early recognition and support which is a key issue for all children's nurses and those working with children and young people who have mental health problems. It is imperative that children and young people's nurses have insight and knowledge of complex mental health problems and their causative and contributory factors so that sensitive care can be delivered and the appropriate support offered to enable the child and young person to cope and develop positive mental health (Price et al. 2014; Royal College of Nursing [RCN] 2014a, 2014b).

SUICIDE IN YOUNG PEOPLE

Worldwide, suicide is the second leading cause of non-natural death in young people and is a significant social and public health problem and a matter of national and global concern (Welsh Government 2015; World Health Organization [WHO] 2014, 2016). Suicide accounts for 8.5% of all deaths globally among young people aged 15–29 years. In the United Kingdom in the 15- to 29-year age range 9.1/100,000 males and 2.5/100,000 females committed suicide (WHO 2014). The Samaritans (Scowcroft 2014) state that in 2012 in the 15- to 19-year age range 128 males and 36 females committed suicide, while in the 20- to 24-year age range 339 males and 68 females committed suicide. Six deaths occurred in the 10- to 14-year age range (Department of Health [DH] 2014). Young men are two to three times more at risk of completing suicide than young women. This is undoubtedly because of the fatal methods employed (Lehti et al. 2009; McNamara 2012; WHO 2014; Welsh Government 2015). Young women, however, have been found to favour alcohol and both licit and illicit drugs (Toero et al. 2001; Agritmis et al. 2004; McNamara 2012). It is suggested that teenagers remain a particularly vulnerable group who require specific attention (Welsh Government 2015; WHO 2014, 2016).

This situation is reflected across Europe, especially in the east, where rates of youth suicide are alarmingly high and it is suggested are underpinned by the rapid social, political and economic changes which have taken place (WHO 2014, 2016). It is also suggested that the figures may be significantly higher owing to underreporting or the death being classified as misadventure or open verdict (Scowcroft 2014; Welsh Government 2015; WHO 2014). It is essential that reliable and timely statistics are available so that accurate information can inform and enable services to respond and support those affected by suicide (DH 2015a).

In the United Kingdom several strategic documents have been published in response to public and professional concerns about the youth suicide rate. The documents outline a number of common objectives which are subject to ongoing review; these include reducing risk, increasing support, providing timely access to services, reducing stigma, developing research and knowledge of youth suicide and promoting well-being and resilience using targeted interventions (DH 2011, 2015a, 2015b; Department of Health, Social Services and Public Safety 2014; Welsh Government 2015; WHO 2014; Scottish Government 2013). These discuss the responsibilities of the voluntary and statutory sectors and the multidisciplinary collaboration and communication which must occur in order to reach those young people who are in crisis; these include delivering early intervention, responding to crisis and managing the consequences of suicide (WHO 2014; Welsh Government 2015). The WHO (2014) proposes a 10% reduction in suicide rates by 2020. This is echoed in the UK strategy documents; for example, Scotland has already reduced the suicide rate by 18% since the publication of its initial strategy in 2002 (Scottish Government 2013).

The strategies address the specific cultural and demographic issues of their target populations. The ongoing review and republication of the policies would suggest that there is social and political concern that the underlying contributory factors may not have not been addressed in sufficient detail or with enough funding to ensure that the need to reiterate the objectives is not required (WHO 2014; Welsh Government 2015). Conversely, it can be argued that there is a continuing imperative to reiterate and address the specific cultural and socioeconomic issues pertinent to each of the UK countries following the devolution of government and which continue to deeply affect the lives of children and young people. This also focuses public and professional attention onto what needs to be addressed within communities and the public health arena (DH 2011, 2015; Scottish Government 2013; Department of Health, Social Services and Public Safety 2014; WHO 2014; Welsh Government 2015).

WHY DO YOUNG PEOPLE COMMIT SUICIDE?

Suicide is a complex, highly individual, multifactorial event in which it is difficult to unravel a single contributory factor. There is usually an escalation of life events and other stressors which occur simultaneously and increase cumulatively, oppressing the individual whose resources to cope are compromised by deteriorating mental health. The young person feels they have no control over events and little support is available to them. It can be an explosive, impulsive act (Gaughan 2011b; Tousignant et al. 2013; Welsh Government 2015; WHO 2014).

Make a list of reasons why a young person would contemplate suicide.

CASE STUDY

Joe is 15 years old and was diagnosed with insulin-dependent diabetes 4 months ago. He has been brought into his local accident and emergency department semiconscious, with breathing difficulties. He was found by his best friend hanging from a tree in the local woods. Joe is well liked among his few close friends but has recently been picked on at school for being different. He has experienced cyber bullying and has been 'trolled' over his social media pages about his health issues. He has been unable to play rugby for several weeks because of a sore on his heel which is not healing. His blood sugar levels have not been stable over the last few months. Joe had a girlfriend but they have split up. His friend says he has been 'down' for a while about things and had given him a signed football and photo from his favourite footballer and other possessions he valued.

REFLECTION POINTS

- What may have prompted this suicide attempt?
- Think about the factors or issues involved in this attempt and reflect on why they would affect Joe.

DEVELOPMENTAL ISSUES

Adolescence is a time of rapid physical and psychological development when the capacity to solve and deal with multiple problems is challenged and emotions are experienced on a more heightened level, leading to stress (Coleman and Henry 2011; Bee and Boyd 2012). Thus the adolescent may have fewer resources for resolving difficulties. These issues, coupled with significant life events and conflict within the family about behaviour or development or mental health issues, leave the young person extremely isolated, vulnerable and disenfranchised. Parents may be perceived to be controlling and blocking the developmental needs, leading to conflict, anger, aggression and increased impulsivity (Lehti et al. 2009; McNamara 2012; Tousignant et al. 2013; WHO 2014).

Self-esteem, social desirability and social capital are particularly important in adolescence and are reinforced through belonging to the 'correct' peer group that provides an arena to refine social skills, behaviour, values and beliefs. 'Failure' to gain entry or be accepted leads to a loss of self-esteem and distress that is often not disclosed. Miotto and Preti (2008) in a study of Italian high school students found that there is an inverse relationship between social desirability and psychological distress. Students with high social desirability scores were less likely to report suicidal ideation, whereas those who were acutely distressed had low social desirability but concealed their negative feelings by appearing outwardly positive. They were challenged by dealing with sadness and frustration and felt isolated, which led to negative self-regard and motivated a search to end the psychological pain through suicide. Loss of social capital leads to exclusion, marginalization and a sense of disconnectedness (McNamara 2012).

Self-esteem and confidence are underpinned by a sound body image. A negative or dysfunctional body image in young people can lead to self-hatred and is a predictor of suicidal ideation. At times of distress, harming oneself – the 'object' of hatred and disgust – seems a feasible option to the individual and as a means eradicating self-hatred, depression and hopelessness (Brausch and Muehlenkamp 2007; McNamara 2012).

MENTAL HEALTH ISSUES

Poor mental health is a contributory factor in youth suicide. Anxiety and depression are implicated in and contribute significantly to suicidal behaviour. The young person's coping strategies and ability to seek help can be significantly compromised, leading to increasing social isolation and exacerbation of their deteriorating mental health and well-being (Samm et al. 2010; Gaughan 2011b; WHO 2014; DH 2015a). Also having a conduct disorder and emotional problems exacerbates the distress experienced as these young people can be socially and educationally excluded, as well as becoming involved with the police with the potential to be involved in the criminal justice system (Green et al. 2005; Welsh Government 2012; DH 2015a). Boys with a conduct disorder and alcohol misuse have a ninefold risk of suicide and girls a threefold risk of attempting suicide. Alcohol may be used to palliate the psychological distress but in fact exacerbates deteriorating mental health (Ilomaki et al. 2007; Lehti et al. 2009; McNamara 2012).

This has implications for parents, who need to be able to respond to their children's needs; however, if their mental health is compromised, the risk of suicide increases as they may be emotionally unavailable to their children and may not observe the indicators of suicidal intent. The young person can feel they have no confidante to assist in dealing with complex emotions (Department for Children, Schools and Families and Department of Health 2010; McNamara 2012; Tousignant et al. 2013; DH 2015b). Parents bereaved by the suicide of their children were often unaware of the signals and wished they had been more accessible to their children (Stanley 2005; Lindqvist et al. 2008). When the mother has a history of mood disorders, there is increased conflict and less cohesiveness and emotional expression. Parenting styles may also be compromised with hostility, increased criticism and a high level of negativity. This leaves the young person feeling vulnerable, isolated and unable to communicate their distress, which becomes internalized to avoid exacerbating a difficult situation at home (Tousignant et al. 2013; RCN 2014b; DH 2015b). There is substantial evidence to suggest that suicidal behaviour is transmitted through families; thus the young person may copy this believing it to be an appropriate means by which to deal with the distress and psychological turmoil they are experiencing (McNamara 2012; Welsh Government 2015; WHO 2014).

ETHNICITY

Traditionally, ethnic groups within a different culture have provided a protective influence over young people, ensuring access to support and help specific to their personal and cultural needs. It is suggested that as social change occurs and prompts changes within a particular social structure, traditional and ethnic communities struggle to preserve their identity and heritage. The communities are expected to integrate into the dominant society, leading to acculturation stress as they find themselves adapting to urbanization, new ways of gaining a livelihood and the transfer of authority. Thus as integration occurs young people find themselves becoming distanced from their traditional ethnic groupings, leaving them feeling isolated, displaced and disenfranchised and without a focus as they try to integrate with a different culture. Traditional values, language, support networks and ways of living and viewing the world are significantly eroded and diluted. There may be a divergence from cultural norms, traditions and values which can result in alcohol misuse, parental overprotection and family breakdown, all of which are associated with an increased suicide risk (Hallet et al. 2007; Silviken and Kvernmo 2007; Khan and Waheed 2009; Lehti et al. 2009; McNamara 2012; Tousignant et al. 2013).

This is borne out by McNamara (2012), who found that young people within the indigenous Australian Aboriginal and Torres Strait Islander (ATSI) communities were at a heightened risk for completed suicide. Despite government initiatives to reduce the incidence of suicide the rates remain high. For example between 2004 and 2007 the suicide rate for 10- to 14-year-olds was 17 times higher than that of Queensland children who commit suicide. This was also true of the 15- to 17-year age group which had a suicide rate two and a half times that of their Queensland peers. McNamara points out that suicide was a rare event prior to colonial settlement. In New Zealand Maori youths have a suicide rate almost double that of Caucasian youths (Beautrais and Fergusson 2006; MOHNZ 2011). Higher rates of suicidal ideation, planning and attempts were found in the Maori and Pacific Islander youths than in Caucasian youths (Beautrais 2001).

This is echoed globally. Lehti et al. (2009) found that suicide rates across the Arctic region were alarmingly high among indigenous young people. The rates of suicide in Greenland were 20 times higher than those of the non-indigenous young people. Tousignant et al. (2013) found a similar picture in Quebec and across Canada, with the highest suicide rate in the Inuit population, and the rate for First Nation young people was double that of the general population.

Language and customs are a tangible symbol of the culture and are of immense importance. It is postulated that, when distressed, the use of their original language enables the speaker to fully express their emotions and access support within traditional communities. Hallet et al. (2007) found that as Aboriginal Canadian young people began to move away from their traditional groups and lost their language through integration, the rate of suicide increased. Where over half the community spoke and used their indigenous language the suicide rate was six times lower than in communities who had lost their language (13/100,000 and 96.55/100,000, respectively). Thus without this link, young people are faced with the challenge of constructing a new identity in a modern world while witnessing the disintegration of a way of life, leaving them isolated, unsure, depressed and vulnerable.

FAMILY STRUCTURE

Increasing divorce rates and the nature of modern relationships mean that family life is now more dynamic and unpredictable. As families change so they disintegrate and reconstitute themselves, leading to a loss of roles, support networks, confidantes and friends (Ayyash-Abdo 2002; Samm et al. 2010; WHO 2014). Children and young people from non-intact families reported lower levels of self-esteem, increased anxiety and loneliness, depression and suicidal ideation and attempts (Garnefski and Diekstra 1997; Tulloch et al. 1997). A closer analysis found that boys within step-parent families reported increased negative feelings but reported less anxiety when part of a lone-parent family (Samm et al. 2010). It has been suggested that within the lone-parent family boys found a role as 'head' of the house, having a responsibility and sense of contributing and being independent. This is eroded when a new partner and other children arrive. Roles and functions are realigned and the young person is expected to compromise and conform to a new regime that may corrode their sense of self and independence (Green et al. 2005; Parry-Langdon 2008). However, girls fared better in step-parent families, having higher levels of self-esteem. For the young girls, being in a lone-parent family was stressful as expectations to be involved in the domestic load were high, whereas being in a step-family meant they could share the burden and take on new roles from choice, develop their sense of self and gain support and confidantes by being part of a family. Emotionally they felt safe (Parry-Langdon 2008; Samm et al. 2010; Welsh Government 2015; WHO 2015).

SUBSTANCE MISUSE

Substance misuse in young people has increased and is implicated as a risk factor in suicidal behaviour. The young person who misuses substances becomes integrated with their fellow users but becomes isolated, disconnected and disenfranchised from mainstream society, leading to stigma and increased vulnerability (Fortune and Hawton 2007; Lehti et al. 2009; McNamara 2012). Alcohol is strongly linked with suicidal ideation, attempts and completion. Binge drinking is certainly a specific predictor of attempted and completed suicide (Ilomaki et al. 2007; Swahn and Bossarte 2007; Price et al. 2014). Petrol sniffing, psychoactive substances and helium sniffing are also implicated in increased suicidal ideation and risk (Lehti et al. 2009; McNamara 2012; DH 2015b). It is posited that substance and alcohol misuse may be associated with risk factors that contribute to stressful events, leading to higher levels of depression and isolation, which results in alcohol being misused to palliate the psychological pain and turmoil experienced. In essence, substance abuse appears to be a part of a larger, more chaotic picture in which several other risk factors are implicated, with the young person unable to identify or access sources of help (Lehti et al. 2009; McNamara 2012).

OTHER RISK FACTORS

- Poor school performance
- Marital discord
- Poor health
- High parental expectation
- Socioeconomic deprivation
- Unemployment
- Homelessness
- Domestic violence
- Sexuality issues
- Death of relative/close friend

Source: Department for Children, Schools and Families and Department of Health, *Keeping Children and Young People in Mind: The Government's Full Response to the Independent Review of CAMHS*, DCSF/DH, London, 2010; Welsh Government, *Together for Mental Health: A Strategy for Mental Health and Well-Being in Wales*, Welsh Government, Cardiff, 2012, available at http://gov.wales/docs/dhss/publications/121031tmhfinalen.pdf; World Health Organization, *Preventing Suicide: A Global Imperative*, WHO, Luxembourg, 2014.

RED FLAG INDICATORS

These are the cardinal signs that suicide is being contemplated and help must be provided in order to support and retrieve the young person.

RED FLAG INDICATORS

- History of sexual abuse
- Death of a parent
- Previous suicide in family
- Depression
- Change in appearance – poor hygiene
- Giving away cherished possessions
- Preoccupation with death
- Repeated visits to GP
- Antisocial behaviour
- Describing oneself as worthless
- Changes in school performance
- Social withdrawal
- Dramatic changes in appetite
- Impaired concentration
- Deliberate self-harm – increased frequency and severity

Source: Fortune, S., Hawton, K., *Pediatrics and Child Health*, 17, 443–7, 2007; Welsh Government, *Together for Mental Health: A Strategy for Mental Health and Well-Being in Wales*, Welsh Government, Cardiff, 2012, available at http://gov.wales/docs/dhss/publications/121031tmhfinalen.pdf; World Health Organization, *Preventing Suicide: A Global Imperative*, WHO, Luxembourg, 2014.

PROTECTIVE FACTORS

The importance of protective factors is strongly emphasized within the policy initiatives. The focus is on promoting good mental health and well-being, prevention of poor mental health by taking early action and early intervention so support can be provided. Protective factors are vital in enabling the child or young person to explore coping strategies in a positive manner which can lead to a reduction in vulnerability (Gaughan 2011b; Welsh Government 2015; WHO 2014; DH 2015b).

Protective factors focus on the provision of a warm, caring environment with access to emotional support, building self-esteem and developing resilience. Resilience has been defined as

> a person's capacity for adapting psychologically, emotionally and physically reasonably well and without lasting detriment to self, relationships or personal development in the face of adversity, threat or challenge. (Williams and Drury 2009, p. 294)

Resilience is not static, but is a dynamic range of personal characteristics, experiences and relationships that provide protection in the face of stress. Thus it is about enabling sound problem-solving; having good communication skills, the ability to tolerate negative effect and frustration, and skills to seek out support; and developing good self-esteem and social skills, a strong locus of control and supportive networks (Miotto and Preti 2008; Gaughan 2011b; Welsh Government 2015; DH 2015a). Young people whose self-efficacy is strong appear to be more resilient as they are successful, socially connected and adept at managing their socio-emotional development (Miotto and Preti 2008; McNamara 2012; WHO 2014; DH 2015).

The development of a sound value and belief system is also associated with resilience in young people, enabling them to develop self-awareness and a sense of identity within their community. McNamara (2012) points out that the formation and acceptance of a cultural identity, while challenging, also enables resilience to be developed, but it may lead to a disconnection with the family and culture followed by partial or total acceptance.

PROTECTIVE FACTORS

- Warm and caring family environment
- Self-esteem, locus of control, self-confidence and social skills
- Belonging to a faith or religious group
- Someone who will listen to them
- Realistic parental expectation
- Supportive friendships
- Ability to tolerate negative affect and frustration
- Engagement at school
- Positive family relationships
- Access to support, help and treatment
- Individual values
- Self-control of behaviour, thoughts and emotions

Source: Welsh Government, *Talk to Me 2: Suicide and Self-Harm Prevention Strategy for Wales 2015–2020,* Welsh Government, Cardiff, 2015; World Health Organization, *Preventing Suicide: A Global Imperative,* WHO, Luxembourg, 2014.

There is a need to provide effective supportive services which are accessible and facilitate timely help and treatment. This is a key imperative outlined specifically in the policy documents which calls upon services to be more effective and efficient in using existing resources at a time of economic austerity.

The onus is upon the children and young people's nurse to assess the young person's development, lifestyle and exposure to risk factors, and to acquire skills in suicide prevention. This requires a multidisciplinary approach to care which demands liaison with the child and adolescent mental health services so that a care package which transcends professional boundaries is put in place as well as providing ongoing access to support services. Such support should be offered on a whole family basis to enable parents and siblings to meet the needs of the child or young person while coping with their own emotions. They too will require support and help to make sense of the event, deal with the feelings of guilt which may be experienced and learn to survive and move forward (Department for Children, Schools and Families and Department of Health 2010; Lindqvist et al. 2008; Welsh Government 2015; DH 2015a, 2015b).

REFLECTION POINTS

- What are your personal feelings about a young person attempting suicide?
- Do your feelings influence your practice and attitudes toward patients admitted following a suicide attempt?

PRINCIPLES FOR PRACTICE

- Suicide is a multifactorial event.
- Poor mental health and a lack of resilience disable the individual's ability to cope.
- The ability to cope with multiple events is compromised.
- It may be an impulsive act in response to crisis.

SELF-HARM

Self-harm is complex multifactorial behaviour which is underpinned by profound psychological issues and is defined as

any act of self poisoning or injury carried out by a person, irrespective of their motivation.

National Institute for Health and Clinical Excellence 2013a, p. 16

It is important to point out that, although self-harm does not always lead to suicide and those who self-harm are not always suicidal, there is a shared continuum of self-harm behaviour (Mental Health Foundation 2006, 2016; Welsh Government 2015). Suicide is an impulsive, final, aggressive act that has a decreased escape potential, whereas self-harm is carried out in response to personal distress, difficult feelings and emotions as a coping mechanism in order to carry on living (Mental Health Foundation 2006, 2016; Spender 2007). It is an impulsive, but not final, act with many individuals thinking about it for just minutes before acting.

Self-harm is becoming increasingly common in young people and is a major public health concern; it is one of the top five reasons for medical admission in the UK, resulting in significant psychosocial consequences for the young person and their family (Mental Health Foundation 2006; Hawton et al. 2012; Young Minds and Cello 2012; Welsh Government 2015). Self-harm affects 1 in 15 adolescents and is three times more prevalent among young females. The number of presentations to accident and emergency (A&E) departments has risen among those aged 15–24 years (Arkins et al. 2013). It is thought to be responsible for 25,000 adolescents presenting at A&E departments following non-fatal self-harm, yet this may not be an accurate figure as it is estimated that only 1 in 10 young people who self-harm present themselves at hospital following an incident (National Institute for Health and Clinical Excellence 2004a; Young Minds and Cello 2012; Mental Health Foundation 2016). Indeed, in the general population 10% of girls and 3% of boys reported self harming (National Institute for Health and Clinical Excellence 2004a; MHF 2016). The rates of repetition are high, as 10%–15% of young people will repeat the self-harm within 2–3 months (Welsh Government 2015). Arkins et al. (2013) point out that nearly half of the participants in their study had attended the A&E department as a result of self-harm in the previous year. They suggest that repeated presentations may signify an underlying unresolved problem or recurring crisis.

REFLECTION POINTS

- What do you understand by the term *self-harm*?
- What do you feel/think about young people who self-harm?

CATEGORIES OF SELF-HARM

- Self-poisoning: Overdose of drugs, alcohol
- Self-injury: Cutting, mutilation, burning, scalding
- Self-mutilation: Head banging, pulling hair
- Suicide attempts: Hanging, jumping, overdose

Source: National Institute for Health and Clinical Excellence, *Self Harm: The Short Term Physical and Psychological Management and Secondary Prevention of Self Harm in Primary and Secondary Care*, Clinical Guidelines CG16, NICE, London, 2004, available at https://www.nice.org.uk/guidance/CG16; National Institute for Health and Clinical Excellence, *Self Harm: Longer Term Management*, Clinical Guideline 133, NICE, London, 2011, available at https://www.nice.org.uk/guidance/cg133/chapter/Introduction; Mental Health Foundation, *Truth Hurts. Report of the National Inquiry into Self Harm among Young People*, MHF, London, 2006.

WHY DO YOUNG PEOPLE SELF-HARM?

The national inquiry into self-harm, *The Truth Hurts* report, states:

Self-harm is a response to profound emotional pain. It is a way of dealing with distress and of getting release from feelings of self-hatred, anger, sadness, depression. By engaging in self-harm people may alter their state of mind so that they feel better able to cope with the other pain they are feeling. (Mental Health Foundation 2006, p. 15)

Self-harm is characterized by depression, feelings of hopelessness and worthlessness. The pain of self-harm ends emotional numbness, pain and dissociative feelings, transforming them into manageable physical pain (Hawton et al. 2012; Cleaver et al. 2014; McAndrew and Warne 2014). It is suggested that self-harm is a coping strategy which may facilitate self-preservation and relief from internalized stress and distress (Gaughan 2011a; Hawton et al. 2012; McAndrew and Warne 2014). However, self-harm reflects serious, distressing personal, emotional, behavioural and mental health problems. The young person feels guilty and will often go to great lengths to conceal their behaviour, which can lead to difficulties in accessing support (McAndrew and Warne 2014). What emerges from the literature is that accessing support requires significant courage and emotional resources on the part of the young person (Hawton et al. 2012; McAndrew and Warne 2014).

Risk factors fall into distal and proximal factors. Distal factors are associated with self-harm and are ongoing while proximal factors occur closer in time and are more immediate to the event (Arkins et al. 2013).

REFLECTION POINT

What might cause a young person to self-harm?

DEPRESSION AND HOPELESSNESS

Feelings of hopelessness, vulnerability and depression are major psychological features strongly associated with self-harm. In this context, low self-esteem, poor self-concept, despair and self-blame are key emotions (Hawton et al. 2012; McAndrew and Warne 2013; Welsh Government 2015; Mental Health Foundation 2016). A survey of young females found that they felt overwhelmed by a number of issues, such as bullying, teasing, exclusion, academic pressures, family problems, media portrayal of young people and peer pressure to 'be cool'. These left the girls feeling frustrated, isolated and lonely as they felt their independence and autonomy was eroded leading to lower levels of confidence and self-worth (Girlguiding UK/Mental Health Foundation 2008; Hawton et al. 2012; Mental Health Foundation 2016).

The young person who self-harms finds it difficult to handle the complex emotions they are experiencing and is uncertain where to seek help or feels guilty about what they do (National Institute for Health and Clinical Excellence 2004a; Mental Health Foundation 2006; McAndrew and Warne 2014). Hawton et al. (2012) suggest that a common aspect of young people who self-harm is less effective social problem solving which may be inhibited by the depression and hopelessness and dissociation they experience. It is challenging to deal with frustration, problems and life events. Young people may feel defeated, become socially and emotionally isolated, and feel trapped and that they are a burden; thus self-harm becomes the way to relieve the distress (National Institute for Health and Clinical Excellence 2004a; Hawton et al. 2012; Welsh Government 2015). However, guilt and shame are powerful emotions experienced following self-harm. In McAndrew and Warne's study (2014) the participants described the powerful sense of relief brought about by self-harming and then detailed the shame, guilt and feeling 'bad' once the 'buzz' had worn off. They felt that they would be judged by those who knew or they looked to for support. Stigma was a powerful force in preventing them accessing help. This in turn compounded their feelings of distress, low self-worth and hopelessness. Seeking help required levels of courage they may not have had and also knowing where to go for help was problematic.

LIFE EVENTS

The incidence of self-harm increases substantially in relation to the number of negative life events which occur within families, e.g. marital breakdown, trouble with police, death and serious illness. Hawton et al. (2012) found that those who self-harm report more events than their peers. The fear, anxiety and stress become internalized in the absence of external support, leading to the young person feeling isolated, lonely and unable to cope. They then lose sight of their own worth and value and in order to avoid further emotional pain and rejection self-harm (Department for Children, Schools and Families and Department of Health 2010; Hawton et al. 2012; McAndrew and Warne 2014; RCN 2014a, 2014b). Self-harm is linked to a poor sense of self-worth and self-esteem and is viewed by the affected individual as a viable coping mechanism to deal with the emotional hurt and pain being experienced (Arkins et al. 2013; McAndrew and Warne 2014).

Substance misuse has been heavily implicated in self-harming behaviour. Arkins et al. (2013) found that nearly half of the young people in their study had consumed significant amounts of alcohol, six or more drinks at one time, or two to three times per week. Drugs were also consumed illicitly from once to twice per month or every week. This led to feelings of shame and guilt which then led to further self-harming behaviours with possible attendance at the emergency department. Rossow and Norstrom (2014) support this finding in their study which found that heavy episodic drinking had a significant association with an increased risk of self-harm. Alcohol is a proximal factor in self-harm which exacerbates psychological distress and becomes a way of coping with underlying emotional distress. Alcohol inhibits the ability to seek alternative coping strategies (Hawton et al. 2012; Arkins et al. 2013; Rossow and Norstrom 2014).

The incidence and repetition of self-harm also rises in response to living with a chronic condition or ongoing health issues (National Institute for Health and Clinical Excellence 2004a; Mental Health Foundation 2006; Krishnakumar et al. 2011; Hawton et al. 2012; Seminog and Goldacre 2014). Meltzer et al. (2001) conducted a national study which found that those who had tried to self-harm or kill themselves were more likely to have a physical problem or impairment such as speech and language problems, coordination problems, epilepsy and soiling. In the 5- to 10-year-old groups, two-thirds of the children who had tried to harm themselves had special educational needs and were visiting the GP and outpatient clinics more frequently than those children who did not self-harm. One-third of the group had been involved with specialist mental healthcare services.

In the older age group around 40% of the 11- to 15-year-old cohort who had tried to harm themselves had special educational needs or a mental health problem and were at an increased risk of self-harming. This was particularly true of those with anxiety disorders, depression, conduct disorder and hyperkinetic disorder (Meltzer et al. 2001; Mental Health Foundation 2006; Welsh Government 2015; Krishnakumar et al. 2011). Thus anger about their situation is internalized and may only be expressed through self-harming, including neglecting to take essential prescribed treatment (Mental Health Foundation 2006). The young person may feel stigmatized, restricted by the demands of their condition which isolates them physically, socially and psychologically from engaging with family, friends and a typical developmental experience. This has adverse effects on their self-worth and self-esteem and can lead to depression and a sense of hopelessness if support is not available or is difficult to access.

FAMILY

The parent–child relationship is vitally important in protecting the young person from self-harm. The attachment process and quality of this is now being examined for its role in protecting the mental health of the child and young person. Where attachment difficulties occur it is suggested that there is an increased likelihood of self-harm occurring. A secure attachment and warm, supportive parents are needed to enable children and young people to manage and regulate their emotions. A secure attachment also underpins positive self-worth and self-esteem (Gaughan 2011a). The quality of parenting and parenting style also have an impact. Where there is maladaptive parenting, family breakdown and adversity the risk of self-harm increases (Hawton et al. 2012). Conflict with family (parents) was common among those who self-harmed. One study found that three-quarters of respondents had argued with family members in the 24-hour period before attending an A&E department. Cohesive families with open communication are more supportive and protective of the young person (Arkins et al. 2013). Young people who self-harmed were found to belong to families who were dysfunctional, experiencing some form of breakdown and in some cases living with relatives or in the care system (Hawton et al. 2012; Welsh Government 2015). Parental mental health and significant life events disrupt interactions and the parent's availability as a confidante, which is strongly associated with self-harm (Arkins et al. 2013).

Socioeconomic and demographic data strongly suggest that those from poorer socioeconomically deprived backgrounds are more at risk of self-harming because of poverty, which affects them economically, psychologically and socially (National Institute for Health and Care Excellence 2004a; Welsh Government 2015). Consequently, the emotional climate in the house is heightened owing to anxieties and worries concerning day-to-day survival and the burden of care. Expectations of the young person may increase substantially, and materially they are disadvantaged compared with the more affluent members of their peer group. This oppresses the young person, lowering their self-esteem and resilience to cope (Welsh Government 2015; McAndrew and Warne 2014; WHO 2014). Young people who have an internal locus of control are more distressed by life events; thus they experience feelings of self-blame and worthlessness because they feel they should be in control and able to cope. This is exacerbated by poor communication within the family. Those with an external locus of control are less distressed by negative events and can cope in more appropriate ways (Tulloch et al. 1997; Meltzer et al. 2001).

Young people who self-harm are less likely to seek support from family, teachers or friends than their peers who do not self-harm. Those who self-harm also conceal this and feel that even if they did speak out about this their concerns and fears would be dismissed (McAndrew and Warne 2014). Young people who self-harm may be less likely to confide in others leading to feelings of loneliness and a sense that no one else is aware of their problems. It has been suggested that not only may they not seek help, but even if help is offered their response may drive that help away (McAndrew and Warne 2014).

Where parents are aware of the self-harm they may be distressed and anxious about how to provide support. Parents need advice on dealing with this complex and frightening situation (Mental Health Foundation 2006, 2016; Department for Children, Schools and Families and Department of Health 2010; Arkins et al. 2013). If support is not forthcoming, ultimately the young person is left isolated and unsupported within the family; the young person thus seeks help externally through friends or conceals their behaviour, leading to a worsening of the issues they are experiencing (National Institute for Health and Clinical Excellence 2004a; Mental Health Foundation 2006). Roles may become blurred as the young person may feel compelled to protect their parents and friends from further stress as their mental health and coping skills deteriorate (Mental Health Foundation 2006).

SOCIOECONOMIC AND DEMOGRAPHIC FACTORS

- Sex/gender
- Low socioeconomic status
- Parental separation or divorce
- Lone parent
- Adverse childhood experiences
- Low educational attainment
- Unskilled occupation
- Unemployment
- Social deprivation
- Social sector housing

Source: Reprinted from *The Lancet*, 379, Hawton K, Saunders KEA, O'Connor R, Self harm and suicide in adolescents, pp. 2373–82, Copyright (2012), with permission from Elsevier; Welsh Government, *Talk to Me 2: Suicide and Self-Harm Prevention Strategy for Wales 2015–2020*, Welsh Government, Cardiff, 2015.

ABUSE

Abuse, both physical and sexual, is highly correlated with suicide and self-harm in young people (National Institute for Health and Clinical Excellence 2004a; Mental Health Foundation 2006; Gaughan 2011a; Hawton et al. 2012; Welsh Government 2015). Where there is frequent use of physical chastisement, the incidence of reported self-harm increases (Hawton et al. 2012). It is suggested that physical abuse increases the risk of self-harm 5-fold, and emotional abuse increases the risk 12-fold. Sexual abuse is a risk factor regardless of socioeconomic and demographic factors (Zoroglu et al. 2003; Green et al. 2005) and where this had occurred, the rate of self-harming behaviours was found to increase. Dissociation is a key feature exhibited by young people who feel disconnected from the world and emotionally numbed. Thus young people may engage in destructive behaviours, allowing their psychological distress to be managed as physical pain and the young person to 'reconnect' with their feelings (Hawton et al. 2012; Arkins et al. 2013; McAndrew and Warne 2014).

PSYCHOSOCIAL RISK FACTORS

- Family/friends/school
- Unable to problem-solve
- Bullying
- Cycles of hopelessness
- Depression in pre-pubertal age groups
- Sexuality
- Illness
- Personal loss
- Family dysfunction
- Suicides of close friends/family members
- Substance misuse
- Perfectionism
- Poor problem solving
- Impulsivity

Source: Reprinted from *The Lancet*, 379, Hawton K, Saunders KEA, O'Connor R, Self harm and suicide in adolescents, pp. 2373–82, Copyright (2012), with permission from Elsevier; Welsh Government, *Talk to Me 2: Suicide and Self-Harm Prevention Strategy for Wales 2015–2020,* Welsh Government, Cardiff, 2015.

Thus there is no one single factor which can identify which child or young person is at risk of self-harming. What is clear is that there is a complex combination and interplay of factors which predispose the individual to self-harm.

REFLECTION POINT

What do you say to a young person who has self-harmed?

EATING DISORDERS: ANOREXIA NERVOSA

Eating disorders are among the most common of all psychiatric disorders. They are highly complex, multifaceted disorders encompassing physical, psychological and social features which have a significant impact on children and young people (National Institute for Health and Clinical Excellence 2004b; Nicholls et al. 2011; Royal College of Psychiatrists 2012a). The most commonly known disorders are anorexia nervosa (AN) and bulimia nervosa, which can significantly affect long-term health and psychosocial functioning. The impact on the family cannot be underestimated as everyone is profoundly affected by this disorder (Honey and Halse 2006, 2007; Halvorsen et al. 2013; McCormack and McCann 2015).

REFLECTION POINT

What are your thoughts, feelings and attitudes about eating disorders?

AN is a serious disorder with life-threatening physical and psychological complications which carries an elevated mortality risk when compared to other psychiatric disorders (Welsh Assembly Government 2009; Royal College of Psychiatrists 2012a; Hartmann et al. 2015). AN literally means a 'loss of appetite'; however, this is too simplistic in describing a highly complex eating disorder with a multifaceted aetiology and with varying approaches to treatment (Royal College of Psychiatrist 2015; Hartmann et al. 2013, 2015). The World Health Organization (2007) defines AN as

> a disorder characterized by deliberate weight loss, induced and sustained by the patient. The disorder is associated with … a dread of fatness and flabbiness of body contour persists as an intrusive overvalued idea, and the patients impose a low weight threshold on themselves.

Young people with AN will restrict their food intake becoming preoccupied with their eating pattern, food consumed, a fear of gaining weight and body image (National Institute for Health and Clinical Excellence 2004b; Boughtwood and Halse 2008). The fundamental causes remain elusive, but the behaviours are symptomatic of underlying complex and intersecting biological, psychosocial and cultural issues which have an impact on a vulnerable personality (National Institute for Health and Clinical Excellence 2004b; Royal College of Psychiatrists 2012a, 2015).

PREVALENCE

AN commonly starts in adolescence, with the risk of onset highest at the ages of 14–18 years. Girls are 10 times more likely to develop AN and it is suggested that, of those aged 15 years, one in 150 girls and one in 1000 boys are affected by AN. AN is 8–11 times more common in females, although it has been found that 25% of boys aged 7–14 years have AN (Royal College of Psychiatrists 2015). The chance of recovery is less than 50% in 10 years, 25% remain ill and the mortality rate can be up to 25% of sufferers (Morris and Twaddle 2007; Zandian et al. 2007).

Nicholls et al. (2011) in a national survey across the United Kingdom found that while the incidence of eating disorders was stable overall, it appeared to be increasing in the younger age groups (below 13 years of age). They found an incidence of 3/100,000 children with an eating disorder, of whom 80% presented with an AN-like illness. It is suggested that this increase is due to a number of factors. This includes increased awareness of eating disorders and the recognition of AN as a disorder with underlying psychological issues, which have led to it being recognized, diagnosed and treated with specialist interventions much earlier than had been the case previously. Also, perspectives have now shifted to cast a critical eye across modern society and the potential contributing factors which affect young girls and boys, e.g. the media, celebrity-oriented culture and academic expectation. However, it can be argued that the majority of adolescents are subjected to these factors, yet not all develop AN; thus these factors are only a part of the picture, which only illustrates the complexity of the disorder (Orbach 1986, cited in Surgenor et al. 2002; Bryant-Waugh 2006).

CASE STUDY

Amy is 15 years old and has been diagnosed with anorexia nervosa for a year. She has been admitted to the ward for stabilization and re-feeding. Amy is doing well academically. She is a talented ballet dancer who hopes to gain a scholarship to a prestigious ballet school. She is working hard to achieve this goal. Amy is part of a supportive, close-knit family who is very proud of her achievements and have high expectations for her future. However, Amy has become depressed since the death of her grandmother, to whom she was close. She has lost touch with her friends due to her dedication to her dancing. She is losing interest in her school work but practices compulsively believing she isn't good enough to achieve her goals. She has said that she feels ugly, isolated and useless.

REFLECTION POINTS

- Why might Amy have developed anorexia nervosa?
- What are the potential risk factors?

THEORIES OF ANOREXIA NERVOSA

Bruch (1962, 1973) proposed a psychodynamic perspective of AN, identifying that control issues were central to the disorder at a familial and interpersonal level. The young person struggles for control, a sense of identity, competence and effectiveness. Control is exerted in response to a situation whereby the child/young person's development of autonomy is inhibited, yet once reaching adolescence, they need and are expected to function independently at both a familial and a social level. They are, however, ill-prepared to do so and experience low self-esteem, deficits in self-regulation and a sense of inadequacy. The fear of having no control is overwhelming. The control is gained through withstanding hunger; the denial of food and the resultant low weight are the proof (Bruch 1973). Bruch suggests that it is an adaptive mechanism to achieve autonomy, competence and effectiveness. Three perceptual and conceptual disturbances occur. These include body size or image, personal control and interpretation of hunger and satiation signals (Bruch 1973). Bruch's theory was refined giving rise to a cognitive behavioural account of AN (Fairburn et al. 1998). The theory holds that AN is maintained by a set of overvalued ideas about body shape and weight which occur as a result of personal characteristics interacting with sociocultural ideals about the female appearance. Control, fear of weight gain and avoidance of other difficulties have also been identified (Fairburn et al. 1998).

The biopsychosocial model integrates the various factors identified as contributing to AN and examines their role. Sociocultural, familial and individual risk factors are analyzed to provide insight into the complex interplay and multifactorial nature of the causes of AN (Polivy and Herman 2002).

Orbach, in her seminal work (1978, 1986), has proposed that AN is a flight from growth. The individual fails to master his or her biological and psychological experiences accompanying the attainment of adult weight. These require mastery and integration, which the young person cannot achieve or for which they are psychologically unprepared, and so the young person adapts by avoiding puberty, thus gaining control over their development and a sense of safety (Crisp 1997). However, in order to maintain this control over a changing self, it becomes necessary to exert control over the environment and others through 'dominating' the relationship with them.

Orbach (cited in Surgenor et al. 2002) locates AN within a gendered culture and political system. She argues that young women are subject to changes, of both a predetermined biological and culturally determined social nature, which are oppressive, leaving them with a sense of fear, powerlessness and confusion. Orbach (cited in Surgenor et al. 2002) argues that AN restores control and allows the individual to resist the 'controls' placed on them by the external world, thus enabling the self and autonomy to be reasserted.

DISTURBED BODY IMAGE

AN is characterized by severe body image concerns. Young people typically feel that they are overweight despite being dangerously underweight (Hartmann et al. 2013) and see their emaciated body as normal or even fat. They fear being fat and view any attempt to nourish them as an attempt to 'fatten them up'

(Boughtwood and Halse 2007). This distorted image is a cardinal feature of AN (National Institute for Health and Clinical Excellence 2004b) and is a cognitive distortion in which appearance stimuli are given priority and amplified. Sufferers focus on the negative aspects of their appearance that are deemed to be 'ugly' (Jansen et al. 2005; Hartmann et al. 2013). Great value is placed upon the ideal body image, which is transmitted via peers, the media and societal influences. Social notions of beauty and thinness are constantly present. Such social messages have a strong impact on young women with low levels of self-esteem and confidence, who may compare themselves unfavourably with the images they are presented with, yet feel the images are those to aspire to in order to be truly successful. There is a problem with processing self-referential information regarding body image (Benninghoven et al. 2007a; Boughtwood and Halse 2007). The idea that appearance provides confidence, self-esteem and self-worth pervades the social environment, and becomes an overvalued ideal. This adds to the psychological struggle to be accepted in a social world where they are accessed solely on appearance (Boughtwood and Halse 2007).

FOOD PERCEPTION AND HUNGER

Inaccurate and confused perception about food is present. The young person is preoccupied with eating, food preparation and food-related activity, yet derives pleasure from refusing food and partaking in family meals. Fasting and food refusal is viewed as a means to gain control – it is empowering (Dingemans et al. 2006). Hunger awareness is pronounced, yet the individual does not recognize nutritional need and is, it is suggested, unable to assess the amount of food taken or to be consumed (Vinai et al. 2007). However, Vinai et al. (2007) found that their patients with AN did not assess food amounts differently from control subjects. Both groups were incapable of assessing food amounts accurately. Vinai et al. (2007) concluded that this inability to accurately assess food amounts may play a role in the multidimensional nature of the onset and maintenance of AN.

Boughtwood and Halse (2007) found that treatment plans affected food perception. Medical treatment focuses on a reductionist approach to AN where food is quantified, measured, prepared and then served with little involvement of the patient. They suggest that this is removed from reality where the young person would observe food being prepared, may be involved in its preparation and have some choice over what they eat. They suggest that hospital erodes normal eating. Thus the difficulty with food is compounded once discharged into the 'real' world.

PERSONAL CONTROL

The young person may experience a profound paralyzing sense of effectiveness; the individual is convinced that they can only function in response to the wishes and demands of others, rather than making their own choices (Bruch 1973). Potential trigger events can be significant life events seemingly outside the control of the individual, who is overwhelmed by a number of developmental, familial, academic and social pressures (National Institute for Health and Clinical Excellence 2004b; Pike et al. 2008). Depression and anxiety are frequently diagnosed in young people with an eating disorder, who are more at risk of suicidal ideation, attempts and completion (Unikel et al. 2006; Spindler and Milos 2007; Holm-Denoma et al. 2008). This would suggest a spiralling into hopelessness, low self-esteem and an increasing sense of worthlessness, leading to increasing control over eating while contending with the ongoing pressures, which are perceived as threatening and eroding autonomy and a sense of self (Colton and Pistrang 2004; Holm-Denoma et al. 2008).

Family functioning has an impact. It is thought that a negative, conflictual relationship leads to a controlling parent, and verbal and physical abuse lead to interpersonal problems; these, when linked with other life events, have the potential to lead to eating disorders and suicidal behaviour (Unikel et al. 2006; Pike et al. 2008). Individuals with an eating disorder have recounted a disturbed father–daughter relationship, lower paternal care and empathy as well as overprotection (Unikel et al. 2006; Fernández-Aranda et al. 2007). Also, living in a large family with grandparents at home was related to an increase in eating disorders. Eating patterns became chaotic, with grandparents perhaps adopting authoritarian styles of eating, resulting in conflict and a heightened emotional climate around food and its consumption (Fernández-Aranda et al. 2007; McCormack and McCann 2015). Protective factors would appear to be open, honest communication; warm, empathetic parents; and the development of autonomy with less oppressive parental control (Unikel et al. 2006; Duclos et al. 2014).

FAMILY FUNCTIONING

Family relationships are considered to be a key element in AN (Duclos et al. 2014). Several studies suggest that familial conflict and dysfunctional communication patterns are found in families with a child with AN (Lyke and Matsen 2013; Duclos et al. 2014). Lyke and Matsen (2013) found that 'eating-disordered' families were more dysfunctional and had difficulty with appropriate affective functioning. They cite other studies which suggest that families with a child with an eating disorder tend to be poorer at problem solving and have poorer communication patterns, a lack of defined family roles, less affective involvement and interest in family members and difficulties with behavioural control.

The expressed emotional climate also has an impact on the young person's psychosocial functioning. It was found that a higher level of maternal dissatisfaction was associated with the severity of their daughter's clinical state. Anxiety and a lack of understanding about AN were thought to contribute to the rejection of and critical attitudes toward their daughter with AN. Maternal anxiety lowered tolerance for the illness which reflected difficulty in coping and led to criticism of the affected child. Mothers were found to retain their existing parenting style, whereas fathers had adapted to become more involved and had changed their relationship with their child, becoming warmer (Dimitropoulos et al. 2013; Duclos et al. 2014).

It is suggested that such levels of family dysfunction involving control, negative communication styles, negative expression and involvement, together with discrepancies in values and norms, may be a risk factor for the development of body image problems. Thus if the mother is dissatisfied with her body image within this heightened climate, this could then be relayed to the daughter, who would then develop similar ideas leading to an eating disorder to achieve body satisfaction. The dissatisfaction with one's emotional environment and body is mistakenly projected onto weight, which can be easily changed (Jansen et al. 2005; Benninghoven et al. 2007b; Lyke and Matsen 2013).

PARENTING ISSUES

Parental involvement is widely recognized as being important to the success of the treatment interventions. However, parents do need support in order to present a consistent approach to interventions and managing the disorder at home (Unikel et al. 2006; Benninghoven et al. 2007a, 2007b; McCormack and McCann 2015). Parents said they were slow to recognize the impact of the AN, initially thinking the change in their daughter's eating habits was a developmental issue. As a result, they felt guilty, frustrated and angry with their general practitioner who had failed to recognize the condition despite their concerns and was unaware of the services available. Parents wanted to develop knowledge, but also tried to pinpoint the cause in order to rationalize its appearance (Cottee-Lane et al. 2004; McCormack and McCann 2015). Parents needed support to cope with their own emotions, maintain their partnerships and support their children, which drained them emotionally. They also wanted to be more involved and a part of their child's treatment, asking for improved staff communication and attitudes (Honey and Halse 2006, 2007; Honey et al. 2006; McCormack and McCann 2015).

Parents who spent more time at home with their affected child reported higher levels of conflict with their child and spouse. They felt their child had been taken over and had become 'devious', and that life had changed profoundly for the whole family, which they described as a living nightmare (Honey et al. 2006; Honey and Halse 2007). They also felt stigmatized as felt they were to blame. Guilt was a common emotion. Parents also tried to hide the illness for a variety of reasons – protecting the child and siblings, avoiding stigma. Parents made great efforts to compensate for the disruption, struggling to maintain some normality by protecting their other children from the conflict and distress as well as giving dedicated time to them. They were vigilant for similar symptoms in their well children (Honey and Halse 2006, 2007; Dimitropoulos et al. 2013; McCormack and McCann 2015).

What does emerge on a more positive note is that parents demonstrated resilience and commitment and were determined to access resources and strategies to help their child and family cope with the eating disorder. They found ways to adapt and meet the needs of their child (Honey and Halse 2006, 2007; McCormack and McCann 2015).

The research outlined here illustrates vividly the complexity of parenting a young person who has AN, while the National Institute for Health and Clinical Excellence (2004b) guidelines identify that parents are central to the process of recovery. This can only mean that more support and services must be offered and given to families who are battling to support their child with AN (Department for Children, Schools and Families and Department of Health 2010). Policy documents may be eloquent in describing their vision for services, yet it is mere rhetoric if the reality is not realized.

SIBLINGS

The impact on the siblings was profound as they encountered the conflict, heightened emotions and disrupted routines in the household. In the study by Areemit et al. (2010) the siblings spoke about their confusion, anger and being overwhelmed by the AN. They were acutely aware of the eating behaviours of their sibling and the obsessive behaviours they encountered were more disturbing, leaving them embarrassed and frustrated. The emotional climate was fraught, and secrecy and lies played a role in the communication patterns which they resented. However, they were deeply concerned for their sibling and wanted to protect them. They reported sadness at the loss of a normal childhood and felt left out. Some blamed themselves for what had happened while others blamed the media and society. Every aspect of their lives was affected by the AN (Areemit et al. 2010; Dimitropoulos et al. 2013; Halvorsen et al. 2013).

ATTITUDES TOWARD TREATMENT

Attitudes toward treatment are complex. Young people reported that being with other sufferers was beneficial as they had access to understanding, support and empathy. However, although they understood the value of being an inpatient on the eating disorders unit, which in some respects provided a sense of belonging and kinship, the treatment exacerbated their loss of individuality, the arresting of their development and the rejection they perceived from their families (Colton and Pistrang 2004; Cottee-Lane et al. 2004; Offord et al. 2006). The autonomy which patients wanted was removed and they sensed they were being manipulated. Food choices were removed and the freedom to be themselves often led them into a double-bind situation around food, where if they did eat they were criticized for eating the 'wrong thing' but told off if they did not eat (Boughtwood and Halse 2007). Enforced treatment equalled punishment and, for some, prolonged the inevitable outcome which they wanted. Parents were placed in the invidious position of having to consent to and watch their child undergo enforced life-saving treatment, which they felt further damaged their trust and relationship with their child (Tan et al. 2003). Aspects of treatment served to prolong or exacerbate the symptoms and feelings underpinning the AN (Offord et al. 2006). Not all found the inpatient units a negative experience; the positive aspects meant the adolescents had contact with peers, a sense of community and the opportunity to learn from others in terms of coping (Colton and Pistrang 2004; Offord et al. 2006). Being with other young people in support group settings can be very beneficial. Beat (Beating Eating Disorders) is a UK-wide network of more than 400 support groups for young people, often running in local colleges and universities (Beat 2010).

NURSE ATTITUDES

Although AN is conceptualized as a mental health problem, it affects the physical health of the adolescent, who may require admission to hospital for medical care and stabilization before further interventions or treatments are carried out (Colton and Pistrang 2004; National Institute for Health and Clinical Excellence 2004b). Such an admission will bring the young person into contact with nurses who are trained in the acute care of sick children and young people – nurses who may not have a mental health background and whose experience with mental health issues is limited. Nurses have reported they find it challenging to care for young people with AN, believing that, over time, they challenged their core values as nurses. They found the patients challenging and found themselves making judgments and resenting their patients. Nurses felt they were in emotional turmoil, feeling angry, disheartened and inadequate. The study found that they reached a point of not being able to cope and 'turned off', distancing themselves from the patients. This is a bleak scenario that erodes the therapeutic relationship the nurse can develop with the young person to begin the process of recovery (King and Turner 2000; Colton and Pistrang 2004; Ramjan 2004; National Institute for Health and Clinical Excellence 2004b). The difficulty arises as nurses reported that their knowledge base was poor, and they struggled to understand a complex disorder. This required new ways of working which challenged the nurses who wanted control rather than to work in partnership. Some nurses did begin to view the situation from the patient's perspective, which refreshed their attitudes and care delivery, making it a more positive experience for both them and their patients.

However, it should be borne in mind that the young person with AN who is admitted to an acute children's ward may be critically ill and require life-saving treatment (Royal College of Psychiatrists 2012b). Thus for staff the physical needs, care and treatment may have overwhelmed and taken precedence over considerations of psychological care. However, what emerges with distinct clarity is that there is real need for cross-field education in these issues and an urgent need to provide ongoing multidisciplinary education at the post-registration level (Department for Children, Schools and Families and Department of Health 2008, 2009; Welsh Assembly Government 2009). The children and young people's nurse is a linchpin and has a pivotal role to play in coordinating and delivering compassionate care via a multidisciplinary approach, building therapeutic relationships with the patient while empowering them to take control in their initial care (National Institute for Health and Clinical Excellence 2004b; Welsh Assembly Government 2009).

PRINCIPLES FOR PRACTICE

- Anorexia nervosa occurs in response to a lack of perceived control in the individual's life.
- Body image and perception are distorted, leading to body dysmorphia.
- Hunger perception is altered.
- It is multifactorial, but may be triggered in response to a traumatic event.

NEURODEVELOPMENTAL DISORDERS

AUTISTIC SPECTRUM DISORDER

Autistic spectrum disorder (ASD) is the term used to describe children who have particular characteristics in common and may have difficulties:

- Understanding and using non-verbal and verbal communication
- Interpreting social behaviour, which affects their ability to relate to others
- Thinking and behaving flexibly

The autistic spectrum of disorders comes under the umbrella term of *pervasive developmental disorders* (WHO 2007), with ASD first being described by Wing (1976), who defined the triad of impairments that are experienced (National Autistic Society 2016a):

- *Social interaction* (difficulty with social relationships, e.g. appearing aloof and indifferent to other people)
- *Social communication* (difficulty with verbal and non-verbal communication, e.g. not really understanding the meaning of gestures, facial expressions or tone of voice)
- *Social imagination* (difficulty in the development of play and imagination, e.g. having a limited range of imaginative activities, possibly copied and pursued rigidly and repetitively)

The range of cognitive, language, emotional and behavioural problems that young people experience may include a need for routine and mean that they have difficulty understanding other people, including their intentions, feelings and perspectives (National Institute for Health and Clinical Excellence 2014).

There has been confusion around the different diagnostic criteria and terminology that define ASDs. ASD is a complex developmental disability, which can make diagnosis difficult, but families do greatly benefit from a timely diagnosis and access to appropriate services and support. Children with ASD may be quite different from each other in terms of their abilities and their areas of strengths and weaknesses.

There are a number of categories within the spectrum. In the 1940s, autism was first described in the US by Kanner (1944), with Asperger's syndrome identified by the Austrian physician Hans Asperger (Frith 1991). Children of all levels of ability can have an ASD, and it can occur in conjunction with other disorders, including sensory loss, language impairment and Down's syndrome. Children with an ASD have a different perspective and experience of the world from ours. It is important to value and develop their particular interests and activities and not to focus solely on trying to change them (Mental Health Foundation 2001).

In practice, a diagnosis of an ASD might be given by a paediatrician, psychiatrist, speech and language therapist, clinical or educational psychologist or GP. Others who see the child and family regularly, such as preschool staff and teachers, may already have suspected that the child has an ASD and referred them for further assessment. An autism strategy has been implemented in England and provides guidance as to how local authorities, the NHS and other agencies need to work together (Autism Act 2009). The strategy highlights the need for planning in relation to the provision of relevant services for young people with autistic spectrum conditions as they move from being children to adults.

Wales was the first country in the world to develop a cross-cutting national strategic action plan for people with autism and has put £1.8 million into driving forward its key actions (Welsh Assembly Government 2008).

Northern Ireland also developed an action plan and strategy (Northern Ireland Executive 2014). These action plans aim to give all children and adults with autism every opportunity to fulfil their potential, by putting a plan in place to address the needs of all ages, involving individuals and their families and carers in the decision-making process (Welsh Assembly Government 2008). It is noted that a lack of access to appropriate services and support at an early stage can lead to children and adults with autism developing additional difficulties such as mental health problems, which can have devastating effects. There are now specific multiagency groups in all local authorities with named leads responsible for developing and implementing local ASD action plans in line with the ASD strategic action plan (National Autistic Society Cymru 2010). These actions will go a long way to address the omissions of the past, as care of children with ASD has been a much neglected area, with families often isolated and unsupported.

BEHAVIOURS THAT PROFESSIONALS LOOK FOR IN DIAGNOSING AN AUTISTIC SPECTRUM DISORDER

- Delay or absence of spoken language
- Unusual uses of language (e.g. pronoun reversal – saying 'you' instead of 'I')
- Repeating others' words beyond the usual age
- Difficulties in playing with other children or sharing interest with others
- Inappropriate eye contact with others
- Unusual play activities and interests
- Failure to point with their index finger to communicate
- Resistance to changes in familiar routines

Source: NICE (2011) *Autism in under 19s: recognition, referral and diagnosis.*

SUPPORTIVE INTERVENTIONS FOR CHILDREN WITH AUTISTIC SPECTRUM DISORDER

- Behavioural interventions: Designed to change behaviour
- Diets and supplements: Based on the deliberate selection of foods and supplements
- Medical interventions: Use of prescribed drugs and other medical treatments
- Physiological interventions: Based on the mechanical, physical and biochemical functions of the body
- Relationship-based interventions: Seeking to encourage attachment and bonding
- Service-based interventions: Including education and parental support services
- Skills-based interventions: Aiming to develop, maintain or support specific skills

Source: National Autistic Society, 2016b, available at http://www.autism.org.uk/about.aspx

In order to communicate effectively, observation is the key to the autistic child's world and is not something that can be learned quickly, as it takes time to anticipate and interpret the meaning of the slightest gesture (Brown 2006). Considering how you approach a child is important; there is no use demanding that they do this or that, as in most instances you will get a negative response. It is important to speak slowly, clearly and to keep language simple. Tell the child what to do ('Put your knife and fork down please'), as it is easier for a child to do something than to stop doing something (Brown 2006). Give the child time to work out what it is you have said, what it means and what you want him or her to do. Be prepared to wait, and wait a little longer, which can be very effective (Brown 2006). Further information can be obtained from the world's first national website resource for autism (Autism Cymru 2009), which provides information on autism services, treatments and therapies including an online library.

Children and young people's nurses can play a key role by problem-solving with families and negotiating healthcare, education and a range of resources to improve the life of the child and his or her family, and are ideally placed to help families access resources (Giarelli et al. 2005).

PRINCIPLES FOR PRACTICE

- Children with autistic spectrum disorders have difficulties with social interaction, social communication and flexibility in thinking and behaving.
- Think carefully when you communicate with a child who has autism; speak slowly, clearly and be specific.
- Value the child's interests and activities to promote their self-esteem.

ATTENTION DEFICIT HYPERACTIVITY DISORDER

Attention deficit hyperactivity disorder (ADHD) is the most common behavioural disorder that starts in childhood. In the UK, ADHD affects 6% of children (Schachar 1991), whereas in the US 3%–7% are affected (Salmeron 2009). It is referred to as both a neurodevelopmental disorder and a heterogeneous behavioural syndrome that is characterized by core symptoms of inattention, hyperactivity and impulsivity (Biederman and Faraone 2005). It should not be confused with normal childhood behaviour that is excitable or boisterous. Although it was initially thought that children outgrow ADHD, it is now known that 60% of children continue to have significant symptoms as adults (Harpin 2005).

CHILDREN WITH ADHD

Children with ADHD have been described as:

- Restless, fidgety and overactive
- Continuously chattering and interrupting people
- Easily distracted without being able to finish things
- Inattentive and unable to concentrate on tasks
- Impulsive, suddenly doing things without thinking first
- Having difficulty in waiting their turn in games, in conversation or in a queue

Source: Royal College of Psychiatrists, *Mental Health and Growing Up: Attention Deficit Hyperactivity Disorder and Hyperkinetic Disorder*, RCP, London, 2012a, available at http://www.rcpsych.ac.uk/healthadvice/parentsandyouthinfo/parentscarers/adhdhyperkineticdisorder.aspx

References to children with ADHD-type symptoms date back to the nineteenth and early twentieth century, initially with Hoffman, a German physician, who in 1865 described 'fidgety Philip' (cited in Barkley 2006) as one who 'won't sit still, wriggles, giggles, swings backwards and forwards, tilts up his chair – growing rude and wild'. This was shortly followed by others who described children with similar behaviours (Still 1902; Tredgold 1908, cited in Barkley 2006), who they said could not sit still, maintain attention or learn from consequences of their actions.

While symptoms may appear irritating, if they are ignored or left untreated, the persistent effects of ADHD can have a negative impact. Children with ADHD have an increased risk of academic failure, social isolation and involvement with deviant peer groups (Harpin 2005). Research suggests ADHD occurs as a result of a combination of environmental and genetic factors (Furman 2005) that have an impact on brain chemistry. The current theory that tries to explain ADHD implicates the frontal cortex and its importance in response inhibition, as ADHD sufferers have difficulty in suppressing impulse (Myttas 2001). Such children respond to all impulses, being unable to exclude those unnecessary for a situation. Rather than failing to pay attention, they pay attention to everything, meaning they become overwhelmed with information that they cannot process. Children then find it difficult to think about a situation, to 'put the brakes on' and think through possible consequences before they act.

Children will show different symptoms of ADHD and may have limited control over what they do or say (as they tend to act impulsively). ADHD does not always have a negative impact on academic ability. However, half of all children with ADHD also have a learning difficulty, such as dyslexia. ADHD may have an impact on speech, language and coordination. Children and adults with ADHD are also more likely to experience depression, anxiety and obsessive thoughts or behaviours. Children with ADHD have been shown to prompt negative parenting, which becomes reinforced in a vicious circle, as parents and children maintain each other's negative patterns of interaction, highlighting the need for parenting programmes to be a key part of treatment.

A diagnosis of ADHD may be given by a paediatrician or a psychiatrist, after a period of comprehensive assessment. There needs to be clear evidence of a significant impairment in the child's functioning in social or school settings. New developments in brain imaging technology are assisting with diagnosis in the US, as professionals have a clearer picture of the underlying physiology of the brain (Amen 2010). There has been much debate around the role of diet in children with ADHD, and although high-protein, low-carbohydrate diets are being discussed in the US (Amen 1998), in the UK, the National Institute for Health and Clinical Excellence guidelines simply stress the value of healthcare professionals promoting a balanced diet, good nutrition and regular exercise for children and young people with ADHD (National Institute for Health and Clinical Excellence 2016). Benefits found in omega-3 fatty acids and the elimination of artificial colouring and additives from the diet are, at the time of writing, still subject to large-scale trials.

MANAGING THE MAIN SYMPTOMS OF ADHD

The National Institute for Health and Clinical Excellence Quality Standard (2013b) states that all children and young people with symptoms of ADHD need to be referred to an ADHD specialist for assessment. This should include an assessment of parents'/carers' mental health, and parents/carers being referred to a parent training programme as first-line treatment.

ADHD cannot be cured, but a variety of treatments are available to support the child and his or her family. Although the ethical issues associated with long-term stimulant medication use in children have been much debated (Daley 2006), there is further debate around parents' motivations for the use or non-use of such medication (Taylor et al. 2006). The rationale for medication is that it can improve children's concentration, but emotional and educational support are essential care components too. A treatment plan should be developed according to the individual needs of each child. Usually, a specialist will decide initial treatment, liaise with the GP and regularly review progress. Current UK guidelines recommend that everyone diagnosed with ADHD should receive information and advice about all aspects of ADHD, so informed choices about the treatment options can be made. It is worth noting that in the US, 60% of children receive medication for ADHD, while in Finland less than 1% are prescribed medication and fare similarly both socially and academically as peers without ADHD (Smalley et al. 2007). If drug treatment is used, this should always form part of a comprehensive treatment plan that includes psychological, behavioural and educational advice and interventions.

When working with families, it is essential to understand what parents know and believe about their child's ADHD, and because there is no cure, parents often seek a magic intervention, rather than realizing that successful treatment involves a variety of educational, behavioural and parenting interventions (Cormier and Harrison Elder 2007). As children's self-esteem is shaped by their thinking, expectations and experiences of how others think and feel about them (in terms of how they are treated), ADHD can have an enormous impact. Many children with ADHD have problems in school, including relationships with teachers and peers. Children with ADHD find people often do not understand their behaviour and judge them. They may experience punishments for being disruptive, but find it easier not to bother trying to fit in, and do not engage in schoolwork. This can mean that children with ADHD feel they are a failure and have low self-esteem. Engaging with such children to find out how they feel about themselves is a vital skill.

PRINCIPLES FOR PRACTICE

- Children with ADHD are usually restless, easily distracted, impulsive and find concentration difficult.
- Children with ADHD are at risk of academic failure, social isolation and further mental health problems.
- Current UK guidelines recommend a comprehensive needs assessment and a treatment plan that includes psychological, behavioural and educational advice and interventions.

CONCLUSION

This chapter has reviewed a number of complex mental health problems with which children and young people may present within a variety of healthcare settings from a national and international perspective. There is no one single predisposing factor which precipitates the development of these problems. It would appear that there is a complex interplay of social, psychological and biological factors and issues which contribute to the development of complex mental health problems at a time when the child or young person is vulnerable and in need of positive easily accessible support.

It is self-evident that just as children and young people have physical health problems they may also have mental health problems, and both should receive the same levels of attention, care and ongoing support to them and their families (DH 2011; Welsh Government 2015). It is essential that truly holistic care takes place because, as has been pointed out in Chapter 10, physical health is closely linked with mental health and well-being. This chapter has sought to reiterate this point in relation to the problems reviewed. The children's nurse needs to have well-honed knowledge of the potential risk factors which may precipitate the development of suicidal thinking and behaviour, self-harm and AN, and can play a pivotal role in educating fellow practitioners about mental health issues. Such insight is also required with regard to suicide prevention, self-harm, AN, ASD and ADHD, for which families require support and help to cope with problems that can often take time to diagnose and for the appropriate support and service to be put in place.

Personal and professional attitudes must also be examined in relation to care delivery so that collaborative working with the mental health professionals does occur, and the multidisciplinary team and voluntary agencies can be strengthened in order to deliver high-quality care and support to the child and young person in distress.

This chapter has discussed and highlighted the research evidence underpinning care delivery as well as addressing the key issues that children and young people's nurses need to critically consider for practice when caring for children and young people with complex mental health problems.

SUMMARY OF PRINCIPLES FOR PRACTICE

- Children and young people's nurses need to value and support their patients who present with complex mental health problems so that children and young people feel their problems are being taken seriously.
- Children and young people's nurses must develop knowledge of complex mental health issues and their contributory factors to inform the care they deliver.
- Children and young people's nurses need to develop insight into their own knowledge, skills and attitudes regarding complex mental health issues through ongoing education and training in the care of children and young people with complex mental health problems.
- Children and young people's nurses are in a prime position to provide support, care, reassurance and access to helping services for children, young people and their families.
- Care needs to be collaborative and multidisciplinary in nature and all members of the multidisciplinary team need to liaise clearly with one another.

REFERENCES

Agritmis H, Yaci N, Colak B, Aksoy E (2004) Suicidal deaths in childhood and adolescence. *Forensic Science International* **142**: 25–31.

Amen D (1998) *Change your brain, change your life: the breakthrough program for conquering anxiety, depression, obsessiveness, anger and impulsiveness*. New York: Three Rivers Press.

Amen D (2010) *Images of attention deficit disorder*. Available at http://www.amenclinics.com/brain-science/spect-image-gallery/spect-atlas/images-of-attention-deficit-disorder-addadhd/.

Areemit RS, Katzmn D, Pinhas L, Kaufman M (2010) The experience of siblings of adolescents with eating disorders. *Journal of Adolescent Health* **46**: 569–76.

Arkins B, Tyrell M, Herlihy E, Crowley B (2013) Assessing the reasons for deliberate self harm in young people. *Mental Health Practice* **16**(7): 28–32.

Autism Act (2009) London: Stationary Office. Available at http://www.legislation.gov.uk/ukpga/2009/15/section/3.

Autism Cymru (2009) *AWARES*. Available at http://www.awares.org/homepage.asp?languageID=0.

Ayyash-Abdo H (2002) Adolescent suicide: an ecological perspective. *Psychology in the Schools* **39**: 459–75.

Barkley R (2006) *Attention-deficit hyperactivity disorder: a handbook for diagnosis and treatment*, 3rd ed. New York: Guildford Press.

Beat (2010) *Support groups*. Available at http://www.b-eat.co.uk/get-help/get-support/support-groups/.

Beautrais A, Fergusson DM (2006) Indigenous suicide in New Zealand. *Archives of Suicide Research* **10**: 159–68.

Beautrais AL (2001) Child and young adolescent suicide in New Zealand. *Australian and New Zealand Journal of Psychiatry* **35**: 647–53.

Bee H, Boyd H (2012) *The developing child*, 13th ed. New York: Pearson.

Benninghoven D, Raykowski L, Solzbacher S, et al. (2007a) Body images of patients with anorexia nervosa, bulimia nervosa and female control subjects: a comparison with male ideals of female attractiveness. *Body Image* **4**: 51–9.

Benninghoven D, Tetsch N, Kunzendorf S, Jantschek G (2007b) Body image in patients with eating disorders and their mothers, and the role of family functioning. *Comprehensive Psychiatry* **48**: 118–23.

Biederman J, Faraone S (2005) Attention-deficit hyperactivity disorder. *Lancet* **366**(9481): 237–48.

Boughtwood D, Halse C (2008) Ambivalent appetites: dissonances in social and medical constructions of anorexia nervosa. *Journal of Community and Applied Psychology* **18**: 269–81.

Brausch AM, Muehlenkamp JJ (2007) Body image and suicidal ideation in adolescents. *Body Image* **4**: 207–12.

Brown M (2006) Communicating with the child who has autistic spectrum disorder: a practical introduction. *Paediatric Nursing* **18**: 14–17.

Bruch H (1962) Perceptual and cognitive disturbances in anorexia nervosa. *Psychosomatic Medicine* **24**: 187–94.

Bruch H (1973) *Eating disorders.* London: Routledge and Kegan Paul.

Bryant-Waugh R (2006) Recent developments in anorexia nervosa. *Child and Adolescent Mental Health* **11**(2): 76–81.

Cleaver K, Meerabeau L, Maras P (2014) Attitudes towards young people who self harm: age, an influencing factor. *Journal of Advanced Nursing* **70**(12): 2884–96.

Coleman JC, Henry L (2011) *The nature of adolescence,* 4th ed. London: Routledge.

Colton A, Pistrang N (2004) Adolescents' experiences of inpatient treatment for anorexia nervosa. *European Eating Disorders Review* **12**: 307–16.

Cormier E, Harrison Elder J (2007) Diet and child behaviour problems: fact or fiction? *Pediatric Nursing* **33**: 2.

Cottee-Lane D, Pistrang N, Bryant-Waugh R (2004) Childhood onset of anorexia nervosa. *European Eating Disorders Review* **12**: 169–77.

Crisp AH (1997) Anorexia as a flight from growth: assessment and treatment based on the model. In Garner DM, Garfinkel PE (eds.) *Handbook of treatment for eating disorders,* 2nd ed., pp. 248–77. New York: Guildford Press.

Daley D (2006) Attention deficit hyperactivity disorder: a review of the essential facts. *Child: Care, Health and Development* **32**: 193–204.

Department for Children, Schools and Families and Department of Health (2008) *Children and young people in mind: the final report of the National CAMHS Review.* London: DCSF/DH.

Department for Children, Schools and Families and Department of Health (2009) *Healthy lives, brighter futures: the strategy for children and young people's health.* London: DCSF/DH.

Department for Children, Schools and Families and Department of Health (2010) *Keeping children and young people in mind: the government's full response to the independent review of CAMHS.* London: DCSF/DH.

Department of Health (2011) No health without mental health: a cross-government mental health outcomes strategy for people of all ages. London: DH. Available at https://www.gov.uk/government/uploads/system/uploads/attachment_data/file/213761/dh_124058.pdf.

Department of Health (2014) *Statistical update on suicide.* London: DH.

Department of Health (2015a) *Preventing suicide in England: two years on.* London: HM Government.

Department of Health (2015b) *Future in mind.* London: HM Government. Available at https://www.gov.uk/government/uploads/system/uploads/attachment_data/file/414024/Childrens_Mental_Health.pdf (accessed 14 July 2015).

Department of Health, Social Services and Public Safety (2014) *Development of a new suicide prevention strategy for Northern Ireland: pre-consultation engagement summary report.* Northern Ireland: DHSSPS, Belfast. Available at https://www.dhsspsni.gov.uk/sites/default/files/publications/dhssps/suicide-prevention-new-strat-preconsultation-summary-report.pdf.

Dimitropoulos G, Freeman V, Bellai K, Olmsted M (2013) Inpatients with severe anorexia and their siblings: non-shared experiences and family functioning. *European Eating Disorders Review* **21**: 284–93.

Dingemans A, Spinhoven P, Furth EF (2006) Maladaptive core beliefs and eating disorder symptoms. *Eating Behaviours* **7**: 258–65.

Duclos J, Dorard G, Berthoz S, Curt F, Faucher S, Falissard B, Godart N (2014) Expressed emotion in anorexia nervosa: what is inside the 'black box'? *Comprehensive Psychiatry* **55**: 71–9.

Fairburn CG, Shafran R, Cooper Z (1998) A cognitive behavioural theory of anorexia nervosa. *Behaviour Research and Therapy* **37**: 1–13.

Fernández-Aranda F, Krug I, Granero R, et al. (2007) Individual and family eating patterns during childhood and early adolescence: an analysis of associated eating disorders factors. *Appetite* **49**: 476–85.

Fortune S, Hawton K (2007) Suicide and deliberate self harm in children and adolescents. *Pediatrics and Child Health* **17**: 443–7.

Frith U (ed.) (1991) *Autism and Asperger syndrome,* pp. 37–92. Cambridge: Cambridge University Press.

Furman L (2005) What is attention-deficit hyperactivity disorder (ADHD)? *Journal of Child Neurology* **20**: 994–1002.

Garnefski N, Diekstra RF (1997) Adolescents from one parent, stepparent and intact families: emotional problems and suicide attempts. *Journal of Adolescence* **20**(2): 201–8.

Coughan M (2011a) Self harm. In Claveirole A, Gaughan M, *Understanding children and young people's mental health*, Chapter 4, pp. 64–86. London: Wiley Blackwell.

Gaughan M (2011b) Suicide. In Claveirole A, Gaughan M, *Understanding children and young people's mental health*, Chapter 6, pp. 108–131. London: Wiley Blackwell.

Giarelli E, Souders M, Pinto-Martin, et al. (2005) Intervention pilot for parents of children with autistic spectrum disorder. *Pediatric Nursing* **31**(5): 389–99.

Girlguiding UK/Mental Health Foundation (2008) *A generation under stress*. London: MHF. Available at http://www.mentalhealth.org.uk/.

Green H, McGinnity A, Meltzer H, et al. (2005) *Mental health of children and young people in Great Britain 2004 (a survey for the Office for National Statistics)*. London: Palgrave Macmillan.

Hallet D, Chandler M, Lalonde C (2007) Aboriginal language knowledge and youth suicide. *Cognitive Development* **22**: 392–9.

Halvorsen I, Ro O, Heyerdahl S (2013) Nine year follow up of girls with anorexia nervosa and their siblings: retrospective perceptions of parental bonding and the influence of illness on their everyday lives. *European Eating Disorders Review* **21**: 20–27.

Harpin V (2005) The effect of ADHD on the life of an individual, their family, and community from preschool to adult life. *Archives of Disease in Childhood* **90**: 12–17.

Hartmann A, Thomas J, Greenberg JL, Rosenfield EH, Wilhelm S (2015) Accept, distract, or reframe? An exploratory experimental comparison of strategies for coping with intrusive body image thoughts in anorexia nervosa and body dysmorphic disorder. *Psychiatry Research* **225**: 643–50.

Hartmann A, Thomas JJ, Wilson AC, Wilhelm A (2013) Insight impairment in body image disorders: delusionality and overvalued ideas in anorexia nervosa versus body dysmorphic disorder. *Psychiatry Research* **210**: 1129–35.

Hawton K, Saunders KEA, O'Connor R (2012) Self harm and suicide in adolescents. *Lancet* **379**: 2373–82.

Holm-Denoma JM, Witte TK, Gordon KH, et al. (2008) Deaths by suicide among individuals with anorexia as arbiters between competing explanations of the anorexia-suicide link. *Journal of Affective Disorders* **107**(1–3): 231–6.

Honey A, Clarke S, Halse C, et al. (2006) The influence of siblings on the experience of anorexia nervosa for adolescent girls. *European Eating Disorders Review* **14**: 315–22.

Honey A, Halse C (2006) The specifics of coping: parents of daughters with anorexia nervosa. *Qualitative Health Research* **16**: 1611.

Honey A, Halse C (2007) Looking after well siblings of adolescent girls with anorexia: an important parental role. *Child: Care, Health and Development* **33**: 52–8.

Ilomaki E, Rasanen P, Viilo K, Hakko H (2007) Suicidal behaviour among adolescents with conduct disorder: the role of alcohol dependence. *Psychiatry Research* **150**: 305–11.

Jansen A, Nederkoorn C, Mulkens S (2005) Selective visual attention for ugly and beautiful body parts in eating disorders. *Behaviour Research and Therapy* **43**: 183–96.

Kanner L (1944) Early infantile autism. *Journal of Pediatrics* **25**(3): 211–7.

Khan F, Waheed W (2009) Suicide and self harm in South Asian immigrants. *Psychiatry* **8**(7): 261–4.

King SJ, Turner DS (2000) Caring for adolescent females with anorexia nervosa: registered nurses' perspective. *Journal of Advanced Nursing* **32**: 139–47.

Krishnakumar P, Geeta MG, Riyaz A (2011) Deliberate self harm in children. *Indian Pediatrics* **48**(5): 367–71.

Lehti V, Niemela S, Hoven C, Mandell D, Sourander A (2009) Mental health, substance use and suicidal behavior among young indigenous people in the Artic: a systematic review. *Social Science and Medicine* **69**: 1194–203.

Lindqvist P, Johansson L, Karlsson U (2008) In the aftermath of teenage suicide: a qualitative study of the psychosocial consequences for the surviving family members. *BMC Psychiatry* **8**(26): 1–7.

Lyke J, Matsen J (2013) Family functioning and risk factors for disordered eating. *Eating Behaviours* **14**: 497–9.

McAndrew S, Warne T (2014) Hearing the voices of young people who self harm: implications for service providers. *International Journal of Mental Health Nursing* **23**: 570–9.

McCormack C, McCann E (2015) Caring for an adolescent with anorexia nervosa: parent's views and experiences. *Archives of Psychiatric Nursing* **29**: 143–7.

McNamara P (2012) Adolescent suicide in Australia: rates, risk and resilience. *Clinical Child Psychology and Psychiatry* **18**(3): 351–69.

Mental Health Foundation (2001) *All about autistic spectrum disorders: a booklet for parents and carers*. London: MHF.

Mental Health Foundation (2006) *Truth hurts. Report of the national inquiry into self harm among young people*. London: MHF.

Mental Health Foundation (2016) The truth about self harm. Available at https://www.mentalhealth.org.uk/publications/truth-about-self-harm.

Ministry of Health New Zealand (2011) *New Zealand mortality and demographic data*. Available at http://www.health.govt.nz/publication/mortality-and-demographic-data-2011 (accessed 14 July 2015).

Miotto P, Preti A (2008) Suicide ideation and social desirability among school aged young people. *Journal of Adolescence* **31**: 519–33.

Morris J, Twaddle S (2007) Anorexia nervosa. *British Medical Journal* **334**: 894–8.

Myttas N (2001) Understanding and recognising ADHD. *Practice Nursing* **12**(7): 278–80.

National Autistic Society (2016a) *Patients with autistic spectrum disorders: guidance for health professionals*. Available at http://www.autism.org.uk/professionals/health-workers/guidance.aspx.

National Autistic Society (2016b). Available at http://www.autism.org.uk/about.aspx.

National Autistic Society Cymru (2010) *Progress on the implementation of the Welsh Assembly Government autistic spectrum disorder (ASD) strategic action plan*. Available at http://www.google.co.uk/url?url=http://www.autism.org.uk/~/media/NAS/Documents/Get-involved/Campaign%2520for%2520change/The%2520ASD%2520strategic%2520action%2520plan.ashx&rct=j&frm=1&q=&esrc=s&sa=U&ei=6fe4VK_MHNXbas7wgaAO&ved=0CBsQFjAB&sig2=4hro8g2u_fE3ntGGQUor9g&usg=AFQjCNFtUqY_aHWc58Ey6uUW7HqclJ5RoA.

National Institute for Health and Clinical Excellence (2004a) *Self harm: the short term physical and psychological management and secondary prevention of self harm in primary and secondary care*. Clinical guidelines CG16. London: NICE. Available at https://www.nice.org.uk/guidance/CG16.

National Institute for Health and Clinical Excellence (2004b) *Eating disorders*. Clinical guidelines CG9. London: NICE. Available at http://guidance.nice.org.uk/CG9/Guidance/pdf/English.

National Institute for Health and Clinical Excellence (2016) *Attention deficit hyperactivity disorder: diagnosis and management of ADHD in children, young people and adults*. Clinical guidelines CG72. London: NICE. Available at https://www.nice.org.uk/guidance/cg72.

National Institute for Health and Care Excellence (2011) *Autism in under 19s: recognition, referral and diagnosis*. NICE Guidelines CG128 London: NICE Available at https://www.nice.org.uk/guidance/CG128/chapter/Key-priorities-for-implementation.

National Institute for Health and Clinical Excellence (2013a) *Self harm*. Quality Standard 34. London: NICE. Available at https://www.nice.org.uk/guidance/qs34.

National Institute for Health and Care Excellence (2013b) *Quality standard for attention deficit hyperactivity disorder*. Available at https://www.nice.org.uk/guidance/qs39.

National Institute for Health and Care Excellence (2014) *Quality standard for autism*. Available at http://www.nice.org.uk/guidance/qs51/chapter/introduction.

Nicholls DE, Lynn R, Viner RM (2011) Childhood eating disorders: British national surveillance study. *British Journal of Psychiatry* **198**: 295–301.

Northern Ireland Executive (2014) *The autism strategy 2013–2020 and the action plan 2013–2016*. Northern Ireland: Northern Ireland Executive, Belfast. Available at https://www.dhsspsni.gov.uk/sites/default/files/publications/dhssps/autism-strategy-action-plan-2013_0.pdf.

Offord A, Turner H, Cooper M (2006) Adolescent inpatient treatment for anorexia nervosa: a qualitative study exploring young adults' retrospective views of treatment and discharge. *European Eating Disorders Review* **14**: 377–87.

Orbach S (1978) *Fat is a feminist issue*. London: Hamlyn.

Orbach S (1986) *Hunger strike: the anorectic's struggle as a metaphor for our age*. London: Faber and Faber.

Parry-Langdon N (2008) *Three years on: survey of the emotional development and well-being of children and young people*. Newport: Office for National Statistics.

Patton GC, Coffey C, Romaniuk H, MacKinnon A, Carlin JB, Degenhardt L, Olsson CA, Moran P (2014) The prognosis of common mental disorders in adolescents: a 14 year prospective study. *Lancet* **383**: 1404–11.

Pike KM, Hilbert A, Wilfley DE, et al. (2008) Toward an understanding of risk factors for anorexia nervosa: a case-control study. *Psychological Medicine* **38**: 1443–53.

Polivy J, Herman CP (2002) Causes of eating disorders. *Annual Review of Psychology* **53**: 187–213.

Price S, Knight T, John A (2014) *Research evidence review report for Child Death Review: deaths of children through suicide*. Cardiff: Public Health Wales.

Ramian J M (2004) Nurses and the 'therapeutic relationship': caring for adolescents with anorexia nervosa. *Journal of Advanced Nursing* **45**(5): 495–503.

Rossow I, Norstrom T (2014) Heavy episodic drinking and deliberate self-harm in young people: a longitudinal cohort study. *Addiction* **109**(9): 930–6.

Royal College of Nursing (2014a) *Children and young people's mental health – every nurse's business.* Available at http://www.rcn.org.uk/professional-development/publications/pub-004587.

Royal College of Nursing (2014b) *Mental health in children and young people: an RCN toolkit for nurses who are not mental health specialists.* London: RCN.

Royal College of Psychiatrists (2012a) *Mental health and growing up: attention deficit hyperactivity disorder and hyperkinetic disorder.* London: RCP. Available at http://www.rcpsych.ac.uk/healthadvice/parentsandyouthinfo/parentscarers/adhdhyperkineticdisorder.aspx.

Royal College of Psychiatrists (2012b) *Junior MARSIPAN: management of really sick patients under 18 with anorexia nervosa.* Report from the Junior MARSIPAN group. London: RCP. Available at http://www.rcpsych.ac.uk/files/pdfversion/CR168nov14.pdf (accessed 14 September 2015).

Royal College of Psychiatrists (2015) *Eating disorders.* London: RCP. Available at http://www.rcpsych.ac.uk/mentalhealthinfoforall/problems/eatingdisorders/eatingdisorders.aspx.

Salmeron P (2009) Childhood and adolescent attention-deficit hyperactivity disorder: diagnosis, clinical practice guidelines, and social implications. *Journal of the American Academy of Nurse Practitioners* **21**: 488–97.

Samm A, Tooding L, Sisak M, Kolves K, Aasvee K, Varnik A (2010) Suicidal thoughts and depressive feelings amongst Estonian schoolchildren: effect of family relationship and family structure. *European Child and Adolescent Psychiatry* **19**: 457–68.

Schachar R (1991) Childhood hyperactivity. *Journal of Child Psychology and Psychiatry* **132**: 155–91.

Scottish Government (2013) *Suicide prevention strategy 2013–2016.* Edinburgh: Scottish Government. Available at http://www.gov.scot/Resource/0043/00439429.pdf.

Scowcroft E (2014) *Suicide statistics report 2014.* Samaritans. Available at http://www.samaritans.org/sites/default/files/kcfinder/files/research/Samaritans%20Suicide%20Statistics%20Report%202014.pdf (accessed 16 March 2015).

Seminog O, Goldacre M (2012) Risk of intentional self-harm in young people with selected mental and chronic physical conditions in England. *Journal of Epidemiology and Community Health* **66**: 59.

Silviken A, Kvernmo S (2007) Suicide attempts among indigenous Sami adolescents and majority peers in Arctic Norway: prevalence and associated risk factors. *Journal of Adolescence* **30**(4): 613–26.

Smalley S, McGough J, Moilanen I, et al. (2007) Prevalence and psychiatric comorbidity of attention-deficit/hyperactivity disorder in an adolescent Finnish population. *Journal of the American Academy of Child and Adolescent Psychiatry* **46**: 1575–83.

Spender Q (2007) Assessment of adolescent self harm. *Pediatrics and Child Health* **17**(11): 448–53.

Spindler A, Milos G (2007) Links between eating disorder symptom severity and psychiatric comorbidity. *Eating Behaviors* **8**: 364–73.

Stanley N (2005) Parents' perspectives on young suicide. *Children and Society* **19**: 304–15.

Still GF (1902) Some abnormal psychical conditions in children. *Lancet* **1**: 1008–12, 1077–82, 1163–8.

Surgenor LJ, Horn J, Plumridge EW, Hudson SM (2002) Anorexia nervosa and psychological control: a reexamination of selected theoretical accounts. *European Eating Disorders Review* **10**: 85–101.

Swahn MH, Bossarte RM (2007) Gender, early alcohol use and suicide ideation and attempts: findings from the 2005 Youth Risk Behaviour Survey. *Journal of Adolescent Health* **41**: 175–81.

Tan JO, Hope T, Stewart A, Fitzpatrick R (2003) Control and compulsory treatment in anorexia nervosa: the views of patients and parents. *International Journal of Law and Psychiatry* **26**: 627–45.

Taylor M, O'Donoghue T, Houghton S (2006) To medicate or not to medicate? The decision-making process of Western Australian parents following their child's diagnosis with an attention deficit hyperactivity disorder. *International Journal of Disability, Development and Education* **53**: 111–28.

Toero K, Nagy A, Sawaguchi T, et al. (2001) Characteristics of suicide among children and adolescents in Budapest. *Pediatrics International* **43**: 368–71.

Tousignant M, Vitenti L, Morin N (2013) Aboriginal youth suicide in Quebec: the contribution of public policy for prevention. *International Journal of Law and Psychiatry* **36**: 399–405.

Tulloch AL, Blizzard L, Pinkus Z (1997) Adolescent-parent communication in self harm. *Journal of Adolescent Health* **21**: 267–75.

Unikel C, Gomez-Peresmitre G, Gonzalez-Forteza C (2006) Suicidal behaviour, risky eating behaviours and psychosocial correlates in Mexican female students. *European Eating Disorders Review* **14**: 414–21.

Vinai P, Cardetti S, Ferrato N, et al. (2007) Visual evaluation of food amount in patients affected by anorexia nervosa. *Eating Behaviours* **8**: 291–5.

Welsh Assembly Government (2008) *The autistic spectrum disorder (ASD) strategic action plan for Wales.* Cardiff: WAG.

Welsh Assembly Government (2009) *Eating disorders: a framework for Wales.* Cardiff: WAG.

Welsh Government (2012) *Together for mental health: a strategy for mental health and well-being in Wales.* Cardiff: Welsh Government. Available at http://gov.wales/docs/dhss/publications/121031tmhfinalen.pdf.

Welsh Government (2015) *Talk to me 2: suicide and self-harm prevention strategy for Wales 2015–2020.* Cardiff: Welsh Government. Available at http://gov.wales/topics/health/publications/health/reports/talk2/?lang=en.

Williams R, Drury J (2009) Psychosocial resilience and its influence on managing mass emergencies and disasters. *Psychiatry* **8**(8): 293–6.

Wing L (1976) Diagnosis, clinical description and prognosis. In Wing L (ed.) *Early childhood autism,* pp. 15–48. Oxford: Pergamon.

World Health Organization (2007) *International statistical classification of diseases and related health problems,* 10th ed., vol. 2. Geneva: WHO. Available at http://apps.who.int/classifications/apps/icd/icd10online/.

World Health Organization (2014) *Preventing suicide: a global imperative.* Luxembourg: WHO.

World Health Organization (2016) *Suicide.* Geneva: WHO. Available at http://www.who.int/mediacentre/factsheets/fs398/en/.

Young Minds, Cello (2012) *Talking self harm.* London: Young Minds. Available at http://www.youngminds.org.uk/for_children_young_people/whats_worrying_you/self-harm/what_self-harm (accessed 15 July 2015).

Zandian M, Ioakimidis I, Bergh C, Sodersten P (2007) Cause and treatment of anorexia nervosa. *Physiology and Behaviour* **92**: 283–90.

Zoroglu SS, Tuzun U, Sar V, et al. (2003) Suicide attempt and self mutilation among Turkish high school students in relation with abuse, neglect and dissociation. *Psychiatry and Clinical Neurosciences* **57**: 119–26.

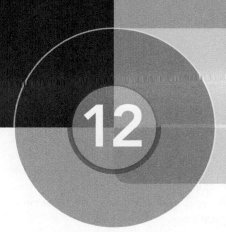

Transitional care for children and young people with life-threatening or life-limiting conditions

KATRINA McNAMARA-GOODGER

OVERVIEW

This chapter covers the need for nurses to work with young people who have a life-threatening or life-limiting condition and their families; to develop an integrated person-centred approach; to guide and support young people, their families and professionals through the transition maze; and to help services to better support young people to adjust to, prepare for and move on to adult services.

INTRODUCTION

Due to improved medical treatments, technology and support, an increasing number of young people live with a life-threatening or life-limiting condition, and many know that they will face a premature death during their teenage years or early adulthood. These young people have a wide range of conditions, some congenital or genetic and apparent from a young age, and others developed later in childhood or adolescence. Their journey through adolescence into adulthood is compounded by facing a complex and often bewildering transition from children's palliative care to adult services, very often at the same time as their condition starts to deteriorate. Young people with palliative care needs should be recognized as a distinct care group as they have physical, psychological and developmental needs that are significantly different from those experienced by children and adults.

A person-centred approach aims to ensure that young people, their families and carers experience a coordinated approach to person-centred care throughout their care journey. It requires clear and open communication and support to enable the young person to build up and maintain access to an appropriate network of support, wherever they are cared for – whether that is in their own home, in their family home or in alternative residential placements such as supported or communal housing or educational settings. Services for young people with palliative care needs should be multidisciplinary and multiagency and should provide a flexible approach to service and care provision, recognizing individual needs. This chapter explores the complex and challenging issues in relation to this and, in doing so, demonstrates how use of an integrated approach can promote a smooth and effective transition for young people.

WORKING WITH YOUNG PEOPLE

Those involved in the care of young people often find themselves working within an organizationally led, arbitrarily set, chronological, restrictive definition set somewhere between adolescence and adulthood. Adolescence is described as a recognizable phase of life and it has a wide range of definitions; some recognize chronological descriptions, or phases, of adolescence, ranging from 10 to 24 years, but most reflect an understanding that adolescence is essentially 'a stage, not an age' – a developmental stage described by the time period between the beginning of puberty and adulthood, which also enables a recognition that adolescence is a period of development unique to the individual rather than a specific age.

At the beginning of adolescence, the parents of young people are generally still mainly responsible for all aspects of the young person's care, but, by the end of adolescence, care issues will be mainly the responsibility of the young person, as they develop their autonomy, although there will probably still be involvement of parents/carers in that care. Other parents, for example those of young people with conditions such as severe cerebral palsy or severe developmental delay, will recognize that their child will never attain full independence, although the young person may choose to seek other care from paid carers to promote as much independence as possible and sometimes in recognition of the impact that caring for them has on their parents.

Work with this broadly defined age group requires an understanding of physical, emotional, social and cognitive development and a recognition that development continues in all or some of these areas for all young people, despite the impact of a life-threatening or life-limiting condition. During adolescence there are a number of developmental phases which lead to young people forming an understanding of their personal identity and value system and accepting a new body image, along with the development of skills and abilities and taking responsibility for their own behaviour. For young people with life-threatening or life-limiting conditions, adolescence may also bring concerns about physical appearance and mobility and a reliance on parents and others in relation to decision making, which delays the development of independence, and there may also be limited opportunities for social interaction with peers or a sense of lack of acceptance or fear of rejection by peers. Young people may experience discrimination in employment or education opportunities and planning for the future has to begin much sooner to deal with the complexity of plans; at the same time, there is the threat of their condition changing or deteriorating and adversely affecting the plans, combined with the possibility of dying.

KEY POINT

A life-limiting or life-threatening diagnosis adds complexity to a normal stage of development.

YOUNG PEOPLE'S PALLIATIVE CARE

Palliative care for young people with life-limiting conditions is described by Together for Short Lives (a UK organization for children and young people's palliative care) as

> an active and total approach to care, from the point of diagnosis or recognition, embracing physical, emotional, social and spiritual elements through to death and beyond. It focuses on enhancement of quality of life for the child/young person and support for the family and includes the management of distressing symptoms, provision of short breaks and care through death and bereavement.

Together for Short Lives 2013, p. 38

Care is provided for young people for whom curative treatment is no longer the main focus of care and therefore the care may extend over a relatively short period, for example for a young person who has a sudden traumatic episode for which no curative option is available, or may extend over many years, such as for those with Duchenne muscular dystrophy. The common factor to be reflected in their care is that they are expected to die prematurely, and plans have to be made to meet their individual and family needs.

Life limiting or life-shortening conditions are those for which there is no reasonable hope of cure and from which a child or young person will die. Some of these conditions cause progressive deterioration rendering the child increasingly dependent on parents and carers. Life-threatening conditions are those for which curative treatment may be possible but can fail, such as cancer (Together for Short Lives 2013). In all cases, the degree of threat to life will be a significant factor.

Young people's palliative care has a number of similarities to children's palliative care and benefits from the core values of all services to children, including openness, honesty, respect and working in partnership with children, young people and families. It also has similarities to the palliative care of adults, such as self-help and support; user involvement; information giving; and social and spiritual support; as well as its own unique aspects of care with a focus on the impact of life-threatening or life-limiting conditions on young people's lives and how professionals deal with this.

Young people's palliative care is often provided by a variety of service providers from health, social care and education as well as from across the statutory, private and voluntary sectors (Price and McNeilly 2009).

Active palliative care approaches to support young people and their families to lead as normal lives as possible include:

- Partnership between the young person and family and professionals, to identify and meet the young person's needs in an individualized and flexible way
- Listening to and responding to young people and their families
- Services which are integrated and reflect the longer-term continuing care required by an increasing number of young people
- Delivering care where the young person and family want it to be, e.g. in the home, hospital or hospice, school or education/employment setting
- Symptom management
- Psychological and social support, including formal counselling and therapy
- Attention to cultural, spiritual and practical needs
- Multiprofessional and multiagency teamwork and partnership
- Supporting young people and their families and education professionals to enable children to continue to access education
- Easy access to services and information; some minority groups may need extra assistance to enable this to happen, including translation services
- Services appropriate to the age and development of the young person
- Good communication

PRINCIPLE FOR PRACTICE

Palliative care is an active, holistic approach to care, not simply a care process.

DEFINING TRANSITION

Blum et al. (1993, p. 573) usefully defined *transition* as 'the purposeful, planned movement of adolescents and young adults with chronic physical and medical conditions from child-centred to adult-orientated health care systems'.

However, for the transition of young people with life-limiting or life-threatening conditions to adult services to be successful, the process needs to include a much wider range of services than just the healthcare services mentioned in the definition above. It needs to reflect the services required to meet the needs of the individual young person, from across the statutory and voluntary sector and a range of support which may include health, social, leisure, housing and education services.

The Together for Short Lives Transition Taskforce has identified the way that the five key agencies should work together as a 'pentagon of support'. This pentagon is underpinned by health and social care working closely together to provide a foundation for all the other provisions, with work/leisure and education being the two 'enabling agencies' on either side and independent living as the 'capstone' at the top.

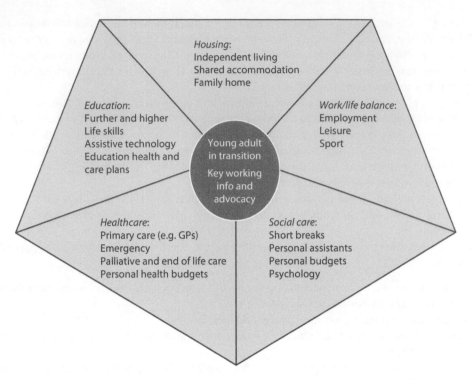

Housing:
Independent living
Shared accommodation
Family home

Education:
Further and higher
Life skills
Assistive technology
Education health and
care plans

Work/life balance:
Employment
Leisure
Sport

Young adult
in transition

Key working
info and
advocacy

Healthcare:
Primary care (e.g. GPs)
Emergency
Palliative and end of life care
Personal health budgets

Social care:
Short breaks
Personal assistants
Personal budgets
Psychology

(From Together for Short Lives, *Stepping Up: A Guide to Enabling a Good Transition to Adulthood for Young People with Life-Limiting and Life-Threatening Conditions*. London: Together for Short Lives, 2015.)

McGrath and Yeowart (2009) describe a series of transitions that young people face:

- From school to further or higher education
- From living at home or at school to living elsewhere
- From education to employment
- From children's services to adults' services

Transition may describe the move from children's to adults' services or may represent the move from child to adult status within society, e.g. moving from school to work. Likewise, services may describe transition as occurring at a specific point, e.g. on a certain birthday or stage or on completion of education. Transition is unique to each individual and, in the context of this chapter, this term is used to describe the move from children's to adults' services. Effective transition must also allow for the fact that adolescents are undergoing changes far broader than just their clinical needs.

Although transition recognizes that young people strive to develop independence from their parents, many young people with life-limiting or life-threatening conditions remain dependent on their parents/carers for their everyday needs at the same time that they are striving to develop this level of independence.

The report *From the Pond into the Sea* (Care Quality Commission 2014) recognizes a health and social care system that is not working, and that is letting down many young people at a critical time in their lives. It shows that we have put the interests of a system that is no longer fit for purpose above the interests of the people it is supposed to serve.

Transition is recognized as a process rather than a single event; government documents recommend that transition should be a guided, educational, therapeutic process rather than an administrative one (Department of Health and Department for Education and Skills 2004).

PRINCIPLE FOR PRACTICE

Transition should be an effective, efficient, timely process, working with young people and their families to transfer the young person's care from child-focused, family-centred children's services to patient-centred adult services.

Lost in Transition (Royal College of Nursing 2007, revised 2013) identified that services need to be flexible and based on the needs of the young person rather than focused on the needs of the service. This requires services to work in partnership and examine what they provide – and do not provide – for young people and their families; this may lead to a service redesign or development. For palliative care services, this exploration will mean working across traditional boundaries and across statutory and voluntary sectors and considering how to overcome barriers in service provision and develop the flexibility and accessibility required to meet the needs of young people and their families, friends and carers.

The criteria described in *You're Welcome Quality Criteria: Making Health Services Young People Friendly* (Department of Health 2011) are based on examples of effective local practice working with young people aged under 20 and cover 10 topic areas:

1. Accessibility
2. Publicity
3. Confidentiality and consent
4. Environment
5. Staff training, skills, attitudes and values
6. Joined-up working
7. Young people's involvement in monitoring and evaluation of patient experience
8. Health issues for young people
9. Sexual and reproductive health services
10. Specialist child and adolescent mental health services (CAMHS)

CASE STUDY

Jenny, aged 20, and Jessica, aged 21, were sisters who both had a rare genetic condition; they remained in the special school system until they were 18 and 19 years old, respectively. It appeared to their mother that when the transport for Jessica ceased, the system seemed to 'lose sight' of Jenny too; their mother became reliant on the local children's hospice for short-break care as the only support she received. Her husband worked long hours and they had two younger sons. Following a review by the children's hospice, plans were put into place to discharge the two young women as they had reached the age limit set out in the hospice's registration documents. The hospice referred the sisters to adult social services. Social services tried to refer the sisters to the adult hospice service but the referrals were not accepted as the hospice focused on end of life care. With no equivalent service easily identified, the sisters were cared for wholly by their mother; when she injured her back lifting one of her daughters, the father gave up work to care for the family. A short time later, the family was referred to social services as the boys were truanting to work in local shops to help support the family financially. The lack of transition arrangements had led to a lack of any support for the family, including benefits advice, leading to severe financial difficulties, two other children missing education and two young women being totally reliant on their family for care.

KEY POINTS

- Transition is a process which affects the whole family.
- The specific needs of siblings should also be considered.

REFLECTION POINT

When should transition planning have started for this family in this case study?

IMPLEMENTING AN INTEGRATED APPROACH TO EFFECTIVELY MANAGE TRANSITION

In 2015, Together for Short Lives published *Stepping Up: A Guide to Enabling a Good Transition to Adulthood for Young People with Life-Limiting and Life-Threatening Conditions,* which aims to provide a generic framework that can be implemented locally to plan and provide multiagency services for young people with life-limiting or life-threatening health conditions as they become adults and move into adult service provision. This builds on the earlier work of the Association for Children's Palliative Care (ACT), which published the first edition of the Transition Pathway setting out a generic pathway for planning services around the needs of young people, but recognizing the need for an even more holistic approach to supporting these young people into adulthood.

Stepping Up recognizes that partnership working between agencies is crucial and must involve all the agencies that need to be in place around a young person: health, social care, education, employment and housing.

The framework focuses on enabling young people to maximize their potential, rather than focusing on service responses to the process of transition between services. It describes a multiagency approach, enabling young people to live their lives to the fullest extent possible, including health, social care, education, employment and housing/independent living.

There is also attention to adult service providers' perspective and how they can support young people through transition and enable them to feel settled in adult care, focusing on the need for a partnership between children's and adult service providers to enable transition to be achieved for all young people, enabling an individualized planning approach. The framework also focuses on the need for parallel planning throughout transition, so that plans are reviewed to meet the young person's ongoing care and support needs as well as their plans for end of life care.

It sets out five standards that should be developed as a minimum, supported by key goals to help achieve those standards, with service examples throughout the young person's transition process.

Each young person will take his or her own unique, individual care journey that reflects his or her own needs and circumstances. The framework provides a template to enable local services to work together to develop essential components to underpin more detailed local and individual pathways. There is a focus on ensuring that the young person is central to the planning process, and the framework aims to ensure that the young person receives integrated, personalized services to meet his or her individual needs.

NUMBER OF YOUNG PEOPLE IN NEED OF PALLIATIVE CARE AND EFFECTIVE TRANSITION

Fraser et al. (2013) identified that the numbers of young adults living with life-limiting and life-threatening conditions in UK are much higher than previously thought and are increasing. Over the 10 years of data collection (2000–2010) the prevalence had increased from 26 to 34.6 per 10,000 population, an increase of 33% (Fraser et al. 2013). In 2009–2010 there were 55,721 young adults aged 18–40 living with a life-limiting or life-threatening condition in England, and 12,827 of these were in the 18- to 25-year age group (Fraser et al. 2013).

It is widely recognized that, as new technologies emerge, an increasing number of children with life-limiting or life-threatening conditions are surviving into adulthood. New developments in the care of young people with Duchenne muscular dystrophy including non-invasive assisted ventilation mean that the life expectancy for this group of service users has risen to 25 years, compared with 14 years during the 1960s, with further predictions that this will rise further to 40 years. Children and young people with cystic fibrosis (CF) are currently not typical users of children's palliative care services, although a study by Jaffe and Bush (2001) reported that the median estimated life expectancy of children with CF born in 1990 is now predicted to be 40 years, which represents a doubling in the last 20 years.

Currently, many palliative care services are considering how to widen access to their services, including developing services for people with cardiac and neurological conditions, with patterns of service changing to care for patients who deteriorate over a long period of time, and then death coming quite unexpectedly and suddenly when compared with patients with cancer who require terminal and end of life care.

In addition to the more typical 'graduates' from children's palliative care services, there are also those who develop a life-threatening or life-limiting condition in early adulthood. 'Second cancers' are the leading cause of death in long-term survivors of Hodgkin's disease, with exceptionally high risks of breast cancer among women treated at a young age. One in three people will be diagnosed with cancer during their lifetime. Although cancer is a disease that affects mainly older people, with 64% of cases occurring in those aged 65 and over, in young men aged 20–39 years testicular cancer is the most frequently occurring cancer. There is also evidence that the use of anthracyclines can cause congestive cardiac failure in later life, with adverse effects increasing over time (Scottish Intercollegiate Guidelines Network 2004).

However, current usage of palliative care services is low for children with malignant conditions, and it is unknown whether this would be different in the young person's group; anecdotal evidence suggests an increasing use from within this care group.

Such predictions include young people who will die prematurely as a result of the life-limiting nature of their illness or disorder. Most of the young people will fall into one of the following groups (Together for Short Lives 2013):

1. Young people with life-threatening conditions for which curative treatment may be feasible but can fail. Palliative care may be necessary during periods of prognostic uncertainty and when treatment fails. Examples include cancer or irreversible organ failures such as heart, liver and kidney.

2. Young people with conditions where there may be long periods of intensive treatment aimed at prolonging life and allowing participation in normal activities, but where premature death is still possible or inevitable. Examples include cystic fibrosis, Duchenne muscular dystrophy and HIV/AIDS.

3. Young people with progressive conditions without curative treatment options, where treatment is exclusively palliative and may commonly extend over many years. Examples include Batten disease and mucopolysaccharidosis.

4. Young people with severe neurological disability, which may cause weakness and susceptibility to health complications leading to premature death. Deterioration may be unpredictable and not usually progressive. Examples include severe multiple disabilities following brain or spinal cord injuries and severe cerebral palsy.

These four categories are described as a guide to the young people who are likely to have palliative care needs; many young people with chronic progressive conditions reach a crisis in terms of physical deterioration in adolescence or early adulthood, with a number dying in their late teens or twenties. It should be noted that this age group has a higher proportion of those needing palliative care than do younger children or 'young adults' – a term used by the Office for National Statistics (2008) for those under the age of 65.

KEY POINT

The lack of real-time data, as more young people survive into adulthood, leads to an inability to plan services to meet needs and a subsequent gap in care.

For professionals working with young people, there is also the potential challenge of working with individuals across a wide spectrum of cognitive ability: some will have severe cognitive impairment related to their underlying disease, whereas others will have no cognitive delay. Identifying the actual number of young people with palliative care needs is problematic because of the lack of statistical information. The prevalence of young people who are ill and who have palliative care needs is much higher than the mortality rate.

IMPROVING TRANSITION: POLICY AND PRACTICE

Over recent years, a number of policy levers for change in children's services have emerged, building from the *Learning from Bristol* report (Department of Health 2001), which recognizes the need for children and young people's needs to be appropriately addressed and touches on staffing issues.

An increasing number of children with life-limiting or life-threatening conditions are surviving into adulthood, and smooth transition to adult services requires cooperative planning across services well ahead of the time when transfer to other services is anticipated. A number of reports identify common themes to be considered in the transition to adulthood, including:

- Apprehension of young disabled people
- Changing roles of families
- Failure of different agencies to work together
- Recognition that children's services for rare conditions are usually more highly developed than adult services
- Insufficient time for transition planning

INVOLVING YOUNG PEOPLE AND THEIR PARENTS/CARERS IN THE TRANSITION PROCESS

In the UK, growing importance is given to the involvement of young people in decision making about their care and service developments within local government and the NHS.

Growing evidence regarding poor transition planning processes and poor outcomes of transitions for disabled young people has meant that improving the transitions to adult services and adulthood for disabled

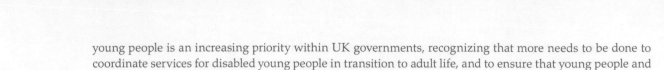

young people is an increasing priority within UK governments, recognizing that more needs to be done to coordinate services for disabled young people in transition to adult life, and to ensure that young people and families can access high-quality information at key transition points.

The National Council for Palliative Care and Together for Short Lives (2015) identifies that all young people want to be seen first and foremost as individual young people with their own views and aspirations, not to be defined by their health condition, and they confirm that every young person will have individual plans and wishes, although there are many priorities in common:

- Independence
- Friendships
- Relationships and intimacy with partners
- Information they can easily access and understand
- Education or vocational training
- Access to meaningful work opportunities
- Suitable housing
- Involvement in decision making, with parental support if requested
- Short breaks, holidays, fun and leisure time
- Reliable and comfortable transport and wheelchairs
- To have an advocate or key worker who can coordinate their transition
- Emotional support and a trusted professional to talk to about issues such as end of life planning, when the time is right for them

Beresford (2004) identified services which successfully manage the challenge of moving from children's to adults' services:

- For young people:
  - Specific service provision
  - Development of skills of self-management and self-determination
  - Supported psychosocial development
  - Involvement of young people
  - Peer involvement
  - Support for changed relationships with parents/carers
  - Provision of choice
  - Provision of information
  - Focus upon the young person's strengths for future development
- For parents:
  - Support for adjustment to changed relationships with young people
  - Parental involvement in service planning
  - Family-centred approach
  - Provision of information

McGrath and Yeowart (2009) identified the following problems if transition is managed badly:

- A lasting negative impact on young people's well-being and chances in life.
- Increased costs of care.
- The benefits of early work with disabled children will be lost.
- Disabled young people can become socially and economically excluded.
- The development of psychological and physical problems.
- Lack of help leading to greater support needs later on in life.
- Distress and disruption to families.
- Possible increased reliance on health and social services.
- Significant financial repercussions.

PRINCIPLE FOR PRACTICE

Young people, wherever possible, and their parents/carers must be involved in the transition process as partners with professionals.

MODELS OF CARE

A number of different models of care have evolved over recent years to provide young people's palliative care, often reflecting the services available in the local setting, as very little additional, directed funding has been made available for service development. Most service developments have emerged from children's services; however, with the establishment of the widening access agenda in adult palliative care and with hospice services considering how to provide better equity of services for people with palliative care needs, services are being developed which provide more appropriate services for younger people. In children's services and at the beginning of the transition process, young people with life-limiting conditions usually remain under the care of a paediatrician, often a community paediatrician or a disease-focused specialist such as a paediatric oncologist, neurologist or metabolic specialist, with input from a multiprofessional team, including therapists and psychology services and social care (McNeilly and Gilmore 2009).

Community teams, often nurse led, provide ongoing care; such services continue to gradually grow in number and provide a key focus for care delivery. Within adult services, the young person's care is overseen by a specialist, with coordination from generalists such as GPs and district nurses. Children's community nursing teams are regarded as the bedrock for children's palliative care, but, in adult services, district nursing services are seen as a more generic support to specialist palliative care services.

The care of young people is delivered in many settings such as home, school or educational placements and short-break settings, of which hospice services and other voluntary services provide an important component of residential care.

The ideal service model for young people is one which brings together all players to deliver individualized packages of care to meet assessed needs and formalizes standards and quality assurance. If such models are going to be developed, commissioning and delivering palliative care to young people needs to be planned in partnership within the NHS, and with social services, education and the voluntary sector, to take account of the lifelong and changing developmental needs of young people, based on accurate, real-time data to recognize the needs of service users.

Beresford et al. (2013) recognized that small changes in practice can make a big difference in the experiences of young people and their families within adult health care settings, this related to the young person and their parents' involvement; the importance of getting it right early in the process and introduction to adult services; helping young people deal with uncertainty and starting conversations around end of life.

The following models of care illustrate how a whole system of support to the young people and family can be based on choice and access.

- Local multidisciplinary palliative care teams often include community nurses, hospital specialists, hospices, social workers, psychologists and therapists to deliver community-based care.
- Outreach nurse specialists work from a tertiary or shared care centre.
- Cardiac centres often provide good transition services which enable the young person to be supported by familiar carers (in a key worker role) as they bridge the gap between children's and adults' services.
- There is medical backup from a variety of services, including oncologists, general paediatricians, GPs and, sometimes, adult or paediatric palliative care consultants. It is essential to ensure that GPs and their teams are kept informed about the care of their patients to facilitate the provision of seamless care and services.
- Paediatricians with an interest in disability and long-term conditions are increasingly involved in the local clinical management of young people with life-limiting conditions, supporting the primary care team for whom the young person's condition may be rare and unfamiliar. This support can also be provided to adult palliative care services to ensure that their expertise can be adapted to meet the needs of the young person.
- Clinical nurse specialists based in specialized service centres, supporting a particular life-limiting condition, can work effectively with families through close liaison and coordinated working with local community nursing teams and work across children's and adults' services.
- Services to support the siblings of young people who are dying are an important part of supporting the whole family.
- Bereavement support for parents, family, siblings and other carers involved with the young people is also a part of palliative care.

> **KEY POINT**
>
> There are a number of models of care which can be combined to provide the care needed by young people.

USING AN INTEGRATED CARE APPROACH TO EFFECT SUCCESSFUL TRANSITION

There are a variety of different models of care that can provide support to meet the needs of young people with life-limiting or life-threatening conditions. The key challenge is to find a coordinated process which can be adapted to differing circumstances to ensure that the needs of the young person are systematically considered to ensure their care needs are met throughout their transition to adult services, focusing on the needs of the young person regardless of the name of the condition.

The challenge of ensuring that transition planning focuses on the fulfilment of the hopes, dreams and potential of the life-limited or life-threatened young person, enabling them to maximize education, training and employment opportunities, to enjoy social relationships and to live independently, calls for innovative, flexible and collaborative care solutions. For nurses, the professional challenge is to work alongside young people and their families and carers, within health and other settings, to support and provide appropriate young person's services with a view to enabling smooth transition to comprehensive adult multidisciplinary care.

In Doug et al. (2009) there is recognition that there are differing condition-dependent viewpoints on when transition should occur, but agreement on major principles guiding transition planning and probable barriers. Gibson et al. (2014) identified eight factors as benchmarks for transition:

1. Moving to manage a health condition as an adult
2. Support for gradual transition
3. Coordinated child and adult teams
4. Services are 'young people friendly'
5. Written documentation
6. Parents
7. Assessment of 'readiness'
8. Involvement of the GP

Improving the Life Chances of Disabled People, published by the UK government's Strategy Unit (Cabinet Office 2005), describes three key ingredients to ensure effective support of disabled young people:

1. Planning for transition focused on individual need
2. Continuous service provision
3. Access to a more transparent and appropriate menu of opportunities and choices

It expects that this will be achieved by

- Putting in place improved mechanisms for effective planning for the transition to adulthood and the support that goes with this.
- Removing 'cliff edges' in service provision.
- Giving disabled young people access to more information for young people. This information should be in a suitable format and should include accessible local and national information on transition processes, services and opportunities.

TOGETHER FOR SHORT LIVES FRAMEWORK FOR TRANSITION

This framework is written to support the transition of young people with life-limiting conditions in all aspects of their life. It provides a multiagency framework to support local planning. It is written from the perspective of health services being the lead agency in this process as the young people often have significant health issues.

The following sections identify how the Together for Short Lives Framework can be used to support young people through each of three phases, underpinned by five standards and supported by key goals which will help practitioners achieve each of the standards.

PHASE 1: PREPARING FOR ADULTHOOD

STANDARD 1

Preparing for adulthood is the first standard. Every young person, from the age of 14, should be supported to be at the centre of preparing for approaching adulthood and for the move to adult services. Their families should be supported to prepare for their changing role.

Key goals

1. Young people are at the centre of planning, using person-centred planning approaches.
2. Parallel planning takes place.
3. Initial conversations about transition take place with the young person and their family at a time and in a place that suits them.
4. A follow-up meeting with the young person and family takes place.
5. The first multiagency and multidisciplinary team meeting takes place.

PHASE 2: PREPARING TO MOVE ON

STANDARD 2

Every young person is supported to plan proactively for their future. They are involved in ongoing assessments and developing a comprehensive holistic plan that reflects their wishes for the future.

Key goals

1. Young people and their parents are helped with the transition from family-centred to young person–centred care.
2. Every young person has a key worker to facilitate continuity of care and prepare the way into adult services.
3. Every young person is supported to consider future plans, supported by ongoing multiagency assessment.
4. Every young person is supported to identify adult services which can meet their needs.

STANDARD 3

Every young person has an end of life plan which is developed in parallel to planning for ongoing care and support in adult services.

Key goals

1. End of life planning:
    a. Transition planning continues to take place even during times of uncertainty.
    b. Every young person has a documented end of life plan running alongside their plan for future life.

2. Time of death:
    a. The young person's pain and other symptoms are dealt with effectively.
    b. Every effort is made to ensure that the young person's death takes place according to their wishes and in their place of choice wherever possible, with the young person's emotional, cultural and spiritual needs met.
    c. Family members and other carers are supported, informed and involved.
    d. The young person has the best quality of life and care to the end.

3. After death:
    a. Parents should retain their parenting role after the death of the young person.
    b. Siblings should be supported and included in all decisions.

c. All professionals and agencies should be informed of the death with the parents' consent.

    d. All family members should be supported according to their individual needs for as long as they need it

STANDARD 4

Child and adult services should be actively working together to enable a smooth transition.

Key goals

1. Child and adult services within health work together so that there is an overlap of care planning and care provision.
2. Services within all agencies should be engaged in planning for the specific needs of the young person.
3. Ongoing reviews (at least annually) with the young person take place.

PHASE 3: SETTLING INTO ADULT SERVICES

STANDARD 5

Every young person is supported in adult services with a multiagency team fully engaged in facilitating care and support. The young person and their family are equipped with realistic expectations and knowledge to ensure confidence in their care and support needs being met into the future.

Key goals

1. A key working function is provided for every young person so that all the agencies providing care and support are coordinated.
2. All agencies ensure that age and developmentally appropriate services are available that address the full range of a young person's needs.
3. Palliative care services may provide a single clinical overview for the young person and link with other specialists involved in their care.
4. There is frequent review and communication across services about care plans and end of life decisions.
5. Primary health care services, including GPs, develop a relationship with the young person and their families/carers.
6. Adult services in secondary care ensure there is an appropriate lead clinician to take responsibility for young adults in their clinics and admissions processes.
7. Short break or respite needs of young people and their parents/carers are considered and provided in the most appropriate setting.
8. Parents are included as appropriate.

CASE STUDY

Samir, aged 15, approached her school nurse to ask how she would be able to arrange her care so that she could attend the local college following her General Certificates of Secondary Education (GCSEs) rather than continuing at school. This care included personal care, assistance with mobility, toileting, feeding as well as assistance with educational activities and using a personal computer. Samir wanted to be involved in the discussions about the plans for her future. A planning meeting was arranged with the local special educational needs and disability (SEND) adviser, as the adviser took a lead in transition planning with the school and health staff, Samir and her parents. At the beginning of the meeting, Samir was asked to outline her hopes for the future and the support she needed to be able to achieve these plans. Samir asked that her teaching assistant could act as her key worker as she had a good relationship with the assistant and trusted her; also, the teaching assistant understood her day-to-day needs and was in regular contact with her and her family. The teaching assistant was willing to act as the key worker, but had no experience in arranging transition; therefore the adviser mentored the teaching assistant in the key worker role and a successful transition took place. Samir achieved her plan to move to college, with an appropriate, personalized plan and transition occurring smoothly.

REFLECTION POINT

What skills can a school nurse bring to key working approaches?

CASE STUDY

Hanna, a 16-year-old newly diagnosed with Wolfram (diabetes insipidus, diabetes mellitus, optic atrophy and deafness [DIDMOAD]) syndrome, has completed her school examinations and wants to plan for a university application. Her parents are reluctant for her to move away from home in the light of her life-limiting diagnosis. A family conference is arranged by the diabetic nurse specialist and includes the family GP and Hanna's head of year at school. During discussions, it is apparent that Hanna is aware of her prognosis, but desperately wants to attain a degree and gain some independence and move away from home. The head of year believes that it is highly likely that Hanna can achieve the educational requirements to go to university. The diabetic nurse specialist is able to confirm that the local hospital in the university town has a good diabetic service. Plans are made for Hanna to progress with university applications, with support from the head of year, and for the diabetic nurse specialist to liaise with Hanna's GP and the family to arrange for healthcare support from the university health service when university placements are being planned.

REFLECTION POINT

How can home and university health services work together to ensure optimal care?

CASE STUDY

Ben, who is 15, is invited to join a transition programme being run by the local children's hospice service. The programme involves a small group of young people arranging a programme of activities for themselves over the year ahead. The programme has a budget for the young people to use. The process is facilitated by one of the hospice staff, who encourages group discussion in the initial stages. During the year, the young people learn and develop negotiating skills, working together to plan budgets and arrange events, including transport; this is a range of skills which can be utilized in other settings. Also during the year, a group for parents of teenagers considers the challenges of parenting teenagers and encourages parents to explore how to support their child as he or she moves toward a more independent lifestyle as a young adult.

REFLECTION POINT

What barriers can there be for young people using hospice services?

CASE STUDY

Mo is 19 years old and is studying information technology at university; he has a 24-hour package of care arranged by the local social services team. He is dissatisfied with the package as carers often change at the last moment and are unwilling to support him socially, leaving him isolated. He decides to arrange his own package of care, supported by his social worker. He creates this using a range of benefits, including direct payments, independent living fund, disability living allowance and local education authority allowances, and employs his own team of carers. He reports that this brings more continuity of care and enables him to employ carers who are willing to support his university lifestyle and meet both the academic aspects and social aspects of his life.

REFLECTION POINT

How can young people access training to develop skills to be able to coordinate their care?

CASE STUDY

Sophie, 16 years old, is admitted to hospital with a chest infection, following a relapse of leukaemia; she is recognized to be approaching the end of her life. Discussions between Sophie's parents and the clinicians caring for her identify that Sophie had not wanted to be admitted to hospital and had expressed her wish to die at home. Her parents are concerned that they may not be able to cope with caring for her at home. A multiagency case conference is arranged and includes the local community children's nurse (CCN) team, local district nursing team, oncology nurse specialists, oncologists and GP. A care plan is developed and Sophie's opinions are sought about where she wants to be cared for. The local CCN team works Monday to Friday, 9:00 a.m. to 5:00 p.m., with cover for end of life care; the care plan ensures that Sophie's parents have 24-hour access to advice from the CCN team and the oncology nurse specialists who have been involved in Sophie's long-term care. The district nursing team offers backup to the CCN team, to ensure equipment availability and support. Sophie's parents do not feel able to work; the oncology unit social worker helps them identify the best way of dealing with their absence from work, which includes Sophie's father taking special leave and her mother getting a medical certificate from the GP. A symptom management plan is developed, with Sophie's parents aware that 24-hour support is available from the oncology team and that their GP is also aware of the plan.

A pharmacy box is arranged so that all the drugs Sophie is likely to need are readily available. Sophie is taken home by ambulance and is cared for by her family, supported by the CCN team and nurse specialists from the hospital, until her death 72 hours later. Following death, she is transferred to the local children's hospice for care in their 'special bedroom', which is chilled and which enables Sophie's family to say their goodbyes to her in their own time, until her funeral.

REFLECTION POINT

Where can the care team access specialist support for symptom management out of hours?

ROLE OF THE CHILDREN'S NURSE IN PROMOTING EFFECTIVE TRANSITION

It has been shown that there are a number of different approaches which can help to achieve effective transition. The role of the children's nurse in ensuring that this happens is discussed here.

- Making the care of children, young people and their parents the first concern, treating them as individuals and respecting their dignity
- Working with others to protect and promote the health and well-being of those in their care, their families and carers, and the wider community
- Providing a high standard of practice and care at all times
- Being open and honest, acting with integrity and upholding the reputation of the profession

When working with young people, this means getting to know the young person as an individual and accepting that all families are different, promoting a need for individualized and collaborative approaches to care. Young et al. (2003) identified the difficulties in managing communication with young people who have a chronic, life-threatening illness and in the role parents take in relation to facilitating and constraining communication between the professional and the young person. They also identified the potential for the parental role to hamper the development of successful relationships between professionals and young patients.

Nurses who work with young people should be aware of the barriers that the young people may face, such as social isolation, and lack of employment or education and leisure opportunities, and work to support them and their families to try to overcome the barriers and the impact they have on the young people's lives and care needs.

Nurses working with young people will need to balance the rights of the young person with those involved in their care. They will need to apply professional codes of practice and legal requirements relating to the care of young people, such as confidentiality, information sharing, consent, service provision, young people's rights, and discriminatory practice and safeguarding issues, to the practical provision of care and support of individual young persons and their families. Nurses have a duty of care to act with appropriate skill and judgment and to take all reasonable steps to ensure that the young person does not suffer harm as a result of their actions or failure to act; nurses should also work within the professional code of ethics regarding working with young people. The care of life-limited or life-threatened young people means the children and young people's nurse must consider the ethical aspects of practice in relation to consent, confidentiality and capacity issues to ensure that the rights of the individual young person are respected in full. The nurse must also be able to communicate effectively about these issues with the individual child and young person as well as all of those involved in their care.

It is recognized that it can be very difficult to predict when a young person is moving into their end of life phase, but forward planning is important and requires nurses and other care team members to have open, honest conversations with parents, families and loved ones. The National Council for Palliative Care and Together for Short Lives (2015) have developed practical guidance for professionals to support them in leading 'difficult' conversations about end of life issues, providing a series of prompts based on feedback from young people's families who had cared for a young person in the past.

Nurses working with young people with life-limiting or life-threatening conditions and their families are ideally placed to act as a care/service navigator to guide and support young people and their families, friends and carers through the transition maze. They can promote an understanding of palliative care approaches and attitudes, within specialist and generalist services. Nurses can help the young person develop skills in communication, decision making, assertiveness, self-care and self-advocacy to assist with the transition process. They are also ideally placed to recognize any gaps in the young person's readiness to move between children's and adults' services and to help address any such gaps, by working with the young person, their family and other supporters, including other professionals, and by making appropriate referrals to other services, when needed. They can also help to manage expectations that young people and their families have about the move to adult services and give the young person time to adjust to the new services. Finally, they have a crucial role in ensuring that the young person has a 'good death', i.e. one which is pain free and dignified, in the environment of their choice and with those they love around them (Davies 2009).

Nurses can also play a key role in helping services establish and develop processes, systems and attitudes to support young people and their families/carers to adjust to, prepare for and move on to adult services, as well as contributing to the commissioning of services for young people.

Social media is an ever-present twenty-first century activity in the lives of many, in particular the lives of young people, and Casella et al. (2014) recognize the need for nurses to embrace changing technology to capitalize on the professional opportunities offered by social media. The UK Nursing and Midwifery Council (2015) published guidance for registrants on the use of social media and set out broad principles to enable nurses to think through issues and act professionally, ensuring public protection at all times.

CONCLUSION

Young people with life-limiting or life-threatening conditions have specific palliative care needs and physical, psychological and developmental needs that are significantly different from those experienced by children and adults. However, although the number of young people who meet the criteria for palliative care has increased significantly, transition for many is poorly managed and this has a detrimental effect not only on the individual but also on their family/carers.

It is clear that young people and their families/carers require an integrated, person-centred approach to guide and support them through what may be described as the transition maze. Such an approach can help ensure that they receive a coordinated and person-centred approach to care and support throughout their care journey. As this chapter has shown, the ACT Transition Care Pathway may be used to plan, implement and deliver effective evidence-based care throughout. In doing so, the role of the children's nurse in ensuring this has been highlighted. Finally, using case studies, it has been shown how the pathway may be applied in practice so that the young person and their family/carers are not lost in the process of transition but have ongoing support from within primary, secondary and tertiary care for long as is needed.

From this discussion several key principles for practice can be clearly articulated.

SUMMARY OF PRINCIPLES FOR PRACTICE

- Children and young people's nurses must be informed that coordinated approaches to care require clear communication and partnership working; this takes time and nurses need to allocate time to the process of transition and to partnership working.
- Children and young people's nurses must understand that continuity of care is essential for young people and their families and requires parallel planning, with the young people and families recognized as equal partners in the planning process; nurses need to develop communication skills to be able to work effectively with young people, families and co-workers.
- Children and young people's nurses must understand that communication provides a firm foundation for a smooth transition and should continue during times of uncertainty.
- Children and young people's nurses must be aware that it is difficult to predict when a young person may enter the end of life phase, but professionals should be honest and open about the probability that the young person's life is nearing an end.

REFERENCES

Beresford B (2004) On the road to nowhere? Young disabled people and transition. *Child: Care, Health and Development* **60**: 581–7.

Beresford B, Harper M, Mukherjee S, et al. (2013) Supporting health transitions for young people with life-limiting conditions: researching positive practice (the STEPP project): research briefing and practice prompts. Available at http://php.york.ac.uk/inst/spru/research/summs/stepp.php?.

Blum R, Garell D, Hodgman C, et al. (1993) Transition from child-centered to adult health-care systems for adolescents with chronic conditions. A position paper of the Society for Adolescent Medicine. *Journal of Adolescent Health* **14**: 570–6.

Cabinet Office (2005) *Improving the life chances of disabled people.* London: Cabinet Office.

Care Quality Commission (2014) *From the pond into the sea: children's transition to adult health services.* London: CQC.

Casella E, Mills J, Usher K (2014) Social media and nursing practice: changing the balance between the social and technical aspects of work. *Collegian* **21**(2): 121–6.

Davies R (2009) Care of the child at the end of life. In Price J, McNeilly P (eds.) *Palliative care for children and families: an interdisciplinary approach.* Basingstoke: Palgrave Macmillan.

Department for Education and Skills (2004) *Every child matters: change for children.* Nottingham: Department for Education and Skills.

Department of Health (2001) *Learning from Bristol: the Department of Health's response to the Report of the Public Inquiry into Children's Heart Surgery at the Bristol Royal Infirmary 1984–1995.* London: Department of Health.

Department of Health (2011) *You're Welcome Quality Criteria: Making Health Services Young People Friendly.* London: Stationery Office.

Department of Health and Department for Education and Skills (2004) *National Service Framework for Children, Young People and Maternity Services: the mental health and psychological wellbeing of children and young people.* London: Department of Health.

Doug M, Adi Y, William J, et al. (2009) Transition to adult services for children and young people with palliative care needs: a systematic review. *Archives of Disease in Childhood.* DOI: 10.1136/adc.2009.163931.

Fraser L, Miller M, Aldridge J, et al. (2013) *Prevalence of life-limiting and life-threatening conditions in young adults in England 2000–2010: final report for Together for Short Lives.* Bristol: Together for Short Lives.

Gibson F, Aldis J, Cass H, et al. (2014) Benchmarks for transition from child to adult health services. Great Ormond Street Hospital for Children, South Bank University and the Orchid Centre for Outcomes and Experience Research in Children's Health, Illness and Disability. Available at http://www.yhscn.nhs.uk/media/PDFs/children/Transition/gosh-benchmarksfortransitionfromchildtoadultservices-2015.pdf.

Jaffe A, Bush A (2001) Cystic fibrosis: review of the decade. *Monaldi Archives for Chest Disease* **56**: 240–7.

McGrath A, Yeowart C (2009) *Rights of passage: supporting disabled young people through the transition to adulthood.* London: New Philanthropy Capital.

McNeilly P, Gilmore F (2009) Interdisciplinary working. In Price J, McNeilly P (eds.) *Palliative care for children and families: an interdisciplinary approach.* Basingstoke: Palgrave Macmillan.

National Council for Palliative Care and Together for Short Lives (2015) *Difficult conversations: making it easier to talk about end of life issues with young adults with life-limiting conditions.* London: NCPC.

Nursing and Midwifery Council (2015) *Social networking guidance: our guidance on the use of social media.* London: NMC.

Office for National Statistics (2008) *Social trends.* Report no. 38. Basingstoke: Palgrave Macmillan.

Price J, McNeilly P (eds.) (2009) *Palliative care for children and families: an interdisciplinary approach.* Basingstoke: Palgrave Macmillan.

Royal College of Nursing (2007, revised 2013) *Lost in transition.* London: RCN.

Scottish Intercollegiate Guidelines Network (2004) *Long term follow up of survivors of childhood cancer: a national clinical guideline.* Edinburgh: SIGN.

Together for Short Lives (2013) *A core care pathway for children with life-limiting and life-threatening conditions,* 3rd ed. London: Together for Short Lives.

Together for Short Lives (2015) *Stepping up: a guide to enabling a good transition to adulthood for young people with life-limiting and life-threatening conditions.* London: Together for Short Lives.

Young B, Dixon-Woods M, Windridge KC, Heney D (2003) Managing communication with young people who have a potentially life threatening chronic illness: qualitative study of patients and parents. *British Medical Journal* **326**(7384): 305.

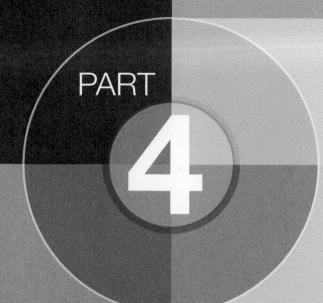

PART 4

DEVELOPING A PROFESSIONAL CHILDREN AND YOUNG PEOPLE'S NURSE

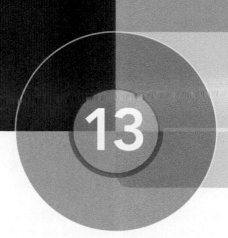

Advanced practice in children and young people's nursing

DAVE BARTON, ALYSON DAVIES AND RUTH DAVIES

OVERVIEW

This chapter provides insight into the issues and debates surrounding the development of the advanced practitioner role within general care settings and specialist areas of practice. The chapter also provides a historical context to set these issues before examining them within current-day nursing practice. The tensions between generalist and specialist practice with regard to children and young people's nursing are articulated and analyzed. That is, should advanced practitioners be generalists with an interest in and some experience in caring for children and young people or should they be educated and qualified as children and young people's nurses? The chapter is contentious, deliberately so, in order to stimulate an informed debate on this vitally important role.

INTRODUCTION

The debate on advanced nursing practice as well as its meaning, value and regulation has been actively ongoing within the UK for well over two decades and continues still (Stilwell et al. 1987; UK Central Council for Nursing, Midwifery and Health Visiting 1998; Farrelly 2014; Rolfe 2014). The level and intensity of this debate increased following the publication of the white paper *Trust, Assurance and Safety* (Department of Health 2007), which was produced as a direct result of the Shipman Inquiry (Smith 2005) and the Francis Report (2013) following the events at the Mid Staffordshire Trust. There was a renewed focus by the government on protecting the public from the potential dangers of health professionals. This resulted in the report of the Centre for Healthcare Regulatory Excellence (CHRE) on the complexity of professional regulatory issues, and the introduction of the new code of practice and Revalidation (2015), as well as noted the Nursing and Midwifery Council's (NMC) continued deliberations and new enthusiasms on advanced nursing practice with regard to definition, regulation and competencies required to practice at this level (Coe et al. 2005). We have also seen the activity and influence of the national *Modernising Nursing Careers*, a review that was published in January 2010 (Department of Health 2010).

It is in this climate of challenge, change and uncertainty that this chapter critically examines the nature of advanced nursing practice both in the broad nursing context and within the specific context of children and young people's nursing. It traces the historical development of the concept and innovation of advanced nursing practice and discusses how this is currently defined and regulated. Differing levels of practice and the resultant array of roles that have emerged are also considered and contrasted alongside the current driving policies and strategies.

The authors of this chapter have deliberately adopted a controversial stance that we hope will engage the reader in some critical and reflective debate regarding children and young people's nursing and the nature of advanced nursing practice. To do this, we have put forward different perspectives on how nurses, particularly those working with children and young people, may advance their practice. In doing so, we have recognized that the boundary between nurses' initial registrant field of practice and others is becoming increasingly blurred, and may even be deemed as irrelevant by some. Likewise, we also recognize and discuss the arguments put forward that the aspiring advanced nurse practitioner, regardless of his or her initial registrant specialist field, needs to attain a generic and generalist standard of practice for advanced practice.

The main purpose of this chapter is to explore and explain the roles and activities of advanced nurse practitioners who are working with children and young people. We believe that such advanced nurse practitioners may arise from any of the current four UK 'fields' or 'branches' of nursing practice to which new registrants are assigned at successful completion of their pre-registration studies (child, mental health, learning disability, adult).

The development of advanced nurse practitioners, as well as their role, activity, scope of practice, education and regulation, has a complex history and is currently an unfinished story. It is fair to say that few areas of nursing activity have been so closely scrutinized and researched (Svensson 1996; Horrocks et al. 2002; Carnwell and Daly 2003; Cady et al. 2014; Farrelly 2014; Rolfe 2014), and yet it remains controversial and challenging. Because of that uncertainty, and because of the main purpose of this chapter, we begin our discussions on advanced nurse practitioners by looking at their historical context, and then apply the concepts that arise from this to the activities of children and young people's nursing.

This chapter reviews and explores the definitions, history and development of advanced nursing practice and advanced nurse practitioners in the general sense and in the widest context. The concepts and principles outlined are then applied and discussed in relation to children and young people's nursing and to the development and status of advanced nurse practitioners in the care of children and younger people. There is discussion on current issues; the relation of children and young people's field competencies to advanced practice competencies, and the modernization of career pathways; and how education must adapt to meet the needs of children's nursing in the future. We then consider specifically the role of the advanced nurse practitioner in some key areas of children and young people's nursing practice.

The chapter concludes with a summary of the current status of children and young people's nursing and advanced nursing practice in the UK.

ADVANCED PRACTICE IN CONTEXT

What is immediately and abundantly clear is that the advanced nurse practitioner has been, and remains, a complex and controversial concept, and an issue that has engendered enormous debate in the nursing profession. In addition it is a concept (a role, a level of practice) that has long been promoted by health strategists as a mechanism to overcome healthcare manpower shortages by enabling new clinical roles that can be used to promote healthcare quality and service delivery (Department of Health 1993; Royal College of Nursing 2014). However, we also believe that, despite the strategists' positive promotion of advanced nurse practitioners, the education of such practitioners has been an erratic and unregulated affair that has lacked any central coherency until most recently. Consequently, the standards of practice and competence held by those who claim to be advanced nurse practitioners varies widely (Hunt 1999; Rolfe 2014). It is this situation that has led to the long debate on how advanced practice may be defined and measured. That endeavour has been grounded in the professional and public concern over the profession's ability to ensure that advanced nurse practitioners are fit for practice within any of the four initial registrant fields of nursing practice, including those working with children and young people.

KEY POINTS

- Advanced practice is a complex and controversial concept that has caused enormous debate in the nursing profession.
- It is a role that has been persistently promoted by health strategists as a mechanism to overcome manpower shortages as well as promote healthcare quality and service delivery.

CONCEPTS AND VOCABULARY OF ADVANCED PRACTICE

First, let us consider the concepts and terminology that have evolved over time, and that are now commonly used when describing issues and themes in the world of advanced nursing practice (Figure 13.1).

Now apply these terms in a conceptual map that visually describes the dimensions of practice (Figure 13.2).

The generalist A healthcare worker/professional (doctor, nurse, support worker, physiotherapist, etc.) working with client groups that have undifferentiated or undiagnosed health needs	*The specialist* A healthcare worker/professional (doctor, nurse, support worker, physiotherapist, etc.) woking with a specific client group or a specific disease or pathology
The advanced generalist practitioner is commonly, but not exclusively, titled a: *nurse practitioner*	*The advanced specialist practitioner* is commonly, but not exclusively, titled a: *clinical nurse specialist*
The advanced nurse practitioner Some authors see both nurse practitioners and clinical nurse specialists as advanced nurse practitioners, simply with different foci of role or client group *However* Others see advanced nurse practitioners as possessing skills and attributes above and beyond those of nurse practitioners and clinical nurse specialists This hierarchy may be linked to the 'level' of academic study and clinical preparation for these roles (undergraduate, master, doctoral) as advanced practice competencies OR May be linked to known competency frameworks (e.g. NMC, RCN, KSF) OR *BOTH!*	

Figure 13.1 Concepts and vocabulary of advanced practice.

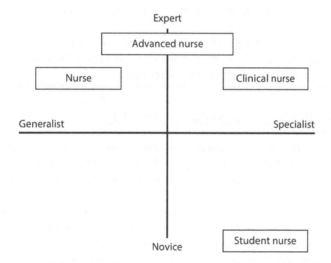

Figure 13.2 Clinical specialists and generalists – novice to expert.

It is now generally acknowledged in the UK that there are dimensions of practice that range horizontally from the novice student through to the most expert practitioner, and laterally from the generalist practitioner to the specialist practitioner. The Advanced Nursing Practice Toolkit (Scottish Government 2008) arose from the *Modernising Nursing Careers* initiative (Department of Health 2006) and promotes this concept as a national guideline. Thus it is entirely credible to suggest that, as we have pre-registrant fields of practice, student nurses are novice specialists, whereas advanced nurse practitioners may be working in generalist environments or specialist environments.

KEY POINT

Dimensions of practice range horizontally from the novice student through to the most expert practitioners, and laterally from the generalist practitioner to the specialist practitioner. Advanced nurse practitioners may be working in generalist environments or specialist environments.

HISTORICAL PERSPECTIVES AND THE INTERNATIONAL VIEW OF ADVANCED PRACTICE

The first specialist nurses are referred to in the literature as early as the late nineteenth century (Manton 1971) and the use of the title *specialist* became increasingly evident in healthcare practice in the US during the 1930s and 1940s (Peplau 1965; Storr 1988). However, it was during the 1960s that clinical nurse specialists were widely introduced into the American nursing profession (Storr 1988; Hamric and Spross 1989; Fenton 1992). The development of the specialist nurse in the US was mainly an uncontroversial one and reflected a general perception of the clinical nurse specialist role as one that lay comfortably within the domains of nursing practice as they were understood at that time.

The origins of modern advanced clinical roles in nursing can be traced to the introduction of the specialist nurse in the US. The title *specialist nurse*, with all that it implied, was intimately related to the notion that nurses could develop advanced levels of clinical *nursing* expertise and skill above and beyond that of their initial registration (Hamric and Spross 1989). Thus the clinical nurse specialist role presented no threat to the established order and stability of the boundary between nursing and medicine.

Today, clinical nurse specialists abound in all sectors of care, and they are engaged in an array of clinical areas and specialties. They represent a huge resource to care delivery and they are commonly and intimately linked to concepts of advanced nursing practice. Nevertheless, how they are prepared for their roles may vary considerably. As we have indicated in our conceptual models, *specialist* should not be confused with *expert* – and although there are multiple competency frameworks in use there is no one universally agreed national standard of competence for the clinical nurse specialist.

KEY POINTS

- The first specialist nurses may be traced back to the late nineteenth century with the title *specialist* being used in the US from the 1930s onward.
- In the US the role of a specialist nurse was based on the notion that they could develop advanced levels of clinical nursing expertise and skills above and beyond those of their initial qualification, a stance which did not threaten the boundary between nursing and medicine.

NURSE PRACTITIONERS: AMERICAN ORIGINS

In contrast to the development of specialist nurses, the introduction of the nurse practitioner role in the US in the late 1960s not only was founded on the principles of the specialist nurse concept but also openly incorporated traditional medical skills. This inevitably led to concerns about and scrutiny of the implications of this professional boundary transgression on the future scope of nursing practice.

Interestingly for children and young people's nursing the earliest origins of the nurse practitioner role lay in the work of Ford and Silver (1967) and their implementation of a new primary healthcare paediatric nurse practitioner role in 1965 in the US. During this development of nurse practitioner practice in the US, Zola and Croog (1968) commented on the professional status of nursing at that time. Zola and Croog (1968, p. 15) described nursing as having an uncertain professionalism, and that this was an 'age old question' that was difficult to resolve as the role of the nurse 'would not stand still long enough'. However, this role mobility also suggested that the professional nurse of that time was adaptable, and accommodating of new role developments. Thus nursing was an occupation well situated, and well motivated, to extend its professional identity and authority, and Dingwall and Lewis (1985, p. 6) observed that enhancement of professionalism was possible if a profession could 'reconstruct its license and win acceptance of an enlarged mandate'.

Ford and Silver (1967) had extended the nursing profession's mandate by their introduction of an advanced clinical nursing role that explicitly used traditional medical skills. However, this transgression of the occupational boundary between nursing and medicine disturbed some professional contemporaries, who saw this as potentially harmful to traditional nursing practice (Fondiller 1995). Some also viewed it as detrimental to the development of a unique occupational identity that would enhance the professional status of nursing (Shaw 1993; Deloughery 1995). These views reflected nurses' preoccupation during the 1960s and 1970s with their professional identity, and their preoccupation with nursing having a greater autonomy and distance from the traditional dominance of medical authority. This wish to distance nursing from medicine underpinned and directed much of the prevailing nursing ideology of the time (Walby and Greenwell 1994), although that ideology conflicted with the introduction of new clinical roles that had a significant component of traditional medical skills associated with them. Thus the introduction of nurse practitioners was a controversial and challenging development affecting nursing and its relationship with other healthcare professions (Fondiller 1995).

However, we must also acknowledge that the development of nurse practitioners in the US arose not only in response to a professional innovation but also in direct response to other social issues of the time:

Several social phenomena of the 1960s provided impetus for the nurse practitioner movement. Health manpower shortages especially of paediatricians and family practice physicians, lack of primary healthcare for many rural and urban poor populations, escalating healthcare costs, and the desire of nurses to achieve professional autonomy were stimuli for the nurse practitioner movement.

Marchione and Garland 1980, p. 37

These social, economic and professional causes all had their part to play in the development of the nurse practitioner role during its introduction into clinical practice in the US in the 1960s. It is true to say that these influences were and are also factors in the development of advanced nurse practitioner roles in the UK.

During the 1970s, the nurse practitioner concept gained considerable momentum and support in the US, but it was a development with associated difficulties. Marchione and Garland (1980) had observed a proliferation of education programmes for nurse practitioners that arose during the 1970s. This typified an unregulated and fragmented expansion of the nurse practitioner role in the US. It would take time before evidence became available that gave basis to the new role, and it was not until the 1990s that regulation and standardization of nurse practitioner education became more widely introduced in the US (Campbell-Heider et al. 1997):

There is now standardisation in terms of educational and certification requirements for NPs [nurse practitioners] in the United States. National certification for NPs is available for the areas of pediatric, family, adult, geriatric, school, women's health, and acute care.

Campbell-Heider et al. 1997, p. 338

However, Campbell-Heider et al. (1997) also noted that inconsistencies remained and that barriers to nurse practitioner practice persisted despite the efforts to regulate and standardize nurse practitioners' activity in the US:

Individual state nurse practice acts dictate the degree of autonomous practice of NPs in terms of prescriptive privileges, reimbursement, and independence. The 50 states vary greatly in terms of title protection, authority over practice, autonomy of practice, and prescriptive privileges.

Campbell-Heider et al. 1997, p. 339

Thus the certification and regulation of nurse practitioners in the US during the 1990s was developing (Hodnicki 1998). By the early 2000s it was more established, although it remained a fairly complex process (Ponto et al. 2002). Today, to become a licensed nurse practitioner in the US, the candidate must first be a registered nurse (RN) and meet several other criteria. Requirements to become a registered nurse vary between states and may include an associate degree in nursing (ADN), a Bachelor of Science degree in nursing (BSc Nursing) or a nursing diploma programme. In most cases, the BSc Nursing is a minimal requirement for prospective nurse practitioners, and some states require this. Once registered as a nurse, the prospective nurse practitioner must then further complete a state-approved advanced training programme, most usually a master-level degree. After completing an advanced education programme, the nurse practitioner then has to be licensed by the state in which he or she plans to practice (Ponto et al. 2002).

Thus the US state boards of nursing regulate nurse practitioners, and each state has its own licensing and certification criteria. Because state board requirements differ, nurse practitioners may also have to fulfil additional requirements, such as certification by the American Nurses Credentialing Center (ANCC). These license periods vary in duration between 2 and 3 years. After receiving state licensing, the nurse practitioner can also then apply for national certification from the American Nursing Association (ANA) or other professional nursing boards such as the American Academy of Nurse Practitioners (AANP). This rather complex process is evident in the guidelines on advanced practice nursing outlined by the American Association of Colleges of Nursing (1999):

Advanced Practice Nurse is an umbrella term appropriate for a licensed registered nurse prepared at the graduate degree level as either a Clinical Specialist, Nurse Anaesthetist, Nurse-Midwife or Nurse Practitioner. Advanced Practice Nurses are professionals with specialized knowledge and skills that are applied within a broad range of patient populations in a variety of practice settings.... All Advanced Practice Nurses should hold a graduate degree in nursing and be certified. Each existing and future professional nursing specialty certifying entity must meet uniform national standards when certifying nurses for advanced practice.

American Association of Colleges of Nursing 1999, p. 130

Thus it is evident that the introduction of nurse practitioners in the US, and the related regulation and standardization of advanced nursing practice that had commenced in the late 1960s and early 1970s, was still developing and topical in the 1990s and 2000s (Dunn 1997; Ponto et al. 2002). Unsurprisingly, aspects of the US experience, for example the complex social background and the subsequent early lack of regulation, were mirrored in the UK in the 1990s and early 2000s as nurse practitioner roles, and clinical nurse specialist roles, became widely implemented in clinical practice (Hunt 1999; Carnwell and Daly 2003).

KEY POINTS

- From the 1960s, the introduction of an advanced clinical nursing role that explicitly used traditional medical skills became the subject of much debate.
- Some nurses viewed this role as detrimental to nursing and reflecting nurses' preoccupation of time with professional identity as well as their desire for greater autonomy and to distance themselves from medical dominance.
- From the 1970s onward, social, economic and professional issues played a part in the development of the nurse practitioner in the US, and by the early 2000s regulations were being established.
- Regulation and standardization of the advanced nurse practitioner role remains contentious.
- Regulations are stringent with variation between states, but in most cases BSc Nursing is a minimal requirement for prospective practitioners.
- Nurse practitioners may also have to fulfil additional requirements including completion of a recognized specialist nursing degree programme, usually at the master level.

UK DEVELOPMENT OF ADVANCED NURSE PRACTICE

The origins of the nurse practitioner role in the UK arose from the work of Stilwell and colleagues (Stilwell et al. 1987; Stilwell 1988) with her introduction of a nurse practitioner role into primary healthcare in the late 1980s. Stilwell (1988) viewed the nurse practitioner role as undertaken by an experienced nurse who would use existing nursing skills in combination with health assessment and diagnostic skills in autonomous patient management. Subsequent to her landmark work, during the 1990s and early 2000s, nurse practitioner roles increasingly emerged in clinical practice (Hunt 1999; Carnwell and Daly 2003).

Stilwell's (1984) work provided an impetus for the development of nurse practitioner role competencies. The Royal College of Nursing (RCN) with a collaborative of universities took the established American competencies (Royal College of Nursing 2008) and adapted them for UK use. Those competencies were based on consultancy skills, disease screening, physical examination, chronic disease management, minor injury management, health education and counselling. Essentially, they required nurses to advance their clinical skills via an apprenticeship model based on collaborative time spent with clinically active doctors. During this clinical mentorship, the novice nurse practitioner observed and participated in consultations and learned skills and techniques of medical history taking and physical examination (Stilwell 1988).

From an educational perspective, the RCN in the early 1990s established the first formal training/education programme for prospective nurse practitioners in the UK. The programme unequivocally demanded that the students develop advanced skills in health assessment and differential diagnosis and they were assessed on these in clinical examinations, often with medical practitioners present. This programme set the stage and universities around the UK quickly developed their own programmes of nurse practitioner education. Initially at the diploma level, these evolved to full undergraduate programmes, and today many are at the master level. Indeed, today the Advanced Nursing Practice Toolkit (Scottish Government 2008, 2010) and *Wales Guidelines for Advanced Practice* (2010) point clearly to master-level education as a requisite for the advanced nurse practitioner.

KEY POINTS

- By the 1980s the nurse practitioner role had been introduced into primary care and they became widely accepted and established in clinical practice.
- By the early 1990s the first formal training/education programme for prospective nurse practitioners had been introduced and developed by universities across the UK; initially at the diploma level, these evolved to the degree level and today most are at the master level.
- The Advanced Nursing Practice Toolkit (Scottish Government 2008) points clearly to master-level education as a requisite for advanced practitioners.
- This is reiterated by *Advanced Nursing Practice Roles: Guidance* (Scottish Government 2010).

The evolution of these educational programmes was constantly confronted with a significant barrier to their development. Hockey (1983) had early on pointed to the paradoxical situation associated with the early development of specialist and advanced nurses in the UK. Although it was evident that the UK healthcare service needed and wanted specialist and advanced nurses, it totally misunderstood the nature of those roles because of the lack of a legitimate clinical career structure to accommodate them. The service providers wanted 'right here, right now' quick fixes to skill shortages. They saw little value in expensive 2- or 3-year 'academic' education programmes that took their staff out of the workplace for a day a week. What they wanted was quick, tightly focused skills training packages that would meet their needs in months, or even weeks. We remember clearly being contacted by an accident and emergency nurse manager who wanted a 2-day clinical module on 'assessment of lower limbs', and her frustration and irritation when we explained that lower limbs did not exist in isolation from the rest of the body.

This problem persisted throughout the 1990s and into the 2000s. Many will recognize the concerns raised when statutory non-medical prescribing identified such little time for formal education, and the hurdles that were placed in the way of educationalists when they tried to tie non-medical prescribing to wider programmes of advanced practice to ensure a depth and breadth to the practitioners' practice.

However, a clinical career structure for nursing was developing internationally, identified from the research on nurse practitioners and their place in nursing (Offredy 2000; Ketefian et al. 2001; Pearson and Peels 2002). Yet, in the UK, early research had focused mostly on client satisfaction and the workforce resource implications of nurse practitioners (Spitzer and Sackett 1990; NHS Executive South Thames 1994; South Thames Regional Health Authority 1998), and not on the demand for clear, structured career pathways in the nursing profession. Consequently, and in the most basic sense, advanced clinical practice became articulated not by actual clinical role or competence but by an array of nebulous titles.

The key to the problem was not simply the result of the major organizational and structural changes to healthcare that began in the 1980s (and which continue unabated to the present day), but that the nursing profession in the UK had an undeveloped career structure. Undeniably there were attempts to restructure clinical nursing, as demonstrated by the introduction of the clinical regrading exercise of 1988. This was introduced just before other NHS reforms came into place in the 1990s (Holliday 1995), and it was an attempt to provide a clinical hierarchy based on role and responsibility. It was a framework which failed not only because employers manipulated it to control costs, ignoring the clinical rationale for the change, but also because no one was able to explain what an advanced clinical role was. Nevertheless, its failure acted as the spur for nursing to continue to seek a wider and more professionally relevant structure of clinical career development. The introduction of the Knowledge and Skills Framework (KSF) (Agenda for Change) in the 2000s was more significant and far reaching (Department of Health 2004). Yet even this comprehensive competency framework did not fully describe a clear career framework for nursing, with it still being essentially service driven as opposed to professionally conceived, and in its brave attempt to be all embracing.

Three other important professional developments that had implications for advanced nursing practice in the UK occurred during the 1990s: the introduction of the scope of nursing practice principles (UK Central Council for Nursing, Midwifery and Health Visiting 1992), the introduction of the Specialist Practice Award (UK Central Council for Nursing, Midwifery and Health Visiting 1996) and the exploration of the Higher Level of Practice (HLP) Framework (UK Central Council for Nursing, Midwifery and Health Visiting 1998). These in different ways contributed to the slow evolution of a more refined clinical hierarchy in nursing and mirrored the parallel uptake of specialist titles by nurses (Read et al. 2000; Carnwell and Daly 2003) and the proliferation of clinical programmes for qualified nurses that sought to enable specialist and advanced skills. There was even an apparent political will to support such developments, which was evident in the government's promotion and funding of consultant nurses (Waller 1998).

From an educational perspective, it is important to note the emergence in the UK during the early 2000s of the Association of Advanced Practice Educators (AAPE) (formally the Association of Advanced Nursing Practitioner Educators [AANPE]). The AAPE was and is an influential lobby of 47 UK universities that sought to represent the collective view of the education of advanced nurse practitioners. Their terms of reference pointed to collaborative curriculum development and standard setting, and advising and establishing the role and status of nurse practitioners and advanced practice through interface with other professions, professional and statutory bodies, commissioners, employers and relevant government bodies. The AAPE established close links with the RCN accreditation unit, the RCN Nurse Practitioner Association and the NMC.

The origins of the AAPE lay in the US National Organization of Nurse Practitioner Faculties (NONPF). NONPF was established in 1980 following the introduction (outline previously) of nurse practitioners to clinical practice in the US in the mid-1960s. It arose as a direct result of the wish of American universities to ensure that there was a forum for dialogue on nurse practitioner education issues across the US. NONPF's mission was and is the provision of leadership in promoting quality nurse practitioner education at a national and international level. Its mission would, by the early 1990s, provide a foundation to the very early development of a UK-wide network of nurse practitioner educators. Indeed, it was in the 1990s that the first education collaborations arose as a result of the implementation and franchise of the RCN 'nurse practitioner' diploma. That franchise brought together a small group of UK university representatives, and they began to meet on a regular basis, and shared their educational experiences and expertise. As the 1990s progressed, and as programmes of nurse practitioner and advanced clinical practice education proliferated, the number of universities involved in this early network slowly grew. In October 2000, the fledgling educational network called a general meeting of UK university representatives (all of whom were providing some form of nurse practitioner education) at the RCN in London. The attendees of that meeting concluded that a formal education forum was needed in the UK to facilitate the sharing of good practice and standard setting for nurse practitioner education in the UK.

The inaugural meeting of UK NONPF took place in November 2001, a decade after the first RCN nurse practitioner diploma course had began. Membership of the UK NONPF slowly increased during 2002 and 2003, and by late 2003 a series of key meetings led to the establishment of a formal network link with the extensive national RCN Nurse Practitioner Association. In 2005, the UK NONPF changed its name to the Association of Advanced Nursing Practice Educators (AANPE) and was formally relaunched as a new independent association. By early 2007, the AANPE had forged a collaboration of universities that was unprecedented in scale and nature in the UK, with formal membership from 47 UK universities and 107 academics and other senior health professionals in its membership. The NMC has publicly acknowledged the influence of the AANPE. In 2015 the association renamed itself Association of Advanced Practice Educators (AAPE), acknowledging the now increasingly multi-professional context of advanced practice. From its beginnings in the early 1990s, the AAPE has evolved to become a national, influential and powerful voice in the world of advanced practice.

KEY POINTS

- Barriers to the development of advanced nurses included a misunderstanding about their role and those of specialist nurses, and most pertinently the lack of a legitimate career structure.
- Important professional developments during the 1990s paved the way for a more refined clinical hierarchy and there was a proliferation of clinical programmes for both specialist and advanced nurses.
- By early 2007, the Association for Advanced Nursing Practice Educators, a consortium of 47 UK universities, had been established to represent the educational requirements of advanced nurse practitioners.

REFLECTION POINTS

- Do you have advanced nurse practitioners working in your healthcare setting?
- If so, how many are there?
- Which areas do they work in?
- Are they generalists or specialists?

CURRENT STATUS OF ADVANCED NURSING PRACTICE

The *Modernising Nursing Careers* initiative of 2007–2010 (Department of Health 2006) was initiated by the four nursing officers of the UK. For advanced practice, its most significant product was the Advanced Nursing Practice Toolkit. We urge readers to visit this web-based resource (http://www.advancedpractice.scot.nhs. uk/home.aspx). The toolkit's principle is that there are many entirely appropriate and accurate definitions of advanced practice, and as such it is somewhat fruitless to continue to seek the 'ultimate' definition.

Nevertheless, we will provide you with a working definition to be used later in the chapter. The International Council of Nurses (2002) definition of advanced nursing practice states the following:

The advanced nurse practitioner is a registered nurse who has acquired the expert knowledge base, complex decision-making skills and clinical competencies for expanded practice, the characteristics of which are shaped by the context and/or country in which s/he is credentialed to practice. A Master's degree is recommended for entry level.

Skills for Health developed the *Career Framework for Health* in 2006 (Skills for Health 2006a, 2006b). The framework placed the 'advanced practitioner' at level 7 (KSF), defining advanced practitioners as

experienced clinical professionals who have developed their skills and theoretical knowledge to a very high standard. They are empowered to make high-level clinical decisions and will often have their own caseload. Non-clinical staff at Level 7 will typically be managing a number of service areas.

The wordier NMC definition of advanced nurse practitioners (Nursing and Midwifery Council 2005) is as follows:

Advanced nurse practitioners are highly experienced and educated members of the care team who are able to diagnose and treat your healthcare needs or refer you to an appropriate specialist if needed.

Advanced nurse practitioners are highly skilled nurses who can:

- Take a comprehensive patient history
- Carry out physical examinations
- Use their expert knowledge and clinical judgment to identify the potential diagnosis
- Refer patients for investigations where appropriate
- Make a final diagnosis
- Decide on and carry out treatment, including the prescribing of medicines, or refer patients to an appropriate specialist
- Use their extensive practice experience to plan and provide skilled and competent care to meet patients' health and social care needs involving other members of the healthcare team as appropriate
- Ensure the provision of continuity of care including follow-up visits
- Assess and evaluate, with patients, the effectiveness of the treatment and care provided and make changes as needed
- Work independently, although often as part of a healthcare team
- Provide leadership
- Make sure that each patient's treatment and care is based on best practice

At the time of this second edition, the NMC is introducing its Revalidation framework (Nursing and Midwifery Council 2015). The impact that this may have on the governance of advanced practitioners is potentially far reaching. Thus it is the NMC's scope of practice that imposes the limits on the extent of any nurse's role or clinical activity, coupled with the local employer's governance of practice. Whether this affords sufficient public protection is a concern for the NMC and is a matter for wide debate.

It is a concern for all of us with a stake in advanced practice that it must look to competency frameworks and metrics. We have alluded to the competency framework evolved by the RCN and collaborating universities. These competencies have been adopted and further modified by the NMC, and they serve as a measure by which advanced practitioners judge their knowledge, skill and competence. Many universities that provide advanced practice programmes use these competencies to tailor their curriculum. In addition, these competencies have been mapped to the KSF. However, we would be remiss if we did not also acknowledge the many other competency frameworks that are available, with Skills for Health, Critical Care and Emergency Care being but a few that are in use.

Modernising Nursing Careers (Department of Health 2006) has also resulted in a major review of the pre-registration nursing curriculum on a UK-wide basis. This has led to the development of generic and field-based competencies (Nursing and Midwifery Council 2009, 2010). Again this illustrates the dynamic nature of nursing. The link between the competency and practice of the newly qualified children and young people's nurse as a result of this new curriculum, and how this will compare and contrast with the existing competencies that are expected of an advanced practitioner, has yet to be tested. Indeed, at the time that this chapter was being rewritten further reviews of nursing pre-registration curriculum are under way. It is to be hoped that, as these innovations establish themselves, the articulation of the transition from novice to advanced practitioner will become more transparent than it is now. In addition, the four countries of the UK have all produced their post-registration career frameworks, each usefully mapping succession planning across the KSF – from 1 to 9.

> ### KEY POINTS
>
> - The *Modernising Nursing Careers* initiative throughout the UK has led to the development of an Advanced Nursing Practice Toolkit.
> - In 2010 the NMC announced its decision to introduce regulations for advanced practice.
> - *Modernising Nursing Careers* and the review of pre-registration nursing education (Nursing and Midwifery Council 2009) have resulted in a major review of the UK pre-registration curriculum and the development of generic and field-based competencies, which has significant implications for all branches of the profession, including children's nursing.

Having laid out the complexity (and uncertainty) of advanced practice in its broadest sense, we move on now to apply this foundation in the context of the care of children and young people.

CHILDREN AND YOUNG PEOPLE'S NURSING

This section is structured in the following way. Although the particular nature of children and young people's nursing has been examined in detail elsewhere in this book, it is necessary to give some brief explanation of what is meant by this to be able to put into context the intimate relationship between advanced practice and children and young people's nursing. The section then examines the current situation of advanced nursing practice in the provision of healthcare to children and young people in the UK. The principal question we are asking here is: Who are the advanced nurse practitioners who are treating children and young people? In responding to this question, we examine the scope of the services being offered and evaluate the knowledge and skills required to provide a professional standard of advanced nursing care for children and young people. Incorporated into this is the application of those concepts and principles of advanced practice identified previously.

The section concludes with a summary of the current status of children and young people's nursing and advanced practice in the UK. It will review the status of the current issues, particularly the relation of children and young people's field competencies to advanced practice competencies, and the modernization of career pathways, service redesign and how education is adapting to meet the needs of children and young people's nursing.

At this point, it is worth noting that children and young people's nurses care for a diverse patient and client group as well as age range, which extends from neonates to young people up to the age of 18 years, as well as those young people who are in the process of transition to adult-based services and may be in their early 20s (see Chapter 12). This is reflected in the evolution of the title *children's nursing* to that of *children and young people's nursing* both informally in clinical and educational practice and more formally at a strategic level (Royal College of Nursing 2003a, 2003b; Nursing and Midwifery Council 2008).

CHILDREN AND YOUNG PEOPLE'S NURSING DEFINED

The RCN (2003a, 2003b) has stated that children and young people's nursing should be underpinned by beliefs that are based on the nature of the child or young person and their status and rights within both the family and society. As well as the functions identified in the RCN's (2004a) definition of nursing, children and young people's nurses focus on assisting children and young people and their families in preventing or managing the physiological, physical, social, psychological and spiritual effects of a health problem or condition and its treatment (Royal College of Nursing 2003a, 2003b).

In a book on children and young people's nursing we are bound to acknowledge that there are healthcare needs for children and young people that are different from those of adults. Indeed, according to the Audit Commission, there are a number of differences between nursing children and nursing adults (Royal College of Nursing 2003a, 2003b; Department of Health and Department for Education and Skills 2004a, 2004b; Nursing and Midwifery Council 2008).

Briefly, there are anatomical and physiological differences between neonates, children and young people, and this group of patients will also have conditions and disease trajectories that are quite different from those of adults. Children and young people's nurses must be knowledgeable about all of this if they are to be safe and effective practitioners in actual clinical practice. Likewise, children and young people's nurses must also be knowledgeable about the different stages of physical, cognitive, psychological and emotional development across this age group if they are to meet their needs safely and effectively as well as in a caring and understanding manner (Royal College of Nursing 2012b). It may be stated that the pre-registration child field programme ensures that students gain competencies and confidence in clinical skills across this age group as well as understanding their particular needs at different stages of development, and importantly, are mindful of the need to work closely with parents who play an important role in their child's care (Nursing and Midwifery Council 2010).

It is also important to note the significant consultancy reviews and recommendations that point to the need for children and young people to be looked after by healthcare professionals who hold a recognized qualification in caring for children, as well as relevant specialist qualifications and expertise (Bristol Royal Infirmary Inquiry 2001; Department of Health 2004; Royal College of Nursing 2003a, 2003b, 2004, 2014).

However, it is equally important to be honest and acknowledge that in the real world this is a difficult aspiration to achieve, with opponents of early pre-registration specialization in nursing pointing to the service need for competent generalists with transferable skills (Clark 1994). This return to a generalist preparation has recently been reiterated by the Willis Commission in the Shape of Caring Review (Royal College of Nursing 2012a; Health Education England 2015). The review advocates a 2 + 1 + 1 preparation for practice, that is 2 years generalist preparation, 1 year specialist preparation with 1 year preceptorship on registering. The unregistered workforce would also undergo educational preparation to care for children.

The operational difficulties of having a children and young people's qualified nurse in every accident and emergency department or in every walk-in unit or community health centre have long been acknowledged. And it is in this reality that we find nurses advancing their practice and working with children when they may not have a formal children's qualification. The question that must be asked is: Is this acceptable? We suggest that the answer may be yes, at least when that practitioner has been appropriately prepared and assessed as competent for the advanced role that they fulfil. This argument is rooted in the belief that the advanced nurse practitioner develops a range of generic advanced skills regardless of his or her initial field registration. However, the question arises as to what constitutes appropriate preparation. If the policy guidelines are followed, then an approved registration should be undertaken in order to gain insight into the needs of the child and young person on all levels – physically, emotionally and psychologically. Also, who assesses the competence of the said practitioner? For if advanced practitioners are scarce in practice generally, and in children and young people's nursing specifically, then who has the expertise to make the judgement. The answer may be the paediatrician; yet he or she may assess medically oriented skills, thus omitting the assessment of nursing competence and skills which underpin this nurse's role. The commitment to family-centred care, education and health promotion will distinguish the advanced nurse practitioner role from a medical role (Bennet and Hughes 2009; Cady et al. 2014; Royal College of Nursing 2014).

Perhaps at this stage we now need to ask how nurses may be developed to become safe and effective advanced practitioners for the actual patient group they care for? There are hard empirical data to show that there has been a huge increase in the number of children and young people's nurses since Project 2000, i.e. direct entry child branch at the pre-registration level, in the 1990s (Davies 2008). This seems to suggest that there is now a sufficient pool from which to develop them to become advanced practitioners. However, it may be claimed that this has and is being significantly challenged by the changes in commissioning of numbers of CYP student nurses, shift patterns affecting uptake of study time and austerity and savings measures which affect staffing levels on the wards.

However, there is no reason why nurses in all fields should not develop their careers horizontally or vertically or even in a 'zigzag' fashion, i.e. by undertaking other field educational programmes. For example, an advanced practitioner with an adult field qualification or mental health qualification who aspires to work with children and young people could access an accelerated child field programme to give them the additional knowledge, skills and clinical experience needed to deliver safe and effective care.

PRINCIPLES FOR PRACTICE

- Children and young people's nursing requires specific knowledge and skills in order to deliver high-quality care to children, young people and their families.
- Children and young people should be cared for by suitably qualified and knowledgeable practitioners.
- Cost and availability may preclude this becoming a reality.

REFLECTION POINTS

- Should advanced nurse practitioners who work with children or young people be generalist nurses or specialist nurses?
- Think about your reasons for your answer.

CHILDREN AND YOUNG PEOPLE'S/PAEDIATRIC ADVANCED NURSE PRACTITIONERS

We have argued above that, as the nurse advances their practice, the boundary between the fields of nursing practice and specialism becomes increasingly blurred and irrelevant. Although such an assertion may be controversial, and indeed fly in the face of policy, we suggest that the interweaving of all field-specific competences at the advanced practice level benefits the user (in this case, the child or young person) and service deliverer. At an advanced level of practice, what matters most is the appropriateness and competence of the practitioners in working with their client groups, not necessarily their initial registrant field of practice. Nevertheless, this is viewed as a perceived transgression of field boundary, and a solution to that view is to provide a commonly understood framework and structure for advanced practice that enables that generic competence. We have noted that the current NMC/advanced nurse practitioner competency framework goes some way to achieve that. It can be argued that the maintenance of such competence may be difficult to sustain if a critical mass of children and young people are not seen or experienced on a regular basis to ensure that skills remain well honed and focused. This begs the question as to whether a generically qualified and experienced advanced practitioner would be able to care for children and young people who are very sick.

An alternative view is that entrenched attitudes are in reality evident and significant traits among the generalists, where their prevailing notion is that 'anyone can care for children', and that generalist skills can be easily augmented to meet the needs of children with additional extra 'specialist' knowledge. However, there is a real danger that this view diminishes and devalues the depth and breadth of knowledge and skill required when caring for children and young people, and consequently it is a risk to the delivery of high-quality, safe and effective services. A more balanced perspective is the one that acknowledges the knowledge base and clinical experience of practitioners in all the fields of practice within the profession that make up the family of nursing and finds the means and resolves to work collaboratively while accepting the demand for diversity.

To that end (overcoming traditional field boundaries), it may be useful to revisit the American model that we reviewed earlier. In the US, prospective advanced practitioners all undertake a generalist programme of education. Usually within a master-level clinical programme, they all learn the generic and common skills of advanced health assessment, consultation, diagnosis and patient management. Inherent in this learning are the foundations of leadership, critical thinking, research skills and evidence-based practice. Once qualified as an advanced practitioner they then 'specialize', in any of the many specialties that are commonly understood, including childcare. Indeed, they can also generalize and deal with undifferentiated health needs at an advanced level of practice. What is important is that they have all learned the same generic skills and thus can communicate effectively with each other. What is even more important is that these generic competencies are the same as those used by other health professions, thus enabling interprofessional communication at a level not previously possible. Advanced practice may be seen to bring a common language.

Nevertheless, there are strong arguments against this approach. The majority of children and young people's nurses in the UK at least would argue that their field is not a specialty but rather generalist nursing in a specialist age group (Bradley 2003; Davies 2010). Also, there must be acknowledgement that not everyone would wish to undertake a generic nursing programme, which is really shorthand for adult nursing, so that they can then undertake a further educational programme to 'specialize' in children and young people's nursing. Indeed, this is not a good use of expensive educational resources and, as has been argued (Davies 2008), would result in a significant reduction over time in the numbers of children and young people's nurses in actual practice. In the estimation of many children and young people's nurses, this would herald a return to the bad old days when the majority of children were cared for by general nurses with no real understanding of their needs. The history of the care of children in hospital (Jolley 2011) illustrates that the majority, prior to child branch/field entry, were cared for by generalist nurses who had no understanding of their psychological and emotional needs. Thus for nearly 30 years, the Platt Report recommendation, which stated that 'parents should be allowed to visit whenever they can, and to help in the care of the child' (Ministry of Health 1959), was firmly resisted by most nurses and resulted in an inhumane hospital environment for many children and their parents (Davies 2010).

In the final analysis, it may be argued that if children and young people are cared for by generalists there is the potential for unsafe practice, especially in acute areas of care, and this may lead to more sentinel events such as the Beverley Allitt case (Clothier et al. 1994) or the Bristol Royal Infirmary Inquiry (2001) in the future. Perhaps the solution, or rather compromise, is to provide generic entry at the undergraduate level with specialization, i.e. field-specific education for child, mental health and, in the few parts of the country where programmes are provided, learning disabilities nursing, in the last year or 18 months of the programme as suggested by Lord Willis (Health Education England 2015). Perhaps, in view of the NMC changes to pre-registration nursing education (Nursing and Midwifery Council 2010) and any potential future consultations, now is the time for educationalists to promote the message that all undergraduate or pre-registration nurses receive a generalist education underpinned by clinical practice placements *before* obtaining a 'specialism' in adult, mental health, learning disabilities or children and young people's nursing, so they are in effect dually qualified.

WHO IS LOOKING AFTER OUR CHILDREN?

Earlier we posed the question: Who are the advanced nurse practitioners who are treating children and young people? The answer is predictably uncertain because, at present, there is mixed evidence available on the provision of advanced nursing care to this group. Some areas have an established body of literature, such as that available for the advanced neonatal nurse practitioner (ANNP), whereas others lack a robust portfolio of published information or evidence base. There are several reasons for this. Some advanced practice roles in children and young people's nursing are relatively well established, whereas others are newly emerging. It is also possible that the success of some advanced practitioners in children and young people's nursing (success brought about by the practitioners themselves) has resulted in a proliferation (domino effect) of similar posts, leaving commentators and researchers struggling to keep up with the change.

Interestingly, the evidence base for advanced practitioners in childcare does not abound. Most textbooks on advanced nurse practitioners (or practice) provide little specific information. Perhaps a notable exception to this is Walsh (2006), who devotes two chapters to the issues involved. You can find evidence in the literature if you look hard and dig deep. For example, Peter and Flynn (2002) describe the introduction of two advanced nursing practice posts to a paediatric department of a district general hospital and explore some of the issues that arose. But, although much has been written in the UK about advanced nursing practice in general terms (often from an adult nursing perspective), very little has been published on how advanced nursing practice has affected children and young people's healthcare. Furthermore, within this small pool of children's literature there is limited empirical research available. Indeed, much of the literature is anecdotal in nature and mirrors those issues covered in the main body of advanced nursing practice articles. This fact in itself may be evidence of the commonality and generic nature of advanced practice skills that we mentioned above.

Nevertheless, it is essential that future research and evidence is generated with regard to the issue of advanced nursing care for children and young people for a number of reasons. There is of course a financial imperative. While many dislike the idea that the health service, and nursing, is subject to fiscal scrutiny, the fact is that the modern health service must demonstrate value for money, particularly in the midst of an economic recession. There is a real demand to develop metrics (Griffiths et al. 2008; Maben and Griffiths 2008) that can measure advanced practitioners' contribution to children's healthcare services and to evaluate the roles practitioners have both financially and from the perspective of effectiveness, quality and safety. However, research also needs to be carried out to inform those who have a legal duty to regulate the nursing profession (the NMC) of the nature and evolution of advanced practice. And, of course, research informs academic institutions responsible for the education of future advanced practitioners (Royal College of Nursing 2014).

Children and young people are being cared for by advanced nurse practitioners with professional qualifications from all three (current) parts of the NMC register:

1. Nursing (adult, mental health, children and young people's, and learning disability)
2. Midwifery
3. Specialist community public health nursing

Many of these practitioners hold qualifications from several parts of the NMC register. Thus we will use the register as a framework to illustrate the variety of advanced nurse practitioners who are caring for children and young people. The issue of whether they have received education or training for their role as advanced practitioners will also be discussed.

KEY POINTS

- Children are cared for by advanced nurse practitioners from various clinical backgrounds and expertise.
- There is a paucity of children and young people's advanced nurse practitioners.
- Further research and scholarship is needed to illuminate the impact of advanced nurse practitioners in children and young people's nursing and healthcare.
- Cost is an issue, and advanced nurse practitioners must be seen to provide value for money.

ADULT NURSING IN RELATION TO ADVANCED NURSING PRACTICE WITH CHILDREN AND YOUNG PEOPLE

Children and young people may come into contact with an advanced nurse practitioner who is based exclusively or predominantly in the adult healthcare field of practice. This may be in the hospital or community sectors. For example, many young women are admitted to gynaecology wards and may be treated by the specialist advanced nurse practitioner. Similarly, a child or young person may be an inpatient on a children's ward but be cared for (at some point) by a predominantly adult ward-based specialist advanced nurse practitioner, e.g. orthopaedic advanced nurse practitioner, night nurse practitioner, emergency nurse practitioner or anaesthetic advanced nurse practitioner. Furthermore, children and young people may have to receive treatment from advanced nurse practitioners based in specialist hospital clinics, such as those for sexual health or renal dialysis. In the community, children and young people are likely to come into contact with advanced nurse practitioners working in GPs' surgeries or in out-of-hours services.

Thus it is clear that adult advanced nurses care for children. What is in question is whether this is acceptable. There are concerns, and these must be objectively noted. Although these adult advanced practitioners are experts in their specialist or generalist fields, and may have considerable experience of caring for children and young people, this may be contrasted by a lack of a formal child's nursing qualification, or formal education or assessment in the foundation skills and knowledge related to the care of children. We would assert that this should not be a case to 'bar' such practitioners from their care, but more a demand to ensure their competency with appropriate education, assessment and governance, and thus make best use of the expertise that they have and the service that they offer.

MENTAL HEALTH IN RELATION TO ADVANCED NURSING PRACTICE WITH CHILDREN AND YOUNG PEOPLE

Mental health nursing usefully demonstrates how blurring of roles and fields is becoming increasingly prevalent. It is now possible for children and young people's nurses to work in the mental health field, gathering the knowledge and skills for this area following registration. The children and young people's nurse contributes specific expertise, knowledge and insight into the development, care and support required by children, young people and their families. In some cases, mental health nurses are now members of the child health team, in which their knowledge, skills and expertise are welcomed. As already identified in Chapters 10 and 11, children and young people's nurses often feel ill-prepared to meet the mental health needs of their patients and require specialist input which can be provided by a mental health nurse as part of the team (Watson 2006; Buckley 2010). Child and adolescent mental health services (CAMHS) are multi-professional and multi-field. Indeed, there is evidence that some centres have included some mental health training in their pre-registration child field curriculum, demonstrating shared learning across the traditional branch/field boundaries (Terry et al. 2009). This input has been provided by mental health nurses who have specialized in CAMHS and who have become advanced nurses.

There are many different roles and functions that CAMHS nurses perform, which reflects the wide range of mental health problems and disorders that children and young people experience. There is often a blurring of professional roles with these children and young people, and in some instances nurses are in a prime position to lead services that meet specific needs. For example, there are a number of key assessment and treatment strategies related to attention deficit hyperactivity disorder (ADHD) that are clearly identified in the National Institute for Health and Clinical Excellence (2008) guidance. Good practice is to restrict the number of professionals in clinical pathways to a minimum. Nurses are able to assess, diagnose and treat children with ADHD providing they have developed the advanced assessment skills and advanced therapeutic skills, including that of prescribing. In Southampton, a nurse-led service was developed and subsequently evaluated. Results showed cost savings of more than 41% over 6 months compared with a traditional model of care involving a range of other (often more expensive) professionals. An ADHD pathway was developed with clear routes to the nurse prescriber and good use of expert parents/patients in support groups was included. Outcomes for children and for schools were measured as positive, and this approach demonstrates very well the benefits of having experienced advanced nurses leading services. There are several other examples of nurse-led services for children with ADHD which can be found across the UK. There are other examples emerging where particular patient groups are benefitting from the use of advanced nurses leading services such as in the field of eating disorders and of emerging psychosis in young people.

Source: Mervyn Townley, Consultant Nurse (retired), CAMHS, Gwent, Wales.

LEARNING DISABILITY AND ADVANCED NURSING PRACTICE IN RELATION TO CHILDREN AND YOUNG PEOPLE

Learning disability is by its very nature a multi-professional, multi-discipline, multi-context-based area of care. Equally, it is an area of care that deals with a spectrum of disabilities, challenging behaviour, autistic spectrum disorders and mental health. The literature (Jukes 1996) suggests that there is a clear part to play for advanced nurse practitioners in learning disability. Strategic and professional health policies seeking de-institutionalization of people with learning disabilities also point to the role of advanced practitioners in enabling this. Consequently learning disability nurses have sought additional skills to enhance their practice in areas of 'challenging behaviour', epilepsy management, non-medical prescribing and psychotherapeutic/educational interventions. More importantly, they have advanced their practice development in the context of a lifespan approach, encompassing learning disabilities in children, adolescents, adults and older adults. Thus the learning disability advanced practitioner role is exceedingly varied, and they have a role in the care of children and young people in secondary and primary care settings. There is a demand placed on them for case management and domiciliary care that makes use of multi-disciplinary and multi-agency teams at primary, secondary and tertiary levels of intervention for children and young people with learning disabilities and their families.

People with learning disabilities are a heterogeneous group with a wide range of health and social care needs. Learning disabilities nurses work across a range of settings and services to meet the ordinary and specific health needs that this group present. There is a reported increase in the prevalence of severe or complex disabilities among children with learning disabilities (Emerson and Hatton 2004). More infants are surviving into childhood and adolescence, often with very complex health and behavioural needs.

Learning disability nurses work with children and their families in a number of settings ranging from schools, home and respite through to multi-agency children's services.

An area where learning disability nurses make a significant impact is in transition services. Children in transition are often leaving a children's service where much of their healthcare has been coordinated through a single healthcare professional (paediatrician) for an adult service which is primary care led and where access is required to a range of specialist healthcare services.

The advanced nurse practitioner in learning disabilities transition nurse provides a vital link between child and adult services and works across professional and organizational boundaries to ensure a safe and smooth transfer to adult services and provide a continuity of care. In-depth knowledge and sophisticated clinical skills are required to work effectively with children, their families and the services that support them. Learning disability transition nursing practice focuses on three broad areas: (1) the promotion and maintenance of good health, (2) the delivery of specialist health and behavioural interventions and (3) the coordination of service delivery. This coordination function is vital if the health and development of the individual is to be maintained.

Source: Christopher Griffiths, Consultant Nurse, Abertawe Bro Morgannwg University Health Board, Port Talbot, Wales.

The following case study from practice sets out how the advanced nurse practitioner transition nurse in learning disabilities can make a real difference to the quality of life and care of a young man with severe learning disabilities by working with him, his carers and all the other agencies involved.

CASE STUDY

David is a 15-year-old boy with severe learning disabilities and complex health and behavioural needs. He has been diagnosed with guanidinoacetate methyltransferase deficiency, an autosomal recessive metabolic disorder characterized by developmental delay, epilepsy, failure of active speech and extrapyramidal movement disorder. David therefore has extremely limited communication, epilepsy, mobility problems, incontinence, poor sleep, self-injurious behaviour and aggression toward others. He was referred to the specialist learning disabilities nurse for management of the transition process between child and adult services, specifically in relation to his healthcare needs.

It was suspected that the self-injury and aggression were in part linked to pain, owing to a build-up of air in the gut, which resulted from his behaviour of 'swallowing' air. Poor communication, mobility difficulties and lack of independence were also considered to be contributing factors. David has a special diet because of his condition, which needs to be administered through a percutaneous endoscopic gastrostomy. This was administered in a single feed over 6 hours, during which he was confined to his wheelchair, and resulted in restricted independence as well as frustration for him.

Because of the complexity of David's condition there is a plethora of professionals and agencies involved (health, social care, education, respite services). The advanced nurse practitioner in learning disabilities transition nurse provides specialist intervention and advice on healthcare and behaviour, and also coordinated his care needs through the period of transition. This involved working across traditional professional and organizational boundaries and between paediatric and adult services.

For David, specific health interventions included:

- A detailed functional analysis of behaviours: This revealed that trapped air was indeed a factor in the pain and discomfort that David experienced, together with reinforcing behaviours from staff. A multi-professional action plan was devised to proactively release the trapped air several times a day and thus reduce the pain this caused. The 6-hour feed regime was split into two 3-hour feeds, thus allowing him more freedom and control over his immediate environment.
- Collaborative work around the management of epilepsy: Specifically the completion of an epilepsy profile and Joint Epilepsy Council care plan for the management of seizures and prevention of status epilepticus.
- The main aim of the specialist nurse's intervention was to ensure the safe and smooth transition between child and adult services. To achieve this, it was necessary that all services worked collaboratively. Common guidelines were drawn up to ensure consistency of approach and all organizations were involved in joint training initiatives.

Source: Christopher Griffiths, Consultant Nurse, Abertawe Bro Morgannwg University Health Board, Port Talbot, Wales.

CHILDREN AND YOUNG PEOPLE'S NURSING IN RELATION TO ADVANCED NURSING PRACTICE

It is perhaps no surprise that the number of advanced nursing practice posts within the field of children and young people's nursing is increasing in a variety of different settings within both the hospital and community sectors. Advanced paediatric nurse practitioners (APNPs) within the hospital environment can be generalist paediatric clinicians or distinct specialists, e.g. in oncology, respiratory, neonatology, neurology or intensive care services.

ROLE OUTLINE OF ADVANCED PAEDIATRIC NURSE PRACTITIONER

I am a registered general nurse and registered sick children's nurse who has worked in various paediatric settings for the past 20 years. I achieved a Bachelor of Science in Nursing degree followed by a 2-year diploma course at St Martin's College, Lancaster, and am also a qualified prescriber. My workplace in Scotland has been altering the boundaries of nursing and entering the field of medicine for more than 4 years now. Advanced practice is aimed at providing holistic, effective, high-quality care to patients and their families. A third APNP will join our team this year. At present, we regularly replace a senior house officer within the inpatient ward and the assessment unit, working autonomously and as part of the multi-disciplinary team. As APNPs we use advanced clinical skills and our in-depth knowledge base to comprehensively assess patients by physical examination and history taking. We initiate investigations, interpret results, and assess and treat children and young people with undiagnosed and undifferentiated medical conditions which entails diagnosing, admitting, discharging, prescribing and referring to other professionals.

Source: Jacqueline (Jacquie) Taylor, APNP, Kirkcaldy, Scotland.

APNPs working in acute areas of paediatric medicine can expedite admission, diagnosis and treatment and even discharge as set out in the following case study.

CASE STUDY

Fiona, an 11-year-old girl, had had tummy pain for 2 days, and her GP referred her for suspected appendicitis to the local paediatric assessment unit, where the APNP assessed her. On arrival, Fiona was very chatty; she was apyrexial and had had no high temperatures at home. She complained that her tummy pain was sharp and only stayed in the lower part of her tummy but her lower back was also sore. The pain came and went all day and sometimes was there at night-time. She did say she needed to go the toilet a few more times than usual. When she did pass urine she said it was 'nippy'.

On examination there was tenderness to the lower abdomen but no guarding or rebound tenderness. Normal bowel sounds were auscultated. She had had constipation in the past, used lactulose to help her bowel movements. Fiona and her mother felt that her stools were normal and she had been passing normal stool daily. Results from a urine sample showed some nitrites, protein and leucocytes. Fiona's pain had since gone and she was 'starving' as she had missed her lunch by being at the GP's surgery. The APNP prescribed trimethoprim for 7 days for a urinary tract infection, advised regular paracetamol and ibuprofen for pain and wrote a prescription for this. Fiona was discharged home, with a view to a follow-up telephone call when the urine culture results came back. No further follow-up or investigation was required as per local and national guidelines and policies. She was also given 24 hours open access to the unit if her symptoms changed or her mother was concerned about Fiona.

Likewise, APNPs working in acute areas of paediatric medicine can expedite admission, diagnosis and treatment and arrange admission of the child and parents to the hospital ward for further observation, as in the following case study.

CASE STUDY

Ryan, a 6-month-old boy, was referred to the paediatric assessment unit at the local district general hospital by his GP. Ryan had had a cold, runny nose and cough for 4 days. Today, he developed a high temperature of 38°C at home, which paracetamol had not helped. He was not keen to take his formula milk or breast milk. His mother felt Ryan was unable to breathe and suck at the same time. On attendance, he was assessed by the APNP. Ryan was very miserable, crying, red all over and hot to touch. His vital signs were temperature, 38°C; heart rate, 172; and respiratory rate, 44; oxygen saturations were difficult to obtain but when recorded were 90%–93% in air. His breathing sounded noisy and snuffly; clear discharge was coming out of his nose.

A more in-depth history was taken. Ryan had been taking breast and formula milk that morning, but half his usual amount. There was no history of ingestion of any foreign object. He was very hot to touch, but his hands and feet were very cold. He did not have any colour changes when coughing, or any sub- or intercostal recession on physical examination. Ryan had had one wet nappy. Capillary refill was less than 1 second centrally and peripherally. Ryan had no allergies and was fully immunized. He is the only child of two professional parents, never unwell and was usually very active and inquisitive. Today, he needed to be cuddled constantly.

On auscultation of his chest there were bilateral crepitations, no wheeze and equal air entry bilaterally. Ambient oxygen was given and no spots or rashes were seen. A nasal pharyngeal aspirate was sent to the laboratory to assess for respiratory syncytial virus. The APNP prescribed ibuprofen, oxygen and advised further antipyretic measures. She also took time to explain to Ryan's parents the complexities and treatments for the diagnosis of bronchiolitis. Chest infection could not be excluded, but as antipyretics had made him less miserable and able to feed he was admitted to the ward for overnight stay, with his parents, where observation and further review would take place.

REFLECTION POINTS

- Do you have any APNPs in your healthcare setting?
- If so, what preparation (education and training) did they undergo for this role?
- Where do they work and with whom?
- If not, then do you think your area needs an APNP?
- To what level should the children's APNP be educated?
- Should they hold a specialist qualification?
- Are they an 'expensive' luxury?

Having considered practitioners from all four of the main parts of the nursing register who may work with children and young people, we will now delve more into the details of the role of advanced practitioners who have a more specific remit. It is important to state that, when reviewing those who provide an advanced nursing practice service for children and young people, the first distinction to be made should be between those from whatever field of nursing who have successfully undertaken some formal advanced nurse practitioner programme and those who have not. This is of particular importance because, currently, there is no regulation in the UK on advanced practice, and thus (technically at least) anyone, anywhere, can call themselves an advanced practitioner. As unlikely as you think that may be, and no matter how robust the local governance, and in spite of the scope of practice, the 'unconscious incompetent' can happen. Years of experience count for nothing without a good education. The old cliché 'experience without knowledge is blind, knowledge without experience is mere intellectual play' is true. Unfortunately, there is a legacy in the UK of badge swapping – staff nurse one day, clinical nurse specialist the next and doing a course next year.

The readers of this chapter must appreciate that the authors would expect any advanced nurse practitioner to have undertaken a rigorous and fully assessed programme of educational and clinical preparation. You will note that in this last sentence we have not specified the 'level', 'duration' or 'content', for by now you should be aware of the great uncertainties and diversity surrounding advanced practice. Currently, there is much discussion on how we can differentiate between a nurse practitioner and an advanced nurse practitioner. Advancing practice suggests a continuum, and perhaps this is a good thing – that practitioners 'advance' their practice from undergraduate to master and doctorate level, and advance their clinical role from nurse practitioner to advanced nurse practitioner to consultant. Whichever programme of education is undertaken, we suggest that a well-tested competency framework should be used to structure it – and several have been alluded to already in this chapter. We also believe that current 'regulation' is insufficient to protect the public from the 'unconscious incompetent'.

Having established the need for a robust education, it may be prudent to explore the nuances of definitions. Many authors writing about advanced nurse practitioners in child health identify the problem of agreeing on a common definition of the role (Peter and Flynn 2002; Myers 2009). Myers (2009) refers to Stilwell (1988, p. 38), in which 'the nurse practitioner is seen as an experienced nurse who combines health assessment, diagnostic and prescribing skills to manage the patient autonomously'. There are other definitions, and we provided these for you earlier, but perhaps we should avoid the trap of seeking the ultimate definition. The very fact that advanced practice is founded in evolution and change indicates that trying to tie it down actually defeats its purpose. The Scottish Government (2008, 2010) and the Royal College of Nursing (2014) in their guidance provide several examples of what is expected of the advanced practitioner role. Thus illuminating such roles is best met by using the example of an established advanced practice role. In this section, we focus on just one such role, although we are quick to note that there are many more. Advanced nursing practices in relation to children and young people's nursing are potentially many and varied, ranging from behavioural therapies, family and community-based interventions (e.g. community children's nurses and school nurses), mental health and learning disability and to those roles with a more specific or technical nature to them.

ADVANCED NEONATAL NURSE PRACTITIONER

By far the most developed advanced nursing practice 'child' role (supported by an established body of evidence) is the ANNP. Dillon and George (1997) reported that the former Wessex region was the first in the UK to initiate an ANNP programme of education. A group of neonatologists, paediatricians and senior neonatal nurses came together in 1990 with the intention to develop an appropriate curriculum and subsequent ANNP appointments. The motivating factors for this development were similar to those of advanced nursing roles elsewhere: predominantly, the underutilization of nursing expertise and heavy dependency on a small number of senior house officers who worked in excess of 80 hours per week as part of a 3- or 6-month rotation which resulted in fluctuations in the quality of care. The course was jointly funded by the Wessex Regional Health Authority and the Department of Health, validated by the English National Board and recognized by the University of Southampton for 60 credit accumulation and transfer scheme (CATS) points. They defined the ANNP as 'a registered nurse or midwife with an established neonatal nurse background who has successfully completed a period of education on a recognised NNP course' (University of Southampton School of Nursing and Midwifery 1992, cited by Dillon and George 1997, p. 260).

In order to undertake this course, nurses were required to have 4 years neonatal experience and to be recommended by a paediatric/neonatal consultant and a clinical nurse manager. The course consisted of 36 weeks of full-time teaching and then 26 weeks of clinical probation on the neonatal intensive care unit (NICU) the practitioners had been seconded from. During this period, practitioners would consolidate the theory learned and gain proficiency in managing the clinical care of sick neonates, including the performance of interventions (Box 13.1) previously conducted by physicians.

The first cohort completed the course in 1992. A follow-up survey and evaluation was undertaken after the third cohort of neonatal practitioners completed the course (Dillon and George 1997). The researchers

- Attending deliveries
- Examination
- Drug therapy
- Optimizing mechanical ventilation, including the insertion and removal of endotracheal tubes
- Instigating and interpreting laboratory investigations
- Arterial blood sampling
- Inserting long and peripheral venous cannulae and umbilical arterial cannulation
- Lumbar puncture procedure
- Suprapubic aspiration of the bladder
- Needle aspiration of the chest
- Insertion of chest drains

interviewed 22 ANNPs (18 face-to-face and 4 via telephone). Although they found that, of the 22, only 11 were practicing as ANNPs, the common opinion was that the introduction of the ANNP had extended the role of the neonatal nurse. They considered the primary function of the ANNP as the delivery of care to the neonate either in the labour ward or on the NICU. The ANNP determined admissions to the unit, started treatment regimens, initiated clinical interventions and ensured that changes in neonates' conditions were responded to appropriately.

Interestingly, the survey revealed that many ANNPs had developed a strong rapport with the senior doctors on the team, and that this relationship contributed to job satisfaction. However, some professional relationships with trainee paediatricians were noted as problematic, specifically when the ANNP's practice (such as taking blood specimens) had the effect of limiting clinical learning opportunities for them. Previously, the trainee paediatricians (in their initial weeks on the NICU) would have sought practical advice from the ANNP on such tasks, not competed for clinical experience. The development of advanced practice roles is often charged with de-skilling medical practitioners. However, this survey also revealed that the teaching abilities of ANNPs were found to be increasingly in demand, and that their skills over time actually enhanced junior doctors' learning opportunities. Not only that, but they also began for the first time to contribute to auditing the development of protocols and research with medical colleagues.

Some ANNPs noted a lack of structure within their units with regard to their role, with some feeling a sense of isolation and lacking direction. The more recent evidence indicates that this sense of isolation was entirely due to the lack of clinical career structure in the nursing profession (Barton 2006a, 2006b). The work of *Modernising Nursing Careers*, and the individual post-registration frameworks of the four countries of the UK, has gone a long way to addressing this.

Over a decade after the Wessex group had instigated the first ANNP course, a further study by Smith and Hall (2003) examined how the role had evolved. During that time, the drivers that had brought about the original innovation had also developed and changed. The workload and number of hours worked by junior doctors had been reduced by *The New Deal* (NHS Management Executive 1991). The Calman Report had brought about changes to the duration of training. Nurses had been encouraged to expand their practice and roles by the UK Central Council for Nursing, Midwifery and Health Visiting (1992), while in 1997 New Labour took power following a general election, and had begun to bring about change in the NHS with an agenda of improving quality, including the introduction of clinical governance. The imperative for ANNPs was now more pressing and relevant than ever before, and they have flourished in practice.

KEY POINTS

- ANNPs are currently the most visible and researched group of advanced practitioners in children and young people's nursing.
- The role has developed in response to economic factors and working time directives as well as a need to extend knowledge and skills.
- ANNPs undertake myriad roles, but feel isolated and lack direction owing to a lack of career structure.
- ANNPs contribute to audit, research and the development of protocols as well as teaching and dissemination of knowledge.

EDUCATION OF ADVANCED NURSE PRACTITIONERS IN CHILDREN AND YOUNG PEOPLE'S NURSING

Despite the strategists' positive promotion of advanced nurse practitioners, in the UK the education of such practitioners continues to be an erratic and unregulated affair. This chapter should have illuminated why this was so: the lack of understanding of key concepts and roles, a 'right here, right now' service demand for educational quick fixes, a lack of regulatory guidance and career structure, traditional boundary hurdles and silos. Consequently, as we have already stated, the standards of practice and competence held by those who claim to be advanced nurse practitioners are unregulated and may vary widely. Thus it must also be accepted that there may be in our population of advanced practice nurses those whose practice is 'unconsciously incompetent'.

However, all is not lost for there are many positive activities and developments under way in the world of educating advanced nurse practitioners. As we stated earlier, the revalidation of the pre-registration programme, bringing new child field competencies, should be viewed as a positive development that will underpin post-registration career pathway planning. Mapping these competencies to the current advanced practice competencies is work not yet undertaken. But that mapping exercise is crucial as it will set the career path for the future of children and young people's nursing by taking a completely new look at the options. It may be stated that the unique nature of children and young people's nursing is only secure if the profession is brave enough to step out of traditional ways of working and consider new ways.

The work of the AAPE, the RCN and the NMC has highlighted the need for national standards for advanced practice from which the efficacy of educational programmes may be measured. We have acknowledged the multiple competency frameworks available, but are mapping these to the RCN and NMC competencies. The Advanced Nursing Practice Toolkit has provided a national information resource. More specifically, forward-thinking employers are now looking carefully at their advanced practitioners and developing mechanisms of governance and practical support. Indeed the NMC Revalidation framework (2015) has considerable implications for the development of advanced practice governance frameworks. This is complemented by the work of the Welsh government in offering guidelines on advanced practice governance (National Leadership and Innovation Agency for Healthcare 2010, 2012).

For those caring for the child or young person, there are now many academic/clinical/professional programmes enabling practice-based learning that may be tailored to the specifics of children and young people's nursing and to the key issues of child development and child protection. Educationalists are alert and responsive to new demands for professional education that is responsive to service demand and is rooted in the workplace. Quality undergraduate, master and doctoral programmes are springing up in response to that demand. Finally, and most importantly, there is now an agreement that these advanced nursing practice roles can only be competently achieved by a detailed and structured programme of education.

KEY POINTS

- The emergence of new child and young person field competencies is a positive development.
- Field competencies will allow mapping of post-registration career pathways. Mapping these to current advanced practice is crucial.
- Children and young people's nurses need to consider new ways of working to meet the needs of children and young people.
- Advanced practice roles can only be achieved by a detailed and structured programme of education.

CONCLUSION

This chapter has sought to illuminate the complex world of advanced (nursing) practice, its origin, its current (still undecided) status and its implications in relation to the care of children and younger people. As this chapter has identified in some detail, the reader will now understand how important, and how fraught with controversy, this subject is. We have stated that we believe that fields of practice are increasingly irrelevant as the nurse develops the generic skills of the advanced practitioner. The consultant paediatrician, the consultant pain specialist (nurse or doctor) and the consultant surgeon will all have their part to play in the care of a child with a serious injury. They all bring something special to that package of care, and it is indeed a truism that the whole is greater than the sum of its parts. Equally, the adult advanced practitioner, mental health advanced practitioner, learning disability advanced practitioner and children and young people's advanced practitioner may all have their part to play in a particular child or young person's needs. Specialization and generalization are key to the function of a complex service such as healthcare – they reveal aspects of the necessary division of labour in a complex service. It may be seen that we need generalists – to sift and sort and prioritize – for they are the autonomous practitioners who manage undifferentiated health needs. In contrast, we need specialists to utilize their specific skills to manage particular client groups, or disease processes. It is the package of care that counts, and that is sought by the service user, and once again we must state that the whole is greater than the sum of its parts.

Children, young people and their families need children and young people's nurses – we would not suggest otherwise – but the service user, i.e. the child or young person, may have many needs, and we bar practitioners from that input at our peril. As nurses develop advanced skills, the common transferability of their generic skills is an essential feature that is demanded by service users and service providers. If there are concerns on this, then those issues should be tackled: additional education and screening – all these are possible. What should not be entertained is the idea that only a children and young people's nurse can direct every aspect of a child or young person's needs. The advanced nurse practitioner, as we have suggested, is moving the boundaries, and transcending the traditional barriers between different departments and disciplines.

SUMMARY OF PRINCIPLES FOR PRACTICE

- Children and young people's nurses need to develop clarity regarding the role of the advanced nurse practitioner for children and young people's nursing.
- Advanced nurse practitioners from a generic background who work with children and young people also require completion of a recognized course in caring for this age group.
- Advanced nurse practitioners working with children and young people have a significant impact on the experience of care by assessing and expediting treatment and discharge.
- All nurses working as an advanced nurse practitioner need to develop political awareness regarding their role and the specialist versus the generalist debate.
- Children and young people's nurses must have a voice in developing national educational standards to ensure that clinically competent advanced nurse practitioners are prepared for the demands of practice across all specialties.
- All practitioners must recognize that registration of advanced nurse practitioners will protect children, young people and their families from the unconsciously incompetent.
- Children and young people's nurses must regard the role of the advanced nurse practitioner as another career opportunity.

REFERENCES

American Association of Colleges of Nursing (1999) Certificate and regulation of advanced practice nurses: position statement. *Journal of Professional Nursing* **15**(2): 130–2.

Barton TD (2006a) Clinical mentoring of nurse practitioners: the doctor's experience. *British Journal of Nursing* **15**: 820–4.

Barton TD (2006b) Nurse practitioners – or advanced clinical nurses? *British Journal of Nursing* **15**(7): 370–6.

Bennet J, Hughes J (2009) The advanced practitioner in emergency and acute assessment units. In Hughes J, Lyte G (eds.) *Developing nursing practice with children and young people*. Chichester: Blackwell Publications.

Bradley SF (2003) Pride or prejudice: issues in the history of children's nurse education. *Nurse Education Today* **23**: 362–7.

Bristol Royal Infirmary Inquiry (2001) *Learning from Bristol, the report of the public inquiry into children's heart surgery at the Bristol Royal Infirmary 1984–1995*. Kennedy Report, Command Paper CM 5207. Bristol: Bristol Royal Infirmary Inquiry.

Buckley S (2010) Caring for those with mental health conditions on a children's ward. *British Journal of Nursing* **19**(19): 226–30.

Cady RG, Kelly AM, Finkelstein SM, Looman WS, Garwick AW (2014) Attributes of advanced practice registered nurse care coordination for children with medical complexity. *Journal of Pediatric Health Care* **28**(4): 305–12.

Campbell-Heider N, Kleinpell RM, Holzemer WL (1997) Commentary about Marchione and Garlands 'An emerging profession?' The case of the nursing practitioners image. *Journal of Nursing Scholarship* **29**(4): 228–9.

Carnwell R, Daly W (2003) Advanced nursing practitioners in primary care: an exploration of the developing roles. *Journal of Clinical Nursing* **12**(5): 630–42.

Clark J (1994) *Graduate status for nurses: does this create an elitist profession? (or: ten heresies about nursing education).* Enfield: Centre for Advanced and International Studies in Nursing, Middlesex University.

Clothier C, MacDonald CA, Shaw DA (1994) *The Allitt Inquiry.* Clothier report. London: Stationery Office.

Coe J, Hetherington A, Keating FA (2005) *Comparison of UK health regulators guidance on professional boundaries.* Project report. London: Council for Healthcare Regulatory Excellence.

Davies R (2008) Children's nursing and future directions: learning from 'memorable events'. *Nurse Education Today* **28**: 814–21.

Davies R (2010) Marking the fiftieth anniversary of the Platt Report: from exclusion, to toleration and parental participation in the care of the hospitalised child. *Journal of Child Health Care* **14**: 6–23.

Deloughery GL (1995) *History of the nursing profession.* St Louis: Mosby Year Book.

Department of Health (1993) *Hospital doctors: training for the future.* Report on the Working Group of Specialist Medical Training. Calman report. London: DH.

Department of Health (2004) *An introduction to the NHS Knowledge and Skills Framework and its use in career and pay progression.* London: DH. Available at http://webarchive.nationalarchives.gov.uk/20130107105354/http://www.dh.gov.uk/prod_consum_dh/groups/dh_digitalassets/@dh/@en/documents/digitalasset/dh_4090861.pdf.

Department of Health (2006) *Modernising nursing careers: setting the direction.* London: DH.

Department of Health (2007) *Trust, assurance and safety: the regulation of health professionals in the 21st century.* London: Stationery Office.

Department of Health (2010) *Modernising nursing careers: achievements and future action.* London: DH.

Department of Health and Department for Education and Skills (2004a) *National service framework for children, young people and maternity services: core standards, standard 3.* London: DH/DfES.

Department of Health and Department for Education and Skills (2004b) *National service framework for children, young people and maternity services young people's version: getting it right for you. Health advice and support.* London: DH/DfES.

Dillon A, George S (1997) Advanced neonatal practitioners in the United Kingdom: where are they and what do they do? *Journal of Advanced Nursing* **25**(2): 257–64.

Dingwall R, Lewis P (1985) *The sociology of the professions: lawyers, doctors and others.* London: Macmillan Press.

Dunn A (1997) Literature review of advanced clinical nursing practice in the United States of America. *Journal of Advanced Nursing* **25**(4): 814–9.

Emerson E, Hatton C (2004) *Estimating future need/demand for supports for adults with learning disabilities in England.* Lancaster: Institute for Health Research, Lancaster University.

Farrelly R (2014) Advanced practice in nursing. *British Journal of Nursing* **23**(8): 445.

Fenton MV (1992) Education for the advanced practice of clinical nurse specialists. *Oncology Nurses Forum* **19**: 16–20.

Fondiller SH (1995) Loretta C. Ford: a modern Olympian, she lit a torch. *N&HC Perspectives on Community* **16**: 6–11.

Ford LC, Silver HK (1967) A program to increase health care for children: the pediatric nurse practitioner program. *Pediatrics* **39**(5): 756–60.

Francis QCR (2013) The Mid Staffordshire NHS Foundation Trust Public Enquiry. London: HMSO.

Griffiths P, Jones S, Maben J, Murrells T (2008) *State of art metrics for nursing: a rapid appraisal.* London: National Nursing Research Unit, King's College London.

Hamric AB, Spross JA (eds.) (1989) *The clinical nurse specialist in theory and practice,* 2nd ed. Philadelphia, PA: W.B. Saunders.

Health Education England (2015) *Raising the bar: shape of caring review: a review of the future of education and training of registered nurses and care assistants.* London: HEE/NMC.

Hockey L (1983) *Primary care nursing.* London: Churchill Livingstone.

Hodnicki DR (1998) Advanced practice nursing certification: where do we go from here? *Advanced Practice Nurse Quarterly* **4**(3): 34–43.

Holliday I (1995) *The NHS transformed: a guide to the health reforms.* Manchester: Baseline Book Company.

Horrocks S, Andersen E, Salisbury C (2002) Systematic review of whether nurse practitioners working in primary healthcare can provide equivalent care to doctors. *British Medical Reviews* **324**: 819–23.

Hunt JAS (1999) Specialist nurse: an identified professional role or a personal agenda? *Journal of Advanced Nursing* **30**(3): 704–12.

International Council of Nurses (2002) *Regulation network bulletin*. Geneva: International Council of Nurses. Available at http://www.icn.ch/.

Jolley J (2011) The development of children's nursing. In Davies R, Davies A (eds.) *Children and young people's nursing: principles for practice*. London: Hodder & Stoughton.

Jukes M (1996) Advanced practice within learning disability nursing. *British Journal of Nursing* **5**(5): 293–8.

Ketefian S, Redman RW, Hanucharurnkul S, et al. (2001) The development of advanced practice roles: implications in the international nursing community. *International Nursing Review* **48**: 152–63.

Maben J, Griffiths P (2008) *Nurses in society: starting the debate*. London: National Nursing Research Unit, King's College London.

Manton DJ (1971) *The life of Dorothy Pattison*. London: Methuen.

Marchione J, Garland TN (1980) An emerging profession: the case of the nurse practitioner. *Journal of Nursing Scholarship* **12**(2): 37–40.

Ministry of Health (1959) *The welfare of children in hospital*. Platt report. London: HMSO.

Myers J (2009) Advanced practice in the management of children with eczema. *Paediatric Nursing* **21**(2): 38–41.

National Institute for Health and Clinical Excellence (2008) *Attention deficit hyperactivity disorder: diagnosis and management of ADHD in children, young people and adults*. Clinical Guidelines CG72. London: NICE. Available at http://guidance.nice.org.uk/CG72.

National Leadership and Innovation Agency for Healthcare (2010) *Wales guidelines for advanced practice*. Cardiff: Welsh Government.

National Leadership and Innovation Agency for Healthcare (2012) *The advanced practice portfolio*. Cardiff: Welsh Government.

NHS Executive South Thames (1994) *Evaluation of nurse practitioner pilot projects*. Touche Ross Report. London: Touche Ross.

NHS Management Executive (1991) *Junior doctors – the new deal*. London: DH.

Nursing and Midwifery Council (2005) *The proposed framework for the standard for post-registration nursing*. London: NMC. Available at http://aape.org.uk/regulator-updates/.

Nursing and Midwifery Council (2008) *Advice for nurses working with children and young people*. London: NMC.

Nursing and Midwifery Council (2009) *Review of pre-registration nursing education – phase 2*. London: NMC. Available at http://www.health.herts.ac.uk/immunology/MentorshipUpdate/N.

Nursing and Midwifery Council (2010) *Standards for pre-registration nursing education*. London: NMC. Available at https://www.nmc.org.uk/globalassets/sitedocuments/standards/nmc-standards-for-pre-registration-nursing-education.pdf.

Nursing and Midwifery Council (2015) Revalidation. London: NMC. Available at http://www.nmc.org.uk/standards/revalidation/.

Offredy M (2000) Advanced nursing practice: the case of nurse practitioners in three Australian states. *Journal of Advanced Nursing* **31**(2): 274–81.

Pearson A, Peels S (2002) The nurse practitioner. *International Journal of Nursing Practice* **8**(4): 5–10.

Peplau H (1965) Specialisation in professional nursing. *Nursing Science* **3**: 268–87.

Peter S, Flynn A (2002) Advanced nurse practitioners in a hospital setting: a reality. *Paediatric Nursing* **14**(2): 14–19.

Ponto J, Sabo J, Fitzgerald M, Wilson D (2002) Operationalising advance practice registered nurse legislation: perspectives from a clinical nurses specialist task force. *Clinical Nurse Specialist* **16**(5): 263–9.

Read SM, Roberts-Davis M, Gilbert P, Nolan M (2000) *Preparing nurse practitioners for the 21st century: executive summary*. Sheffield: School of Nursing and Midwifery, University of Sheffield.

Rolfe G (2014) A new vision for advanced nursing practice. *Nursing Times* **110**(28): 18–21.

Royal College of Nursing (2003a) *Children and young people's nursing: a philosophy of care. Guidance for nursing staff*. London: RCN. Available at https://www2.rcn.org.uk/__data/assets/pdf_file/0003/78573/002012.pdf.

Royal College of Nursing (2003b) *Preparing nurses to care for children and young people: summary position statement by the RCN children and young people field of practice*. London: RCN. Available at www.rcn.org.uk.

Royal College of Nursing (2004) *Services for children and young people: preparing nurses for future roles*. London: RCN. Available at www.rcn.org.uk.

Royal College of Nursing (2008) *Advanced nurse practitioners: an RCN guide to the advanced nurse practitioner role, competencies and programme accreditation.* London: RCN.

Royal College of Nursing (2012a) *Quality with compassion: the future of nursing education.* Report of the Willis Commission. London: RCN.

Royal College of Nursing (2012b) *RCN competencies: core competencies for nursing children and young people.* London: RCN.

Royal College of Nursing (2014) *Specialist and advanced children's and young people's nursing practice in contemporary health care: guidance for nurses and commissioners.* London: RCN.

Scottish Government (2008) *Supporting the development of advanced nursing practice: a toolkit approach.* Edinburgh: Scottish Government, CNO Directorate.

Scottish Government (2010) *Advanced nursing practice roles: guidance.* Edinburgh: Scottish Government.

Shaw MC (1993) The discipline of nursing: historical roots, current perspectives, future directions. *Journal of Advanced Nursing* **18**(10): 1651–6.

Skills for Health (2006a) *A career framework for health.* London: Skills for Health. Available at http://www.skillsforhealth.org.uk/Search-Results.aspx?searchQuery=a+career+framework.

Skills for Health (2006b) *A career framework for health. Section 1. Advanced practitioner roles.* London: Skills for Health. Available at http://www.nsahealth.org.uk/?_ga=1.223893979.1797147935.1461927553.

Smith J (chair) (2005) *The Shipman Inquiry: the sixth and final report.* London: HMSO.

Smith SL, Hall MA (2003) Developing a neonatal workforce: role evolution and retention of advanced neonatal nurse practitioners. *Archives of Diseases in Childhood: Fetal and Neonatal Edition* **88**: 426–9.

South Thames Regional Health Authority (1998) *Evaluation of nurse practitioner pilot projects.* London: NHS Executive South Thames.

Spitzer WO, Sackett DL (1990) 25th anniversary of nurse practitioners: the Burlington randomised trial of the nurse practitioner. *Journal of American Academy of Nurse Practitioners* **2**(3): 93–9.

Stilwell B (1984) The nurse in practice. *Nursing Mirror* **158**: 17–22.

Stilwell B (1988) Patients' attitudes to a highly developed extended role – the nurse practitioner. *Recent Advances in Nursing* **21**: 82–100.

Stilwell B, Greenfield S, Drury M, Hull FM (1987) A nurse practitioner in general practice: working styles and pattern of consultation. *Journal of Royal College of General Practice* **37**(297): 154–7.

Storr G (1988) The clinical nurse specialist: from the outside looking in. *Journal of Advanced Nursing* **13**: 265–72.

Svensson R (1996) The interplay between doctors and nurses: a negotiated order perspective. *Sociology of Health and Illness* **18**(3): 379–98.

Terry J, Maunder EZ, Bowler N, Williams D (2009) Interbranch initiative to improve children's mental health. *British Journal of Nursing* **18**(5): 282–7.

UK Central Council for Nursing, Midwifery and Health Visiting (1992) *The scope of professional practice.* London: UKCC.

UK Central Council for Nursing, Midwifery and Health Visiting (1996) *Standards for education and practice following registration (PREP) transitional arrangements: specialist practitioner title/qualifications.* London: UKCC.

UK Central Council for Nursing, Midwifery and Health Visiting (1998) *Higher level of practice: consultation document.* London: UKCC.

Walby S, Greenwell J (1994) *Medicine and nursing: professions in a changing health service.* London: Sage.

Waller S (1998) Higher level practice in nursing: a prerequisite for nurse consultants? *Hospital Medicine* **59**: 816–18.

Walsh M (ed.) (2006) *Nurse practitioners: clinical skills and professional issues,* 2nd ed. Edinburgh: Butterworth-Heinemann/Elsevier.

Watson E (2006) CAMHS liaison: supporting care in general paediatric settings. *Paediatric Nursing* **18**: 30–3.

Zola IK, Croog SH (1968) Work perceptions and their implications for professional identity: an exploratory analysis of public health nurses. *Social Science and Medicine* **2**: 15–28.

Involving children and young people in research to inform service delivery at home and in hospital

JOAN LIVESLEY AND ANGELA LEE

OVERVIEW

The arguments presented in this chapter are founded on a deeply held understanding that service design and delivery, and nursing and health care practices, aimed at children should be fully informed by children and young people. We begin by offering a critical insight into the historical reasons for non-inclusion of children in research and then consider the contemporary political and policy landscape. We then look at the ethical and legal challenges inherent in research work with children and offer an overview of the research methods that may be used to successfully engage and involve children and young people. This chapter should be read in conjunction with Chapter 1.

INTRODUCTION

Participating with children and young people in research is not an easy task but well worth the effort. Understanding why this is so requires some insight into the meaning of the term *voice* in research.

Researchers often use the word *voice* to denote meaningful contributions from research participants. In health care and nursing practice, the adult proxy voice has most often been invoked to derive meaning and interpretation of children and young people's experiences, wants and wishes. Underlying this is the view that adult commentators can speak on behalf of children and that children and young people are not able to speak on behalf of themselves. It seems to us that this stems from a one-dimensional view of voice – that associated with verbal and written communication. For children and young people, voice is much more than this and includes verbal and non-verbal behaviour, silence and gestures (Livesley and Long 2013). Yet, children and young people's voice has often been silenced due to a common-sense understanding of them being 'incompetent' and unable to speak for themselves.

The last 30 years has seen an increased scholarly interest and publications related to childhood and children. It is a relatively modern phenomenon. Unlike other marginalized members of society, the way in which children are positioned in society means that they have relied on adult proxies to advance their best interests. More recently there has been a shift in policy toward a stance that advocates (rather than legislates) for children and young peoples' involvement in research. However, as argued in this chapter, this requires the development of structures, organizational systems and methods that enable their voices to be heard. In this, research practice is no different to other fields of practice.

In part, this is underpinned by the common use of the terms *child* and *childhood*, though neither has an agreed definition (Alanen 2001). Despite this, any written account concerned with children or childhood must use these terms in order to distinguish the nature and focus of the work. This problem is most usually solved by recourse to social construction. At a simple level social construction implies that members of a group in any given society will invent constructive understandings to arrive at a consensus of what particular terms mean. However, any social construction will always be shaped and limited by the values and mores of the group contributing to the construct. Given this, for the purpose of this chapter we have adopted James and James' (2004, p. 20) view of childhood:

> As a social space [childhood] does remain both constant and universal … [though] its character … changes over time shaped by changes in the laws, policies, discourses and social practices through which childhood is denied.

CHILDREN ARE NOT ALL THE SAME

Undertaking research with children and young people is essential as they are not all the same and, as with adults, individual children and young people derive unique subjective interpretations from their experiences. As indicated by our chosen definition of *childhood* (James and James 2004), there is no universal experience of childhood or a collective way of being a child. Although children account for 25% of the current UK population, evidence of differences between them is stark. One way of thinking about this is to consider the differences between children living in poorer families. For instance, there is little doubt that children from poorer families have qualitatively different experiences to children from better-off homes (Marmot 2010). Yet we have little evidence of how children and young people make sense of this difference. It has been estimated that 26.9% of children living in the UK live in or are at risk of poverty or social exclusion (Chief Medical Officer [CMO] 2012). Again, there is little research work focusing on children and young people's experience and subjective interpretations of living in poverty or being at risk of social exclusion. Yet we know from population studies that they are more likely to suffer from ill health and may expect poorer health outcomes. It has been estimated that children from the poorest families in the UK are 13 times more likely to die, and that children in the UK are more likely to die from avoidable causes than their counterparts in Sweden (CMO 2012). Other evidence reveals that 3 out of 10 school-age children witness domestic abuse, 1 in 10 care for adult relations and 2 in 10 suffer from mental health problems. Still, there is little research evidence derived from the insights of children and young people regarding these matters but strong evidence that service design and delivery are largely driven by adult proxies. This means that those wanting to know about children and young people's lives from the perspective of children and young people need to think carefully about recruitment and sampling and be very aware of whose voice is being privileged in research work.

REFLECTION POINTS

- Try to bring to mind two children of a similar age living in different economic circumstances. What impact do the circumstances have on their day-to-day lives?
- What do you know about these differences and what sources of evidence have informed your understanding?

Some people align with a pessimistic view of childhood in contemporary Britain – a view supported by the UNICEF (2013) report card on child well-being in member states of the Organisation for Economic Co-operation and Development (OECD). While there has been some improvement in Britain's position in the league table, infant mortality in Britain remains in the bottom third. British 11- to 15-year-olds are reported as having the highest rates of alcohol abuse. It is also noted that the current austerity measures and cuts to public services in the UK put any improvements made over the last 8 years at risk. The findings paint a picture of neglect for many of Britain's children. More recently, the *Good Childhood Report* (Children's Society 2015) indicated that children in the UK ranked 15 out of 15 countries for knowledge on children's rights and self-confidence.

Added to this, Britain is one of only five European countries that legislate for corporal punishment. Although under the Children Act 2004 it is illegal to hit a child if it causes bruising, swelling, cuts, grazes or scratches and this is punishable by up to 5 years imprisonment, it is still legal to punish a child in the UK by smacking them. It seems that any alteration to this would be deemed unpopular by parents, yet children also have a view. An example is the work of Willow and Hyder (1998), who were commissioned by Save the Children and the National Children's Bureau to explore the views of 4- to 7-year-old children with regard to smacking. Working with 70 children, they reported that being smacked left them feeling 'horrible inside' and

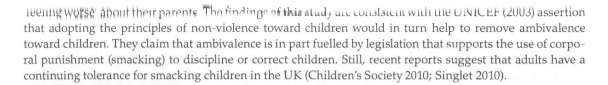

feeling worse' about their parents. The findings of this study are consistent with the UNICEF (2003) assertion that adopting the principles of non-violence toward children would in turn help to remove ambivalence toward children. They claim that ambivalence is in part fuelled by legislation that supports the use of corporal punishment (smacking) to discipline or correct children. Still, recent reports suggest that adults have a continuing tolerance for smacking children in the UK (Children's Society 2010; Singlet 2010).

REFLECTION POINTS

- Thinking about your attitude and views to smacking children may help you to determine how you position children with regard to adults.
- What is your view on smacking children?

CASE STUDY

Imogen is 4 years old and accompanying her mother on a shopping trip. She is clearly bored and despite her mother asking her several times not to crawl under rails of clothes in the department store, Imogen persists. Her mother shouts at her and smacks the back of her hand once. She then tells her that she should listen and do as she is told. Imogen starts to cry.

- What if any actions would you take?
- Would you behave differently if you were in Imogen's home or she was in a health care facility?
- Who has the right to discipline children? What rights do children have?
- Is this a legal or moral right?

In 2008, the United Nations committee report on the implementation of the United Nations Convention on the Rights of the Child (UNCRC) in the UK found a general climate of intolerance and negativity toward children and adolescents in particular. While there has been a shift toward enabling rather than preventing children's involvement in those matters that affect their lives, including their involvement in research (Weil et al. 2015), there continues to be an uneasy relationship in the UK between the state, parents, general public and children. As nurses and researchers working with children are recruited from the public at large, it is highly likely that similar ambiguous attitudes toward children are prevalent.

POLITICAL AND POLICY LANDSCAPE FOR CHILDREN IN RESEARCH

Since the Children Act 1989 (Department of Health [DH] 1989) adults have been encouraged to listen to and involve children in decisions relating to their lives. The importance of listening, consulting with and acting on the views of children was underlined by the UNCRC (1989) and became a defining principle in the National Service Framework (NSF) for Children and Young People (DH 2004b). The principles of effective engagement have been further confirmed in the 'Report of the Children and Young People's Health Outcome Forum 2013/14' (Lewis and Lenehan 2014), in which they set out to put children and young people at the heart of what happens. This involves recommendations to roll out practice such as the friends and family test to children and young people in clinical practice and the Care Quality Commission inclusion of the experience of young people in inpatient settings from 2014. Of note is that until recently, children had been excluded from these research processes. Since then the CMO (2012) has launched a manifesto for children and young people's health and NHS England has started to lead this process by establishing a young person's forum (see http://www.england. nhs.uk/ourwork/patients/public-voice/yth-for/ for more information).

Still, as noted by the Patient Experience Network for NHS England (2013) service development work has centred on adults' views with greater weight attributed to the adults' perspective. This means that with few notable exceptions, knowledge relating to children and young people's experiences of being hospital inpatients needing health care, or their experience of health, has been derived from adults – either through adult interpretation of their observed behaviour or gleaned from interviews with proxy adults. The main problem with this is that the subjective interpretations of children and young people are as unique as those of adults, and often different to those of their parents or carers.

The National Association for the Welfare of Children in Hospital (NAWCH), which changed its name to Action for Sick Children in 1992, indicative of a move toward sick children being cared for at home by their families (Smith et al. 2002), also continues to monitor and report on how the ethos of the Platt Report is being integrated into practice. That said, the Action for Sick Children's charter is dominated by concern for children in hospital rather than those receiving care at home. More recently, the European Association for Children in Hospital (2001) collaborated to draft guidelines on the optimal care for sick children. Action for Sick Children is listed as member from England. These organizations advocate for family-centred care in which families are supported, empowered and offered the opportunity to be involved in their children's care or decisions regarding the care of their children.

In a concept analysis of family-centred care, Smith et al. (2002) argued that the term is used as an all-embracing concept to describe something which has many different attributes. Mikkelsen and Frederiksen (2011) add that family-centred care consists of a set of principles that constitute its meaning. Key among these are the concepts of partnership, involvement and participation (Mikkelsen and Frederiksen 2011). Mikkelsen and Frederiksen (2011, p. 8) continued and defined FCC as

> the professional support of the child and the family through a process of involvement and participation, underpinned by empowerment and negotiation.

The concept of participation is key in this definition, and as McNeish (1999, p. 191) points out, 'participation can be seen as taking part or being present … and the participants' views have real influence on decisions'. However, it is not clear whether Mikkelsen and Frederiksen (2011) intend that it is children and young people or their parents that are the subjects of participation. Others have argued that participation with parents, between parents and the health care team, and the care of other family members alongside that of children, in hospital, are attempts to develop 'family friendly environments' (Franck and Callery 2004; MacKean et al. 2005). However, the meaning of family-friendly is elusive. As noted in Chapter 4, the concept of family-centred care has largely focused on mothers; however, it is evident that little insight from the perspective of children and young people to the development of family-centred care means that it remains adult centric. In turn this means that children and young people are inadvertently removed as the focus of concern as parents and carers become all important.

THINKING POINTS

- Can you remember a time when your view as a child was different to that of your parents?
- Have you witnessed children wanting something different than their parents are prepared to let them have or do?
- How was this resolved?
- Whose perspective was privileged?

Central to the notion of participation and children's rights is that of chronological age as it is age that determines the difference between being a child and being adult (as noted in Chapter 1). Increasingly, the age of majority (right to vote – England and Wales) is seen as problematic, and social and cultural contexts must be acknowledged along with age and developmental criteria when defining childhood. James and James (2004) propose that it is through these cultural and social contexts that 'the child' is defined at any given point in history. The importance of age as a marker of identity has been particularly important for children; it not only sets them out as a particular group in society, but also restricts them from certain activities and the social spaces they can legitimately (or legally) access (James and James 2004, p. 8) – a moot point when considering the involvement of children in research. There is a growing trend to consider those aged 0 to under 25 years as belonging to the category of child and young people (CMO 2012).

WHY IS CHILDREN AND YOUNG PEOPLE'S PARTICIPATION IN RESEARCH IMPORTANT?

Privileging children and young people's voice in research is important if their participation is to be fully realized. If children and young people (defined largely by their chronological age) are seen as less important, less valid and knowing less than adults with whom they share their lives (Coyne 2010) they become marginalized. Arnstein is credited as being the first to advance the argument of meaningful participation in 1969, linking participation to citizenship. She asserted that manipulation and therapy (for instance through education) were both non-participatory means of working with people. She also argued that while important, informing, consulting and placation (inviting a favoured few to participate) were tokenistic participation and less meaningful than delegation or citizen control (Arnstein 1969). Although Arnstein's work was not concerned with children, her ideas on participation were applied to work with children by Hart (1992). While Hart argued that the pursuit of child-initiated shared decisions with adults was the most favoured position for meaningful participation with children, he acknowledged that other forms of participation such as children being consulted and informed or adult-initiated shared decisions with children were also meaningful. What matters most is that children and young people's views are sought, listened to and acted on. Participation Works (2003) has added that there are different cultures of participation. They argue that the first step is for any individual or organization to be clear about their reasons for wanting to engage with children and young people. They also add that significant organizational change is required to sustain meaningful participation, and that this is a process rather than a set of individual activities or events. Being less than clear on the purpose of research work with children is likely to lead to tokenistic approaches.

THINKING POINT

Think about a research report with which you are familiar, which children were excluded?

The Care Quality Commission (2015) reported that children generally had a good experience of hospital care. However, they reported inequality for those children with special needs and mental health problems. Spend some time reflecting on the arguments presented in this chapter thus far and identify why this is the case.

The argument for children's inclusion and involvement in research is now being led by key government figures and departments (CMO 2012; NHS England 2013). However, it is likely that some children may be more easily engaged and involved than others. It seems to us that the next important step is for researchers to work out how to ensure that their efforts to involve children are inclusive and avoid any unintended exclusion of certain groups. There are some children that have been identified as those most likely to have their rights denied and as such most likely to be excluded from research (Shaw et al. 2011). These include the very young; young parents; 16- to 18-year-olds; black and minority ethnic groups; disabled children; looked-after children; children who are refugees and asylum seekers; those in trouble with the law; those living in poverty; those affected by violence, abuse and neglect; lesbian, gay, bisexual and transgendered children and young people; and traveller children and young people. We would add those children and young people that use augmented communication and those with communication difficulties. Added to this, children aged from 12 years onward may be seen as 'close to adult' and dissuaded from engaging in research should they fear disclosure to parents or others with authority.

Clear communication is key. An excellent example of this is the Me First website, funded by the NHS (see http://www.mefirst.org.uk).

CORE PRINCIPLES FOR THE PRACTICE OF RESEARCH WITH CHILDREN AND YOUNG PEOPLE

Children and young people want:

- To be treated with courtesy and respect
- To 'participate in' rather than feel the 'subject of' consultations
- To receive information and direct communication in a clear language they can understand
- To be 'spoken to' not 'through their parents'

CORE ORGANIZATIONAL PRINCIPLES FOR THE PRACTICE OF RESEARCH WITH CHILDREN AND YOUNG PEOPLE

Organizations should ensure that:

- Involvement should be part of the individual or organizational strategic goals and embedded within business plans, ensuring feedback and reporting mechanisms are incorporated in the research proposal.
- Involvement of children and young people is included in strategic planning and identification of research and project priorities.
- Involvement with children and young people requires thorough preparation and planning.
- Tokenistic involvement is counter-productive as it may lead to disillusionment and frustration.
- Involvement requires flexibility to accommodate both children and parents' needs – with scheduling around children's commitments.
- Protection of children and young people from over-involvement through avoidance of repeatedly using the same individual children in different projects.
- Involvement of children and young people in dissemination activities.

While it is evident that children have been given a marginal position in most research concerned with their experiences in hospital and health, a shift away from the practice of asking proxy adults to speak on behalf of children is discernible in research work with children in hospital (see Lambert et al. 2008; Livesley and Long 2013) and the community (Miller 2000). As Franck and Callery (2004, p. 269) note, 'it is a mistake to assume that the objectives of the child and the parents are always the same'.

LEGAL AND ETHICAL ISSUES RELATED TO RESEARCH WITH CHILDREN AND YOUNG PEOPLE

The legal requirements governing the conduct of research with children and young people include the concepts of confidentiality, consent, assent and permission, anonymity and risk of harm, and need careful consideration. Some of these are different when applied to work with children and young people rather than research work with adults. First, children in the UK always live in the context of relationships with adults – usually parents. These relationships are even more complicated in work with looked-after children (Bogolub and Thomas 2005). Regardless, power and generational issues are inherent in child–adult and child–practitioner relationships (Punch 2002). Modi et al. (2014) have recently published comprehensive guidance on research with children on behalf of the Royal College of Paediatricians and Child Health. They have argued that while children's right to protection is vital, this should not preclude children from realizing other important rights such as their right to be involved in matters that impact their lives.

LEGAL AND PROFESSIONAL FRAMEWORK

It should also be remembered that the legal framework on the age of majority for children is country specific. It is incumbent on any researcher to become familiar with the legal framework governing the practice of research in the country in which the research is to be undertaken. Unfortunately there is no single specific case or statute that determines the appropriate conduct of research with children or adults in England; rather there are a number of statutes that apply in certain circumstances (Modi et al. 2014). These include the Family Reform Act (1969), the Children Act (1989, 2004) (DH 1989, 2004a), the Data Protection Act (1998), the Human Rights Act (1998), the Freedom of Information Act (2000), the Human Tissue Act (2004), the Mental Capacity Act (2005), the NHS Act (2006), the NHS Consequential Provisions Act (2006), the Health and Social Care Act (2012) and the NHS Constitution for England (DH 2015). The Medicines for Human Use (Clinical Trials) Regulations (2004) have specific legal conditions that must be met for those involving children in clinical trials related to medicines.

THINKING POINTS

- What differences exist in the age of majority between countries?
- How would this impact the recruitment of children into the same research study?

INFORMED CONSENT

While competent adults can self-determine whether to consent to research, the need to gain permission from parents or those with parental responsibility to approach children to participate in research studies remains a contested matter. According to Alderson (2008), respect for children and young people's views is closely linked to their right to be heard. As noted earlier, this is embedded in the UNCRC (1989), in particular Article 12 (children's views should be given due weight in accordance with their age and maturity) and Article 13 (the right to freedom of expression). However, these rights are conditional and tempered by the capacity of children, responsibilities and rights of parents and other gatekeepers, and national legislation (Alderson 2008). Coyne (2009) argued that children's involvement in research should be driven by children's rights; she drew on the notion of the self-determination principle set out in the UNCRC (1989) to support her argument that it is children and young people that should be consulted first, not adult gatekeepers that may restrict their involvement.

Case law arising from *Gillick v West Norfolk and Wisbech* (1986) provides the basis on which researchers can attempt to assess a young person's competence to consent for involvement in research. Still this is not easy. The Medical Research Council (2004) identified a number of factors that contribute to the assessment of a young person's competence: that they can comprehend and retain information, that they can use and weigh that information to inform their decision-making processes and that they can reach and communicate their decision (Medical Research Council 2004). Yet, drawing on laws governing the NHS, the Research and Governance Framework for Health and Social Care (DH 2005, p. 7) stated:

> Care is needed when seeking consent from children and from vulnerable adults, such as those with mental health problems or learning difficulties. Arrangements must be made to ensure that relevant information is provided in appropriate written or pictorial form, and that the role and responsibilities of parents, carers or supporters are clearly explained and understood.

In addition, despite being at odds with its own guidance on children's competence (DH 2004a), the DH (2009) has stated that

> for consent to be valid it must be given voluntarily, by ... someone with parental responsibility for a patient under the age of 18.

Alongside the legislative framework there is an abundance of guidance published by professional bodies, for instance, the Royal College of Nursing (2009), the Economic and Social Research Council (2010), the British Sociological Association (2002), the Medical Research Council (2004), the National Children's Bureau (Shaw et al. 2011) and the Royal College of Paediatrics and Child Health (Modi et al. 2014). All seek to provide guidance on the high ethical standards required throughout the conduct of research with children and young people.

However, a discernible tension is evident between the inherent ideological view of children as active commentators on their own social situations and the traditional construction of children as 'pre-competent or developing in competence' (Danby and Farrell 2004, p. 36). In spite of the growing acceptance in the UK of the right of children to be involved in matters that impact their lives, and the lives of those that matter to them now or in the future, research activity with children in England, as elsewhere, has been subject to increasing regulation (Danby and Farrell 2004). Some excellent advocacy work has been undertaken with good results by organizations such as INVOLVE (http://www.invo.org.uk) and Participation Works (http://www.participationworks.org.uk), together with the appointment of a children's commissioner for Wales (https://www.childcomwales.org.uk), England (http://www.childrenscommissioner.gov.uk) and Scotland (http://www.cypcs.org.uk). All have added energy and impetus in driving forward children and young people's right to be heard. As noted in the recent guidance from the Royal College of Paediatricians and Child Health (Modi et al. 2014) there is a growing shift toward enhancing the ability of children and young people to participate in research. This shift in intent must be met by researchers and practitioners seeking meaningful involvement from children and young people.

PROCESS CONSENT, ASSENT AND DISSENT

Regardless, all children and young people should be guaranteed that they have the absolute right to withdraw from any study or evaluation at any time, without giving a reason, or the absolute right to dissent from involvement in research. Seeking consent from children is a contested matter. It is generally accepted that once parents have given permission for their children to participate, consent or assent from children should be sought. Some researchers have developed specific means to help children and young people understand what is intended and what their involvement in research activity might be. For instance, games may be used to elicit their assent or consent (Runeson et al. 2000; Bray 2007). Others have argued that seeking assent offers a more comprehensive and inclusive framework than consent for gaining the agreement of children to participate in research, especially those with special needs (Cocks 2006). Cocks' (2006) arguments regarding this seem to rest on the understandings of adult carers who argued that while children were incapable of giving informed consent, they could assent.

Nonetheless, the concept of assent muddies the water somewhat. Coyne (2009) noted that the terms *assent* and *consent* are sometimes used interchangeably and give rise to different interpretations. Balen et al. (2006) defined assent as 'an agreement by a person that something be done to her or him, even where she or he does not understand the purpose behind the act'. English (1995) suggested that assent was 'the affirmative agreement of the child to participate in the research'.

Alderson's (1995) assertion that seeking parental permission is the safest course of action still applies as the existing gatekeeping systems are adult focused and founded on constructions of children as becoming adult, incompetent and in need of protection. It is also evident in the approach taken by most research governance departments in health care organizations that are far more likely to adopt a cautious approach and work through parents in the first instance. It seems advisable then that seeking permission to approach children from parents and legal guardians offers a pragmatic solution. Other researchers have reported taking a similar course (Balen et al. 2006; Coyne 2006; Coyne et al. 2009). A downside to this is that some children who may be interested in taking part may not be able to do so should their parents refuse permission.

CASE STUDY

In one research study, Melissa's mother left a voicemail message stating that her daughter was too ill to be involved in the study and that she wanted no further contact from the research team. Her wishes were respected.

The research team could never know if Melissa had been consulted or her views sought on her involvement.

On the other hand and as noted by Coyne (2009), parents may exert considerable pressure on their children to participate in activities regardless of the children's wishes. Just as adults have the right to decline consent for research, children also have the right to decline to participate in research activity (Alderson 2007).

THINKING POINT

What would you have done?

CASE STUDY

Joseph's father rang the researcher and asked her to persuade his son to be involved in a research study exploring children's experiences of hospitalization. He thought he would have a lot to contribute and was keen for him to join the research study. His son was adamant that he did not want to do so; in this instance the child's wishes were respected.

What matters most is that children and young people's compliance is not taken as assent and that respecting their dissent is paramount. It is also important to remember that children may not express their dissent verbally; they may dissent through behaviour, such as turning away or being silent. Children and young people should also be asked at each stage of their involvement if they wish to continue, as this enables them to take some control of the amount of involvement they have. This may be especially important during any observational stage of research or when children and young people become distressed. That said, involving children and young people in research is a means of giving them control over what they wish to communicate. Sometimes, children wish to continue their involvement even though a topic is sensitive or they appear vulnerable.

THINKING POINT

What would you have done?

CASE STUDY

Sophia had agreed to be interviewed at home, in the evening, with her parents present, to discuss her recent experiences of being in hospital. On two separate occasions during the conversation she became upset and started to cry. On each occasion the researcher switched the digital recorder off and expected that she and her parents would want to end the interview. However, that was not so. Twice Sophia asked for the recorder to be switched on again so that she could continue to tell her story. It was the first time that she had been able to tell someone about her experiences regarding how she felt and how upset she had been by what had happened to her. By acceding to her request the researcher enabled her to take control of the extent to which she could be involved in the research.

CONFIDENTIALITY

The need to maintain confidentiality adds further complexity to research with children. The common law principle (based on precedent laid down in court cases) has established that 'there is an expectation of confidentiality between 2 parties, that confidence will not be broken without the explicit consent of the patient' (Caldicott Guardians 2015). Still, anonymized and de-personalized data can be used for the purpose of reporting research.

Nonetheless, there is a precedent that the safety of children and others remains paramount. This means that researchers are normally obligated to let children, young people and gatekeepers know that should anyone disclose that they are being harmed, at risk of harm or intending to hurt another, confidentiality will be breached and appropriate authorities informed. While it is acknowledged that it is impossible to predict all of the consequences for participants or host organizations involved in any research study, special procedures can be designed to ensure that the names and addresses of participants and signed consent forms are stored separately from transcribed discussions and field notes. The storage of data should be compliant with the Data Protection Act (2008) and securely stored (through password-protected computer hardware and locked cabinets and drawers). Pseudonyms can be used throughout, and any special features that could lead to identification of children through verbatim quotes or detailed descriptions may also be changed. However, not all children will always agree with these measures.

THINKING POINT

What would you have done?

CASE STUDY

Iggy had been involved in an ethnographic research study for more than 2 weeks. The researcher had explained that his name would be changed in any written accounts or reports of the research findings. Iggy disagreed with this and wanted his name to be used. The researcher spent time with Iggy explaining why she thought it would be better to change his name. This was also a condition of the ethics permission for the study to proceed. Iggy accepted this but was disappointed.

Liamputtong (2007) suggested that simple explanations and the avoidance of jargon were mechanisms that sensitive researchers could use to help research participants to understand what was intended. One way of communicating with children about what may be involved is through an information leaflet which they can read or can have read to them. Information leaflets should be attractive, use appropriate language (including Makaton and Braille) for the children being asked to read them and be simple but contain essential information. Pictures can also be used to help younger children or those with communicative challenges to be involved in the decision-making process about their involvement. Different versions of the same information leaflet should be made available for children with different needs and capabilities. Further information can be obtained from the UK National Research Ethics Service (2011), which provides guidance on the development of information leaflets for research with children and young people. Children can also be asked for their help in designing such leaflets as this can assist in the information being written in a language they and their peers understand and ensure that the leaflets are attractive and relevant to their peers.

THINKING POINT

What benefits from including children in the design and development of research information leaflets can you identify?

CASE STUDY

In one research project, the researcher worked with children attending an after-school club. They helped her to design a logo that was used on information leaflets to make them more attractive to children of different ages. The children worked independently and then voted on the best design. The young boy that had designed the winning poster received a prize and a letter of thanks. His parents wrote to say they were delighted that his design had been chosen and that he was able to help other children.

PRINCIPLES OF PRACTICE: EXAMPLE QUESTIONS FOR INFORMATION LEAFLETS

Date xx-xx-xxxx Version x

We would like to invite you to take part in a research study. Before you decide you need to understand why the research is being done and what it would involve for you and your child. Please take time to read the following information carefully. Ask questions if anything you read is not clear or if you would like more information. Please take time to decide whether or not to take part.

Who are you?

Who has reviewed this study?

Why are we being asked to participate in this study?

What do you hope to find out?

What would our involvement be?

Will you record what we say?

Do we have to take part?

What will you do with the findings?

What happens if we become upset?

What happens next?

Can we become more involved in other research like this?

Who do I contact for more information?

You can have a copy of this information sheet to keep. The postal address, telephone, email and contact number for XXXXXXXXXXXXXXXXX, who is leading this study, is listed below. Please feel free to contact me, or ask the xxxxxxxxxx or one of the xxxxxxxxxx to leave a message and she will get back to you.

Thank you for taking the time to read this information leaflet

Principle Investigator (contact details)

POSITION OF THE RESEARCHER IN RESEARCH WITH CHILDREN AND YOUNG PEOPLE

Regardless of the level of children and young people's involvement in research, the first task for any researcher working with them is to consider how they are to position themselves and, as already discussed, the natural power imbalance between adults and children. Gordon et al. (2005) positioned themselves as non-participant observers in schools to observe boys and girls in the classroom. They discussed how their presence had sparked different interactions, and their field notes revealed that their attention was most often drawn by audible and active events. In turn, this led them to turn their attention to those children who were silent and passive. This enabled them to understand more fully the gendered relationship between resistance, an unstable and shifting concept, and power relations in high schools.

Davis et al. (2008) studied the experience of disabled children in the context of a special school. One perceived difficulty related to the field workers' concerns about the expectations that both the children and the staff would have about his behaviour. In his words he

> didn't have a clue how [he] was expected to behave ... and found it extremely difficult to understand if the children were happy with [his] presence in their class. (Davis et al. 2008, p. 221).

He reported that the children did not associate his role with being the same as that of other adults in the school, but they still used his power as an adult to realize their best interests. Some authors have argued that researchers working with children can choose to position themselves as a friend, non-authoritarian adult, least adult or detached adult (Davis et al. 2008). We argue that the position of the researcher should always be that of 'researcher', with the children and young people learning about the researcher's role throughout the process.

RESEARCH CONTEXT

Adults may presume that using existing familiar mechanisms that structure adult–child relationships is the best way to advance research work with children (Christensen 2004). However, better research outcomes may be realized when researchers take the time to observe children and identify their preferences for communications and engagement. Unfortunately, it is not always possible to sit and observe children before working with them in the context of research. For instance, the researcher and child may meet for the first time just before the research encounter is to take place. When this happens researchers can use those things with which the children are familiar to engage them. This is important as the children can use these things (play materials, books, etc.) and people (parents, siblings, friends) to help researchers understand and discover something about their experiences.

Regardless, the first step in any relationship with children and young people requires trust and the development of trust requires time. Time is needed to overcome the unequal power relationship that can exist between child participants and adult researchers (Punch 2002). Giving children the time to understand the processes involved is an important part of being sensitive to the needs of the children and a way of reciprocating the time they are giving.

THINKING POINT

What would you have done?

CASE STUDY

Kamran was 6 years old and lived with his younger sister and his foster parents. The researcher wanted to talk to him about his time in hospital. He was described as having special educational needs, and his foster parents were unsure if he would be able to communicate his views and opinions. Kamran explained that one of his favourite pastimes was drawing pictures and he really enjoyed sticker books. The interviewer began working with Kamran by sitting on the floor with him. Next they started to play with felt stickers and the researcher helped Kamran to make a picture of his choice. Over time he was able to describe his experience of being lonely and frightened in hospital. Although he used one-word responses his views were given equal importance to those of other articulate children that had been interviewed.

Kamran's participation in this work underlined the importance of the supportive role other children can play in helping children to participate in research activities. In a way similar to that of adults, some children are willing to intervene and support other children to enable them to give their account and express their thoughts and feelings.

The importance of the context for research is sometimes too easily overlooked. The place in which any research work takes place may have a significant impact on the quality of what is revealed (Connelly 2008). Alderson (2008) and Mayall (2008) observed how children behaved and responded very differently in different places. Even more important is the understanding that children and young people's

> social experiences and their relative competences as social actors must always be seen as contextualised rather than determined. (Christensen and James 2008, p.171)

Although it is reasonable to undertake research work with children in those places that children and young people normally spend their time, the impact this may have on their participation should never be underestimated. It is necessary for the researchers to consider the children's usual experiences in this environment; i.e. they often associate school as a place to learn and a place that is controlled by adults. They may also feel pressured into giving the 'right' answers (Shaw et al. 2011). The same children may behave quite differently in the absence of teachers or in different places.

CASE STUDY: WORKING WITH CHILDREN IN PRIMARY SCHOOLS

Researchers wanted to find out what local primary schoolchildren thought about the local environment in which they lived. The research had been commissioned by a local voluntary group that was applying for money from a community regeneration fund. The voluntary group commissioned different research teams to undertake wide-reaching consultations, but realized that none had included children. The research team were asked to find out from children attending two primary schools in the area what they thought about their local environment and what, if any, improvement they would like to see.

The researchers worked with a small group of children in a room used for creative craft and play. A classroom assistant was always present. The children spent time drawing and colouring pictures of their houses and the local area. These were used with simple questions such as 'Where is that?' 'What is it like when you go there?' 'What do you like about this place or space?' 'How would you like it to be?'

The children were then asked to undertake a sentence completion exercise in the form of writing and posting a postcard to the local mayor. Once complete, the postcards were posted into a special box. The session concluded with the children drawing or writing (with assistance from the researchers when needed) on a leaf which they attached to a wishing tree. The wishing tree was later deployed in the local councillor's surgery for other residents to see.

Local leaders were very surprised by the children's accounts of the local area and they decided to hold regular meetings in the schools with the children.

Children are not used to being asked for their opinions about the services that they have received, and they are often socialized into giving correct answers to authority figures. It is not always possible to control the location; however, the researcher can be mindful of the effects of different environments and where possible minimize the impact. This can be achieved by creating a relaxed atmosphere and ensuring the children understand that all responses are equally acceptable, that there are no right or wrong answers and that as adult researchers they were different to teachers (Moules 2009).

As noted by Mayall (2008), the home is a private place, with some areas, such as bedrooms, often considered more private than others. Homes are most often dominated by adults who suggest where the interviews take place and who will be present. As a guest the researcher will be subject to the 'house rules'. It may be necessary to adopt or mirror the communication patterns usually used within the house.

THINKING POINT

What would you have done?

CASE STUDY: UNEXPECTED EVENTS

During one interview with a 15-year-old girl, her parents and her older sister, a younger sibling entered the room. She was distressed as she could not find her mobile phone. She insisted on a thorough search which involved looking under sofas and chairs and removing cushions. When she found the mobile phone she left the room and the interview recommenced.

Preparation for research activity with children will always require contingency plans for unexpected events. These may include interruptions such as telephone calls, people arriving unexpectedly, siblings and other family members who want to know what is going on (MacDonald and Greggans 2008), family pets trying to get in on the act, and children and young people becoming distracted or changing their minds.

THINKING POINT

What would you have done?

CASE STUDY

The Smith family, which consisted of the mother, two boys (aged 19 and 12 years) and two daughters (aged 17 and 15), with the daughter of the 17-year-old present (aged 8 months), had agreed to be involved in a family interview at their home. The research was concerned with relationships between service providers and troubled families. The family was described as chaotic. Throughout the interview the family went about their ordinary day-to-day business, walking in and out of the room, joining in when they felt they had something important to say. The interviewer simply went with 'the flow', quickly falling into the family routine of communication, accepting interruptions. However, the multiple conversations revealed the strategies used by individual family members to help them cope with and overcome aspects of their chaotic life.

Some issues are considered to be sensitive by researchers and some populations are considered or described as vulnerable. Yet better understanding and developing an evidence base around sensitive issues with vulnerable populations is extremely important. Engaging vulnerable young people such that they can express their views on sensitive issues requires both sensitivity and creativity. That said, sometimes children and young people will have concerns that they want to be kept hidden from the adults with whom they live or work.

THINKING POINT

What would you do?

CASE STUDY: CONFIDENTIALITY

A young boy asked the researcher, 'Will you tell them what I say?' Another young woman recruited into the same research study also asked if the staff on the ward would find out what she had said. Both were regular ward attenders and knew they would be back at the hospital in the future. Both had opinions and insights that were complimentary to the staff and the work that they did. They also had concerns; both had endured experiences that had left them in pain, feeling ignored and having difficulty in getting the attention of the staff when they needed something. Despite their level of concern, they had felt unable to raise these with the staff.

Some children and young people will automatically, even if reluctantly, accept a subordinate position as they are socialized into doing so and may feared reprisals should they complain. In this they are no different to adults. It is also consistent with Coulborn Faller's (2007a, 2007b) assertion that children and young people's fear of reprisal can limit the extent of what they are prepared to talk about and disclose.

> **CASE STUDY: YOUNG PARENTS LIVING IN SUPPORTED HOUSING**
>
> Young female parents living in a supported housing unit were asked to participate in a service evaluation. The researchers met them in the shared living room of the supported housing unit. They supplied food and drinks and began the research session by sharing lunch with the young women. Some young women had chosen to bring their babies. The young women were then asked to draw simple pictures of their current lives before being asked to draw a picture of their perfect future. The pictures were used to explore the young women's experiences and establish their hopes and aspirations for their and their children's futures. The findings revealed the extent to which the commissioned service was meeting their needs.

Using engagement strategies such as these can provide a successful means of enabling the development of a social relationship that helps children and young people to make a distinction between the researcher and other adults they usually meet in the same place. However, it is also possible to help children establish some control over their engagement with the research activity.

> **CASE STUDY: ENGAGING CHILDREN AND YOUNG PEOPLE IN RESEARCH**
>
> Children that had agreed to work with a researcher over time on a study concerned with their experiences of being hospital inpatients were always offered a toy or craft item at the start of each meeting. The range available included toys and craft activities that were suitable for all ages such as finger puppets, drawing materials, dominoes and stickers. A 15-year-old girl chose a bracelet-making pack and the researcher helped her with this while they chatted about her experience.
>
> Another young boy chose to play dominoes. His mother explained that he had special educational needs and would not be able to play properly. She was amazed to see that he could and said she never knew he could count so well.
>
> Another young girl was very shy, but she took delight in talking to a finger puppet that she named 'princess finger'. Other children drew pictures; one young girl drew a simple picture that showed her confined to bed by her urinary catheter. She would not have been able to articulate this verbally.

GIVING CHILDREN CONTROL

There is little written about researcher's showing respect for children's decisions to dissent from being engaged in research. In some contexts such as hospitals, children have little control over events and what happens to them. Respecting their decision to dissent from research work is an important aspect of trying to re-balance power relations and respect their right to be self-determining. However, researchers should be ready for children and young people to test out if the researchers mean what they say.

> **THINKING POINT**
>
> What would you have done?

> **CASE STUDY**
>
> Kelvin had agreed with the researcher that he would work with her on a particular day at a particular time. When she arrived, she asked Kelvin if he wanted to go ahead. He said no, he had changed his mind. His decision was respected. Later, he approached the researcher and stated that he was now ready to work with her. The researcher thought he was testing her promise to let him decide when and how he would be involved in the research study.

SUPPORTIVE ADULTS AND SUPPORTIVE CHILDREN

Decisions regarding who should be present during research activity with children and young people can be difficult. As noted in the previous section, the context and usual or expected role of adults in that context can influence what children and young people will say or reveal. However, it is not always necessary or desirable to exclude adults or other children that may support their efforts to communicate their views. Supportive adults and children can scaffold children's communicative competence. They do this by being an appropriate supportive presence or through gestures, other non-verbal behaviours and verbal encouragement.

CASE STUDY

At one point during an interview about her experiences of health care, Sarah had asked her parents to confirm her account of having a Jackson Pratt drain removed. She turned to her parents and stated: 'They did, didn't they?'

When they agreed with her she turned back to the researcher, gave me a nod and smiled as though to say I told you so, I'm not lying. It was as though they had boosted her confidence and courage to tell me more. Sarah had also relied on her sister for support on several other occasions during my conversation with her. When she was deciding the extent to which spina bifida was part of her identity, she turned to her sister for confirmation that her ideas were valid. It was not that she needed them to speak on her behalf; rather, she sought and received support from them.

Supportive adults are not those that insist that children behave in a certain way or those who expect children to do what they are told. Rather, supportive adults are those who follow the lead offered by children, affirming, scaffolding and encouraging their efforts. The value of having supportive adults present during conversations with children can be amplified when children and young people opt to speak on their own.

CASE STUDY

When I first arrived at Adam's house his mother had left us in the lounge. She said she would be upstairs if we needed her. At first Adam seemed very nervous about talking to me gleaned from the way he fidgeted with his handheld gaming device. His nervousness may have been underpinned by uncertainty, not knowing what to expect. He may have been nervous about the content of the conversation that we were about to have. Given the nature of his surgery, a circumcision, it is possible that he was simply embarrassed. Embarrassment is known to prevent some children from talking freely about their experience (Coulborn Faller 2007a, 2007b). There are, however, many other possibilities. Adam had not met me before nor had he been involved in any other research interviews. As he had agreed with his mother that he would be interviewed by me on his own (she returned to the room only when the interview was complete), he did not have access to a supportive known adult or advocate during our conversation. However, he may have been less comfortable talking about his circumcision with his mother present. Without further confirmation from Joe, my explanations remain speculative.

CASE STUDY

Christopher had undergone surgery on his penis. He had asked his mother to stay in the room while he was interviewed. He began very reluctantly, asking if I knew what had happened and saying he didn't want to use the right words. His mother was very supportive, and without answering for him would often say, 'It's okay, go on'. At the close of the interview Christopher had become very animated, even asking if I wanted to see the results of the surgery.

Mayall (2008), Roberts (2008) and Maybin (2009) have all illustrated the importance of children's talk in helping them to make sense of their experiences. O'Kane (2008) suggests that creative methods of engagement enable children to focus on events and talk about both abstract and complex matters that are important to them. By doing so, she asserts, 'The methodological problems surrounding interpretation of children's activities' are diminished as children are enabled to speak for themselves and reveal their unique interpretations. We would add to this the need to assist children in overcoming a significant number of hurdles that can limit rather than enhance their communicative competence. These hurdles may include the need to overcome adult explanations of the children's experiences that were different to their own, vocabulary impoverishment, linguistic capacity, nervousness, fear of reprisals and the difficulty inherent in the expression of emotion. Still, there is a constant need to balance the boundary between probing too much, inadvertently oppressing children, and enabling and supporting their communicative competence. It is also possible that the children may speak more freely to other children; however, some children work incredibly hard to keep their difference from other children a secret (Livesley and Long 2012). Researchers should respect their decision to do so.

Sometimes, eliciting children's insights means going beyond verbal communication.

Children may be unable to write, and others are concerned about their ability to spell or draw. Being mindful of this and attuned to the cues (such as reluctance or uncertainty) can help researchers to provide the extensive support needed by some children and young people to enable their participation. We have found finger puppets, drawings, storytelling techniques, reading for children and writing down their thoughts for them, and sentence completion postcards, among other techniques, to be particularly helpful.

All have worked as effective strategies to earn their trust, enable communication and support inclusion in research work.

Researchers can scaffold children and young people's communicative competence by repeating questions, adding contextual information, paraphrasing what has been said, using humour and accounting for silence. As noted by Lewis (2010, p. 3), researchers who work with children are often caught between

the promotion of authentic 'child voice' and a context [of] limited development, time and minimal opportunities for involving 'reluctant children'.

Research work with children with special needs can be painstaking and time-consuming, but is most often very rewarding. However, the impetus to get research work completed on time and the amount of effort that is required to work with some children means that reticence and incapability are inappropriately used to exclude some children. However, children's accounts are at least as reasonable as those of adults. When children are communicating their knowledge about their lives, then their voices deserve to be given precedence. However, it is also important to acknowledge that regardless of any shared characteristics, such as age, gender and culture, subjective interpretation of personal experiences means that individual differences and variations between children always exist. As with adults, in the context of similar experiences, children bring highly subjective interpretations to bear on their accounts of those experiences. In addition, it is incumbent on researchers to be sensitive to the many types of voice that may be presented by children. Determined efforts are needed, not only to recruit children who are usually excluded from research, but also to ensure that their participation is not subverted by participants with yet stronger voices or voices that are more readily heard. There is then no one authentic voice of children, nor one authentic voice for any individual child. Children's voices are contingent on time, place, space and those with whom they interact (Connelly 2008). Individual children, as do adults, have many voices, each one as authentic as any other. The challenge is to work creatively to reveal children's knowledge through the children's choice of voice.

As noted by Shaw et al. (2011), research with children and young people is important as it provides relevant evidence for service development and design, and practice; it respects their right to have a say in their lives and matters that affect them; it can lead to improved cultures of participation; it can help children and young people to reveal something of their authentic selves; and it can enhance their knowledge, skills and capabilities.

METHODS OF UNDERTAKING RESEARCH WITH CHILDREN

While it is increasingly expected that children and young people will be involved in all aspects of research studies, it seems most likely that the starting point will be adult-initiated projects, even when these start by asking children and young people to identify research priorities in any particular area. They may lead the research, develop instruments such as surveys, recruit other children and young people as research participants, collect and analyze the data, write reports and disseminate the findings. However, any methods used in any research study or evaluation will be contingent on the research question, the time available, the context, and the children and young people involved.

That said, some researchers have attempted to determine the most effective way to obtain children's views about specific topics. For instance, Carney et al. (2003) concluded that more information was obtained from a structured verbal questionnaire. This supports Docherty and Sandelowski's (1999) suggestion that children respond to direct and structured questioning. However, structured questions are pre-determined, and when used with children, they have seldom been derived from work with children, though there are some exceptions to this.

Conversely, the advantage of unstructured data collection methods is that they allow for a more authentic representation of the children's thoughts and may be successful in eliciting data about emotions and anxiety (Carney et al. 2003). An alternative method is to use observational research methods, but these may present significant challenges. They are time and resource greedy, but nonetheless valid as a means to engage with children. James (2010) has argued that ethnographic methods are particularly suited for research work with children, but again these can be very time-consuming and expensive. We have found that using a range of methods, simultaneously, with groups or individual children and young people works well.

Whichever methods are chosen, there is good evidence from forensic interviews in support of taking a four step approach to interview with children (by interview we mean any research encounter that seeks to hear and explore children and young people's views). This four-step approach involves developing a rapport, eliciting a free narrative, questioning and closing – a technique first introduced by the UK Home Office and Department of Health in 2007 (Livesley and Long 2012).

CASE STUDY: EVALUATING A DAD'S CLUB

When asked to explore children and young people's views about a dad's club, multiple engagement methods were used. The research event took place in the centre where the children and young people and their fathers met. A small wooden enclosure that contained bean bags and a video camera was set up. The children were invited to paint the enclosure, and they did so by writing on it their thoughts about the club. They were also invited to video their thoughts on the club. At the same time, other children selected drawing activities. Some agreed to digitally recorded conversations about the club while they drew. Others joined in a ball throwing game. One older boy that was initially very reserved asked if he could record interviews with other children. Although resource (researcher) intensive, the strategies used were very successful in ensuring that as many children and young people as possible could contribute to the evaluation of the club and express their views.

CONCLUSION

The children we have worked with as researchers have taught us a great deal. They have allowed us to spend time with them during some very difficult moments in their lives. They were welcoming, tolerant, challenging and always willing to consider our questions, even when to them the answers were obvious. The results of our research work with children and young people have enabled us to document outcomes and impact on their and their families' lives of a range of services and experiences. This work has fuelled our passion to advocate for the involvement of children in all aspects of research, and we are firmly committed to the notion of 'no decision about me, without me' (DH 2010). Our main point, however, is that within any family, the adults, children and young people (regardless of age) have unique perspectives; their views cannot be subsumed into a single voice. The views of children, young people and their parents may, and sometimes do, differ significantly. Eliciting children's and young people's insights is critical in developing authentic understanding, authentic knowledge and an authentic evidence base for the practice of nursing children wherever they require nursing. This means that it is critical to engage with children and young people regarding all issues related to health care and the development and delivery of health care services. Our final point is that any engagement with children should be founded on clear and effective communication.

REFERENCES

Alanen L (2001) Explorations in generational analysis. In Alanen L, Mayall B (eds.) *Conceptualising child-adult relations.* London: Routledge Falmer.

Alderson P (1995) *Listening to children: children ethics and social research.* Ilford: Barnardo's.

Alderson P (2007) Competent children? Minors' consent to health care treatment and research. *Social Science and Medicine* 65: 2272–2283.

Alderson P (2008) Children as researchers: participation rights and research methods. In Christensen P, James A (eds.) *Research with children: perspectives and practice,* pp. 276–290. London: Routledge.

Arnstein S (1969) A ladder of citizen participation. *Journal of the American Institute of Planners* 35(4): 216–224.

Balen R, Blyth E, Calabretto H, Fraser C, Horrocks C, Manby M (2006) Involving children in health and social research. *Childhood* 13(1): 29–48.

Bogolub E, Thomas N (2005) Parental consent and the ethics of research with foster children: beginning a cross-cultural dialogue. *Qualitative Social Work* 4(3): 271–292.

Bray L (2007) Developing an activity to aid informed assent when interviewing children and young people. *Journal of Research in Nursing* 12(5): 447–457.

British Sociological Association (2002) *Statement of ethical practice.* Available at www.britsoc.co.uk (accessed 28 October 2015).

Caldicott Guardians (2015) Caldicott Guardians – principles into practice. Available at http://www.knowledge.scot.nhs.uk/caldicottguardians/caldicott-guardian---principles-into-practice/legal-framework.aspx (accessed 30 October 2015).

Care Quality Commission (2015) Children and young people's inpatient and day case survey 2014. Available at http://www.cqc.org.uk/content/children-and-young-peoples-survey-2014 (accessed 29 October 2015).

Carney T, Murphy S, McClure J, Bishop E, Kerr C, Parker J, Scott F, Shields C, Wilson L (2003) Children's views of hospitalization: an exploratory study of data collection. *Journal of Child Health Care* 7(1): 27–40.

Chief Medical Officer (2012) Annual report our children deserve better: prevention pays Available at https://www.gov.uk/government/publications/chief-medical-officers-annual-report-2012-our-children-deserve-better-prevention-pays (accessed 28 October 2015).

Children's Society (2010) *Public attitudes to safeguarding children.* London: Children's Society.

Children's Society (2015) *The good childhood report.* London: Children's Society.

Christensen P (2004) Children's participation in ethnographic research: issues of power and representation. *Children and Society* 18: 165–176.

Christensen P, James A (2008) Childhood diversity and commonality: some methodological insights. In *Research with children: perspectives and practices*, Christensen P, James A (eds.), pp. 156–172. London: Routledge.

Cocks A (2006) The ethical maze: finding an inclusive path towards gaining children's agreement to research participation. *Childhood* 13(2): 247–266.

Connelly P (2008) Race, gender and critical reflexivity in research with young children. In Christensen P, James A (eds.) *Research with children: perspectives and practice*, pp. 173–188. London: Routledge.

Coulborn Faller K (2007a) Questioning techniques. In Coulborn Faller K, *Interviewing children about sexual abuse: controversies and best practice*, pp. 90–109. Oxford: Oxford University Press.

Coulborn Faller K (2007b) Children who do not want to disclose. In Coulborn Faller K, *Interviewing children about sexual abuse: controversies and best practice*, pp. 175–190. Oxford: Oxford University Press.

Coyne I (2006) Children's experiences of hospitalization. *Journal of Child Health Care* 10: 326.

Coyne I (2009) Research with children and young people: the issues of parental (proxy) consent. *Children and Society* 24: 227–237.

Coyne I (2010) Accessing children as research participants: examining the role of gatekeepers. *Child Health Care and Development* 36(4): 452–454.

Coyne I, Hayes E, Gallagher P (2009) Research with hospitalised children: ethical, methodological and organisational challenges. *Childhood* 16(3): 413–429.

Danby S, Farrell A (2004) Accounting for young children's competence in education research: new perspectives on research ethics. *Australian Educational Researcher* 31(3) 35–49.

Data Protection Act (1998) Available at http://www.legislation.gov.uk/uksi/2008/1592/contents/made (accessed 28 October 2015).

Davis J, Watson N, Cunningham-Burley S (2008) Disabled children, ethnography and unspoken understanding: the collaborative construction of diverse identities. In Christensen P, James A (eds.) *Research with children: perspectives and practice*, pp. 220–238. London: Routledge.

Department of Health (1989) Children Act. Available at http://www.legislation.gov.uk/ukpga/1989/41/contents (accessed 28 October 2015).

Department of Health (2004a) Children Act. Available at http://www.legislation.gov.uk/ukpga/2004/31 (accessed 28 October 2015).

Department of Health (2004b) *Core standards – National Service Framework for Children, Young People and Maternity Services.* London: DH.

Department of Health (2005) Research and Governance Framework for Health and Social Care. Available at https://www.gov.uk/government/publications/research-governance-framework-for-health-and-social-care-second-edition (accessed 26 October 2015).

Department of Health (2009) *Reference guide to consent for examination and treatment.* London: Stationary Office. Available at http://webarchive.nationalarchives.gov.uk/+/www.dh.gov.uk/en/Publicationsandstatistics/Publications/PublicationsPolicyAndGuidance/DH_4006757 (accessed 28 October 2015).

Department of Health (2010) *Equity and excellence: liberating the NHS.* London: DH.

Department of Health (2015) The NHS constitution for England the NHS belongs to us all. Available at https://www.gov.uk/government/publications/the-nhs-constitution-for-england (accessed 28 October 2015).

Docherty S, Sandelowski M (1999) Focus on qualitative methods interviewing children. *Research in Nursing & Health* 22: 177–185.

Economic and Social Research Council (2010) Framework for research ethics. Available at http://www.esrc.ac.uk/funding/guidance-for-applicants/research-ethics/ (accessed 29 October 2015).

English A (1995) Guidelines for adolescent health research: legal perspectives. *Journal of Adolescent Health* 17: 277–286.

European Association for Children in Hospital (2001) EACH charter. Available at http://www.each-for-sick-children.org/each-charter.html (accessed 28 October 2015).

Family Reform Act (1969) Available at http://www.legislation.gov.uk/ukpga/1987/42/contents (accessed 28 October 2015).

Franck L, Callery P (2004) Re-thinking family-centred care across the continuum of children's health care. *Child: Health Care and Development* 30(3): 265–277.

Freedom of Information Act (2000) Available at http://www.legislation.gov.uk/ukpga/2000/36/contents (accessed 28 October 2015).

Gillick v West Norfolk and Wisbech (1986) Available at http://www.nspcc.org.uk/preventing-abuse/child-protection-system/legal-definition-child-rights-law/gillick-competency-fraser-guidelines/ (accessed 28 October 2015).

Gordon T, Holland J, Lahelma E (2005) Gazing with intent: ethnographic practice in classroom. *Qualitative Research* 5: 113–131.

Hart R (1992) *Children's participation: from tokenism to citizenship.* Innocenti Essays No. 4. Florence: Innocenti Research Centre, UNICEF.

Health and Social Care Act (2012) Available at http://www.legislation.gov.uk/ukpga/2012/7/contents/enacted (accessed 28 October 2015).

Human Rights Act (1998) Available at http://www.legislation.gov.uk/ukpga/1998/42/contents (accessed 28 October 2015).

Human Tissue Act (2004) Available at http://www.legislation.gov.uk/ukpga/2004/30/contents (accessed 28 October 2015).

James A, James A (2004) *Constructing childhood theory policy and social practice.* Hampshire: Palgrave Macmillan.

James A (2010) Ethnography in the study of children and childhood. In *Handbook of ethnography* Atkinson P, Coffey A, Delamont S, Lofland J, Lofland L (eds.). London: Sage.

Lambert V, Glacken M, McCarron M (2008) 'Visible-ness': the nature of communication for children admitted to a specialist children's hospital in the Republic of Ireland. *Journal of Clinical Nursing* 17: 3092–3102.

Lewis A (2010) Silence in the context of 'child voice'. *Children & Society* 24(1): 14–23.

Lewis I, Lenehan C (2014) Report of the children and young people's health outcome forum 2013/14. Available at https://www.gov.uk/government/publications/improving-children-and-young-peoples-health (accessed 23 November 2015).

Liamputtong P (2007) *Researching the vulnerable.* London: Sage.

Livesley J, Long AJ (2013) Children's experiences as hospital in-patients – voice, competence and work. *International Journal of Nursing Studies* 50(10): 1292–1303.

Livesley J, Long T (2012) Communicating with children and young people in research. In Lambert V, Long T, Kelleher D, *Clinical skills in children nursing*, pp. 152–170. Oxford: Oxford University Press.

MacDonald K, Greggans A (2008) Dealing with chaos and complexity: the reality of interviewing children and families in their own homes. *Journal of Clinical Nursing* 17(23): 3131–3141.

MacKean G, Thurston W, Scott C (2005) Bridging the divide between families and health professionals' perspectives on family-centred care. *Health Expectations* 8: 74–85.

Marmot (2010) Fair society, healthy lives. Marmot Review. Available at http://www.instituteofhealthequity.org/projects/fair-society-healthy-lives-the-marmot-review (accessed 28 October 2015).

Mayall B (2008) Conversations with children: working with generational issues. In Christensen P, James A (eds.) *Research with children: perspectives and practice*, 2nd ed., pp. 109–124. London: Routledge.

Maybin J (2009) A broader view of language in school research from linguistic ethnography. *Children and Society* 23: 70–78.

McNeish D (1999) Promoting participation for children and young people: some key questions for health and social welfare organisations. *Journal of Social Work Practice* 13(2): 191–203.

Medical Research Council (2004) *Medical research ethics guide: medical research involving children.* London: Medical Research Council.

Medicines for Human Use (Clinical Trials) Regulation (2004) Available at http://www.legislation.gov.uk/uksi/2004/1031/contents/made (accessed 28 October 2015).

Mental Capacity Act (2005) Available at http://www.legislation.gov.uk/ukpga/2005/9/contents (accessed 28 October 2015).

Mikkelsen G, Frederiksen K (2011) Family-centred care of children in hospital – a concept analysis. *Journal of Advanced Nursing* 67(5): 1152–1162.

Miller S (2000) Researching children: issues arising from a phenomenological study with children who have diabetes mellitus. *Journal of Advanced Nursing* 31(5): 1228–1234.

Modi N, Vohra J, Preston J, et al. (2014) Guidance on clinical research involving infants, children and young people: an update for researchers and research ethics committees *Archives of Disease in Childhood* 99(10): 887–891.

Moules T (2009) They wouldn't know how it feels …: characteristics of quality care from young people's perspectives: a participatory research project. *Journal of Child Health Care* 13(4): 322–332.

National Research Ethics Service (2011) Information sheets and consent forms: guidance for research and reviewers. Available from NHS Health Research Authority.

NHS Act (2006) Available at http://www.legislation.gov.uk/ukpga/2006/41/contents (accessed 28 October 2015).

NHS Consequential Provisions Act (2006) Available at http://www.legislation.gov.uk/ukpga/2006/43/contents (accessed 28 October 2015).

NHS England (2013) Everyone counts: planning for patients 2014/15 to 2018/19. Available at https://www.england.nhs.uk/ourwork/forward-view/sop/ (accessed 29 October 2015).

O'Kane C (2008) The development of participatory techniques: facilitating children's views about decisions which affect them. In Christensen P, James A (eds.) *Research with children: perspectives and practices*, pp. 25–155. London: Routledge.

Participation Works (2003) Organisational standards and young people's participation in public decision-making. Available at http://www.participationworks.org.uk/topics/standards (accessed 29 October 2015).

Patient Experience Network (2013) Improving patient experience for children and young people. For NHS England 2013. Available at http://patientexperiencenetwork.org/wp-content/uploads/2013/11/PEN-Improving-PE-for-Children-Young-People-Report-FINAL-Electronic-file.pdf (accessed 26 October 2015).

Punch S (2002) Research with children: the same or different from research with adults? *Childhood* 9(3): 321–341.

Roberts H (2008) Listening to children: and hearing them. In Christensen P, James A (eds.) *Research with children: perspectives and practice*, pp. 260–275. London: Routledge.

Royal College of Nursing (2009) *Research ethics: RCN guidance for nurses.* London: RCN.

Runeson I, Elander G, Hermeren G, Kristensson-Hallstrom I (2000) Children's consent to treatment: using a scale to assess degrees of self-determination. *Pediatric Nursing* 26(5): 16–22.

Shaw C, Brady L, Davey C (2011) *Guidelines for research with children and young people.* London: National Children's Bureau Research Centre.

Singlet R (2010) *Physical punishment: improving consistency and protection.* London: Department for Children, Schools and Families.

Smith L, Coleman V, Bradshaw M (2002) *Family-centred care concept theory and practice.* Hampshire: Palgrave.

UNICEF (2003) The state of the world's children. Available at http://www.unicef.org/sowc03/ (accessed 23 November 2015).

UNICEF (2013) Report card 11: child well-being in rich countries. Available at http://www.unicef.org.uk/Latest/Publications/Report-Card-11-Child-well-being-in-rich-countries/ (accessed 30 October 2015).

United Nations (1989) United Nations Convention on the Rights of the Child. Geneva: United Nations.

United Nations (2008) Committee report on UN Convention on the Rights of the Child in the UK. Available at http://www.ohchr.org/EN/HRBodies/CRC/Pages/CRCIndex.aspx (accessed 29 October 2015).

Weil L, Lemer C, Webb E, Hargreaves D (2015) The voices of children and young people in health: where are we now? *Archives of Disease in Childhood* 100(10): 915–917.

Willow C, Hyder T (1998) *It hurts you inside: children talking about smacking.* London: National Children's Bureau.

Issues in developing an educational and professional portfolio

15

ALYSON DAVIES AND GARY ROLFE

OVERVIEW

This chapter examines the use of portfolios as part of professional development and progression within nursing careers. This includes an overview of their purpose and construction. The chapter also discusses the issues and debates surrounding the use of portfolios and how these tensions may be resolved for post-registration children and young people's nurses as part of their professional development and lifelong learning.

INTRODUCTION

Portfolios have been widely used for many years in a variety of disciplines to demonstrate individual progression and development. These have also become increasingly popular in nursing and healthcare as a means of recording and enhancing learning, analyzing the integration of theory with practice, developing critical thinking and promoting personal professional development (Jasper and Rosser 2013; Byrne et al. 2007; Timmins and Dunne 2009; Hill 2012; Nursing and Midwifery Council (NMC) 2015a, 2015b). Nurses are under a professional obligation to ensure that their knowledge and skills are safe, current and effective (NMC 2015a), and this requires them to engage in appropriate learning and practice-oriented activities that develop and maintain competence and performance (Timmins and Dunne 2009; NMC 2015b). Thus as educational courses move toward more competency-based assessments, so the portfolio has come to play a vital role in making the process and development of learning transparent through its components, including reflective writing (Jasper and Mooney 2013; Jasper and Rosser 2013; Hill 2012; Green et al. 2014; NMC 2015b). Such an approach is based on andragogical principles whereby the learner takes responsibility for the scope and shape of their learning. The learner is recognized as being in control of his or her learning, contributing personal knowledge and experience to the process (Knowles 1990). Thus nurses are responsible for directing their own learning experiences and providing evidence of their competence. This demands a degree of self-directed learning, with the portfolio being used as a dynamic, flexible, highly individualized document of the learner's development (Timmins and Dunne 2009; Garrett et al. 2013; Green et al. 2014; NMC 2015b).

A number of debates surrounding the use of portfolios have emerged during the past decade. Portfolios have been adopted enthusiastically but with little evidence to support their use and the claims made for them (Timmins and Dunne 2009; Hill 2012). Indeed, their use is contentious at a time when there is still considerable debate about defining what is meant by competence and competency-based assessments (Timmins and Dunne 2009; Green et al. 2014). Assessment of the portfolio has proved to be a challenging aspect, with discussion focusing on frameworks, language used to assess the portfolio, standardization of assessment and formalization of the process (Endacott et al. 2004; Scholes et al. 2004; Byrne et al. 2007; Rossetti et al. 2012). Critics have questioned the rigour of the portfolio as well as the reliability and validity of the assessment process. Supporters of their use claim that they enable students to develop reflective skills and take ownership of their lifelong learning following the social, political and professional imperatives placed upon them; that they facilitate the acquisition of skills and knowledge; that they give insight into competence; and that they provide a means of integrating theory with clinical practice, thus developing a practitioner who is insightful and critically aware and who matures professionally with each experience (Jasper and Fulton 2005; Byrne et al. 2007; Kicken et al. 2009; Garrett et al. 2013; Green et al. 2014). What emerges from the literature is that there is little empirical evidence to support such claims, yet educational and clinical assessment is now based on such a method of assessment (McColgan 2008; Timmins and Dunne 2009; Hill 2012; Green et al. 2014).

ORIGINS AND PURPOSE OF PORTFOLIOS IN NURSING

HISTORICAL DEVELOPMENT

The term *portfolio* is derived from the Italian words *portare*, 'to carry', and *foglio*, 'leaf' or 'sheet', and has come to mean both the folder in which sheets of paper are carried and the papers themselves. The concept of a portfolio was formally introduced into nurse education within the United Kingdom during the early 1990s, first by the Welsh National Board for Nursing (WNB) as part of its continuing educational framework, and shortly after by the English National Board (ENB) as part of its 'Higher Award'. The purpose of the portfolio in relation to these initiatives was predominantly a way of demonstrating prior formal and experiential learning within the Credit Accumulation and Transfer Scheme (CATS) and was generally defined in terms of previous learning. For example, Snadden and Thomas (1998) defined a portfolio, in their discussion of their use in general practice, as 'the collection of evidence that learning has taken place'. This retrospective function of recording prior learning was also emphasized by the United Kingdom Central Council (UKCC) governing body for nursing and midwifery in 1995, when it introduced the portfolio as a means for registered nurses and midwives to demonstrate that they had met the UKCC's requirement for a minimum of 5 days of updating.

Portfolios were initially introduced as a statutory requirement and the UKCC could demand to see them at the point of re-registration. Writing at the time, Hull and Redfern (1996) predicted that portfolios were therefore set to 'become an integral part of professional behaviour', and noted the rapidly increasing market in professionally produced portfolios, many of which were little more than binders (hence emphasizing the definition of a portfolio as the folder in which the documents were kept rather than the documents themselves). However, the statutory requirement for nurses and midwives to keep and submit a portfolio ended when the UKCC was replaced in 2002 by the Nursing and Midwifery Council, and the requirement to submit a portfolio was replaced with a requirement to fill in a form asking for 'a brief description of the CPD [continuing professional development] they have undertaken and its relevance to their work' (Hull et al. 2005). While it was not a statutory requirement practitioners were encouraged to maintain a portfolio to record and reflect on their educational attainments and professional development (NMC 2008, 2009, 2010). However, Hull et al. remained hopeful that the portfolio would continue to be an integral part of professional behaviour and pointed out that 'without a Personal Professional Portfolio with clear records of CPD activities to refer back to, the task would be far more difficult' (Hull et al. 2005, p. 3). Despite the positive gloss given to portfolios, it is difficult to escape the implication here that their primary function is as a retrospective record of educational and professional activity kept primarily for the purpose of remaining on the active register of nurses and midwives. This appears to be the case with the new rules on revalidation published by the NMC (2015b) which require a portfolio of evidence to be kept which details the learning, professional development and progression during the 3 years prior to re-registration. In fact, this retrospective documentary nature of portfolios and features in many definitions describe a portfolio in more or less identical words as the collection of evidence that learning has taken place.

Jasper and Rosser (2013) appear at first to agree with this definition of a portfolio when they write that 'a portfolio, when used in a professional context, is simply a collection of documents that present a picture of the practitioner. It is like a photo album, but in word, not visual, pictures' (p. 146). If this were indeed the case, then the purpose and motivation for keeping a portfolio would be extremely limited. However, Jasper and Rosser (2013) elucidate further by pointing out that portfolios are not just recording devices but are used 'to present a record of the practitioner's professional history and achievements ... they are dynamic in nature and constructed throughout a practitioner's working life' (p. 148). This view is in keeping with earlier work undertaken for the ENB shortly before it was disbanded (Webb et al. 2003). That paper took as its starting point the definition of portfolios offered by McMullan et al. (2003, p. 288) as

a collection of evidence, usually in written form, of both the products and processes of learning. It attests to achievement and personal and professional development, by providing critical analysis of its content.

That definition develops from being merely a collection of evidence for prior learning to including a critical analysis of that content. In other words, it provides the opportunity for *ongoing* learning through critical reflective writing – the concept of a portfolio.

PRINCIPLES FOR PRACTICE

- Portfolios are now recognized as a tool for professional and personal development.
- Portfolios provide opportunities to reflect analytically and write critically.
- Portfolios have re-emerged as means of recording professional development and are a statutory requirement.
- Portfolios must be kept as evidence in order to be revalidated and to register as a nurse within the United Kingdom.

PURPOSE OF THE PORTFOLIO

It is acknowledged that portfolios have an educational and professional purpose which relates to educational progress and professional development. Educational portfolios 'attempt to connect and relate the student's learning experiences to professional practice and competencies', while professional portfolios 'demonstrate continuing learning and professional development' (Hill 2012). Jasper and Rosser (2013) also draw the distinction between student portfolios driven by assessment and the professional portfolio demonstrating competence, fitness to practice and ongoing development learning. However, in whichever sphere the portfolio is used the roles seem to be broadly similar. Portfolios have several roles to play in pre- and post-registration education and development. First, they resonate with the aims of adult education insofar as they promote self-directed learning from previous experience of real-life problems. Portfolios are a means of integrating theory and practice in order to facilitate practice development. The development and maintenance of a portfolio can facilitate the development of reflective learning skills which enable the practitioner to learn strategies, attitudes and cognitive processes essential for clinical practice (Neades 2003; Hill 2012; Garret et al. 2013; Green et al. 2014; NMC 2015b). Students are active and engaged in their learning process so that they take ownership of the portfolio, organizing and directing its content so that it is individual and pertinent to the student's clinical practice (Hill 2012; Garrett et al. 2013; Green et al. 2014).

Clearly, these issues which portfolios are seen to address are also issues of concern to *all* qualified nurses, regardless of whether they are formally enrolled in an educational course. Thus although portfolios have a role to play at all stages of a student's progression through a course of study and can be used variously as a means of gaining access to a course or being exempted from some elements of it, as a tool for learning and as a means of assessment, they are also arguably of benefit to all registered nurses, not only as a record of their continuing professional development (CPD), but more importantly as an ongoing part of it. Thus the value of the portfolio lies in the nature of the process, rather than the end product per se (Webb et al. 2003).

This shift in the focus and purpose of portfolios has not been without difficulties. Assessment of pre- and post-registration nursing courses has traditionally been undertaken through prescriptive and highly structured written assignments, and the shift to a portfolio-based system has demanded far greater autonomy and accountability from nurses and students, who are expected to play a leading role in identifying their own learning needs and outcomes as well as self-assessing their development in relation to the objectives or competencies set by the course or regulatory body (Knowles 1990; Endacott et al. 2004; Scholes et al. 2004; Joyce 2005; Rossetti et al. 2012). This in turn should provide the foundations for lifelong learning and continued use of the portfolio to demonstrate development in a number of personal and professional areas (Endacott et al. 2004; Jasper and Rosser 2013; Green et al. 2014; NMC 2015b).

Portfolios are seen as an authentic form of assessment which clearly demonstrates the skills and capabilities of the nurse. It is suggested that portfolios foster a culture of evidence in that the nurse will ascertain the best evidence to underpin practice (NMC 2015b). Portfolio use is increasing in pre-registration undergraduate programmes of nursing as a means to assess learning and achievement of competencies. The portfolio provides a means to assess the student's ability to set their own goals and think critically about their individual experiences to enable new knowledge to be synthesized (Rossetti et al. 2012; Green et al. 2014). Assessment can focus not just on the factual knowledge gained but also on cognitive and affective skills, self-evaluation, peer assessment and reflection, making them student centred (Green et al. 2014).

Rossetti et al. (2012) also suggest that portfolios facilitate the closing of the assessment loop by enabling the teacher to assess the student's learning and progression and in doing so gain insight into whether the education provided is robust and educationally sound. Rossetti et al. (2012) discuss the detailed processes by which the student portfolio is assessed and educational input is evaluated. The practice involves the use of expert assessors who scrutinize a number of areas in the portfolio before feedback to the educators is provided, which discusses the rigour of the programme and its ability to meet the students' learning needs. Thus not only is the programme and teaching assessed, but also the assessment process itself is scrutinized to ensure it is robust (Green et al. 2014).

At the post-registration level portfolios are assuming a greater role in work-based learning and more particularly as part of the revalidation process (NMC 2015b). Revalidation is primarily concerned with promoting good practice. It allows for greater engagement on the part of the registrant in maintaining this, but also facilitates employer engagement by increasing awareness of the NMC's roles and standards and encourages early discussion of concerns raised about an individual's practice. This is to be achieved through the maintenance of a portfolio which contains the requisite information which needs to be verified by a confirmer for revalidation to occur (NMC 2015b). Revalidation will be closely aligned with the employer's professional review.

The guidance while prescriptive is clearly aligned to the Professional Development Review (PDR) or annual appraisal; thus the developmental aspects of the portfolio and its maintenance are inherent in the process. The guidance has evolved to account for this aspect. However, care needs to be taken that the portfolio does not become little more than a collection of incidents and artefacts or descriptions of events and the learning which occurred. It would appear that the vital reflective component highlighted by many writers needs to be emphasized strongly and the requirement to demonstrate the use of underpinning knowledge through reflective writing is apparent. A portfolio that adheres solely to the NMC guidelines and which is not linked to the PDR may not develop in such a way as to demonstrate a progression and maturation of learning and an appreciation of the nuances of practice, which is its primary aim (Bowers and Jinks 2004; Joyce 2005; Jasper and Rosser 2013; NMC 2015b). Thus it is anticipated that portfolios will vary significantly and substantially in quality between practitioners, where some will demonstrate reflective practice and others merely describe incidents, resulting in potential discrepancies and variations in the standard of knowledge acquisition and utilization by registered nurses. While there is a prescribed layout there are no such guidelines for assessing the quality of the portfolio. It also requires confirmers to be cognizant with portfolios, reflective practice and the principles of assessment. This in turn may lead to variations in the quality of the assessment dependent on the confirmer's expertise (Hill 2012; Green et al. 2014).

PRINCIPLES FOR PRACTICE

- Portfolios allow the practitioner to learn from experience.
- Portfolios 'recognize' the individual nature of the learner/practitioner's experience and have the flexibility to reflect this in their construction.
- Portfolios demonstrate lifelong learning.
- Portfolios are an integral part of the revalidation process.

PORTFOLIO CONSTRUCTION

REFLECTION POINTS

- Do you keep a portfolio?
- What is in the portfolio?
- How is it arranged?
- What criteria did you use to organize your portfolio?

Clearly, the purpose for which the portfolio is kept will have an influence on the way that it is structured. If the portfolio is seen merely as a way of recording learning, and if there is no requirement to reflect on or integrate that learning, then there is a danger of producing a 'shopping trolley' or 'toast rack' portfolio rather than a 'spinal column' or 'cake mix' (Endacott et al. 2004), as set out in Box 15.1. This can give rise to tension and confusion in relation to structure. At the pre-registration level portfolios may follow a structured set of guidelines specifying content and layout, e.g. competencies and reflective accounts. Post-registration the portfolio is designed to be increasingly flexible, individual and creative, and thus no particular structure is prescribed. The nurse is free to design the portfolio to meet his or her own professional needs and experiences (Jasper and Rosser 2013; NMC 2015b), but with this freedom comes a number of problems.

First, many nurses may have previously been assessed traditionally through structured essays and may be novices in portfolio construction. Although being capable of studying, thinking and practicing at the post-registration or master's level, they may struggle to produce the requisite cake mix portfolio, which demands well-developed self-directed learning skills, including the ability to diagnose their learning needs in light of performance standards, formulate meaningful goals, diagnose and monitor their own performance, and identify resources and learning strategies appropriate to the competency and knowledge required (Kicken et al. 2009; Green et al. 2014).

Second, some nurses may have great difficulty in fulfilling the requirement to determine the structure and content of their portfolios. The lack of structure becomes frustrating and disorienting as nurses struggle to find direction (Bowers and Jinks 2004). The portfolio must have some structure or framework in order to understand what is to be assessed, and Kicken et al. (2009) point out that if the nurse does not know what knowledge they lack, then it is difficult to identify what needs to be known. Conversely, if the structure of the portfolio is too prescriptive it may cause negativity in the nurse, who may feel it to be restrictive and stifling of creativity (Nairn et al. 2006; Hill 2012). In addition, there is a danger that the portfolio could be assessment driven and focus on the submission of work by specified deadlines; i.e. it could become product rather than process led, in which case the richness and potency of the portfolio as a developmental learning tool may be lost (Scholes et al. 2004; Joyce 2005; Hill 2012). It may be argued that the portfolio then becomes

BOX 15.1: Portfolio models

- Shopping trolley – collection of items
    - Repository of artefacts
    - Chosen by student
    - Little attempt to link evidence to outcomes/competencies
    - Reflective accounts stand alone

- Toast rack
    - Discrete elements assessing theory and practice
    - Placed into separate sections of a binder, e.g. skills log, competencies and reflective accounts
    - Reflective accounts stand alone, not integrated with other elements
    - Different people participate in the assessment

- Spinal column
    - Structured around practice competencies/learning outcomes
    - Evidence slotted in to demonstrate each competency
    - Reflective accounts consider more than one competency
    - Explicit evidence of learning and competence
    - Multiple pieces of evidence for overarching competencies
    - Emphasis on original work

- Cake mix
    - Evidence from theory and practice integrated into portfolio
    - Overarching narrative
    - Reflective commentary
    - Demonstrates critical and analytical skills
    - Reflectivity, practice and professional development are features

Source: Endacott, R., et al., *Nurse Education in Practice*, 4, 250–7, 2004.

an intellectual exercise geared more toward prescribed activities rather than facilitating a critical analysis of practice. This may result in a loss of identity and ownership of the portfolio as it is tailored to suit the needs of the course and practice assessor rather than those of the writer (Endacott et al. 2004; Scholes et al. 2004; Hall 2012; Rossetti et al. 2012; Green 2014).

The available evidence tends to support these concerns. Nairn et al. (2006) in their study of final-year student nurses found they were unsure about the structure and purpose of the portfolio and were less optimistic about its use than first-year students. They were also sceptical about its importance as an aid to communicate learning, but felt that it did provide a cathartic function by enabling feelings and difficult experiences to be explored (Nairn et al. 2006; Williams et al. 2008). Ongoing support and guidance is required to facilitate the development of the portfolio and reflective and critical thinking skills. However, such support and guidance should not be at the cost of relevance, creativity, personal identity and ownership (Endacott et al. 2004; Jasper 2005, 2013; Nairn et al. 2006; Rossetti et al. 2012; Green et al. 2014). While these studies focus on pre-registration students, the arguments can be extrapolated to post-registration children's nurses who are compiling portfolios either as part of a formal course or to provide evidence to ensure they are revalidated and are able to remain a registrant (NMC 2015a, 2015b).

PRINCIPLES FOR PRACTICE

- Portfolios do not have a prescribed structure; thus support may be needed to construct one.
- Portfolios follow one of four models; the cake mix portfolio is the hallmark of an analytical, critical learner/practitioner.

CONTROVERSIES IN PORTFOLIO DEVELOPMENT

It can be seen that although portfolio writing can be a powerful method of facilitating reflection, analyzing practice and recording learning, it is not without its critics. Several writers have raised concerns about the usefulness of portfolios as a means both to develop practice and to assess and evaluate educational or practice developments. Portfolios are used not only to identify and record *theoretical* learning but also as a means of critically evaluating and assessing *clinical* competence. A number of reasons are identified as to why the educational assessment of clinical competence in pre- and post-registration nursing is 'inherently problematic', and many of the concerns apply equally to situations in which the portfolio is being used primarily as a 'reflective diary' for personal CPD reasons (Gannon et al. 2001; Green et al. 2012).

One issue is the lack of standardization with regard to portfolios as well as a number of disagreements about the structure, content and purpose of portfolios (which has already been discussed). Another issue which is particularly problematic is whether the portfolio is primarily a developmental tool (formative), an assessment tool (summative) or both; this question lies at the root of a number of fundamental concerns about the use of portfolios, particularly in relation to honesty and confidentiality (Gerrish 1993; Gannon et al. 2001; Hill 2012; Green et al. 2014).

HONESTY

REFLECTION POINTS

- Are you truly honest in your reflective writing?
- Do you write for yourself (privately) or with an audience in mind (publicly)?
- Think about your answers and the impact on your learning and clinical practice.

It may be argued that if nurses do not write about practice in an insightful, incisive manner, then children and young people's nursing practice specifically and nursing practice generally will not develop in an innovative, dynamic way. Children and young people's nurses need to scrutinize what they do in order to identify innovative practice personally and on a wider professional level to ensure their own CPD, career progression and the development of services and care delivery to the most vulnerable members of society – children and young people (Storey and Haigh 2002; Department of Health 2004a; Welsh Assembly Government 2009; NMC 2015b).

This requires honesty and the confidence to confront those elements of practice and knowledge deficits which make practitioners feel uncomfortable. While positive incidents do facilitate learning, it is often the 'negative' events which provide the richest learning experience and the opportunity to reflect at a deeper level (McMullan 2006). Children's nursing practitioners may begin to question their values and beliefs concerning children's nursing when events or actions appear to conflict with those values. Thus such scrutiny may result in a changed perspective and the development of new practice and new ways of using knowledge.

If the purpose of the portfolio is primarily as a personal means for the writer to explore his or her own practice through a process of critical reflection, then an honest examination of practice is relatively unproblematic. In other words, if the practitioner is writing solely for his or her own benefit and no other eyes are likely to see the contents of the portfolio, then the writer will have no cause to elaborate or fabricate what is being recorded and reflected on. However, in cases where the portfolio is used for assessment purposes, students may feel threatened about expressing their innermost thoughts and feelings and be reluctant and uncertain about engaging in self-reflection, in some cases feeling that the portfolio is an 'invasion of privacy' (McMullan 2006; Byrne et al. 2007; Green et al. 2014). Thus they write for a perceived audience, the assessor, according to their perception of what they think the assessor should read (Scholes et al. 2004; McMullan 2006; Byrne et al. 2007). As Gannon et al. (2001, p. 356) point out:

> there may be an inverse relationship between the use of portfolios in the assessment process and the honesty of the records which the keeper of the portfolio may maintain.

In other words, the pressure on a student to pass a portfolio-based assignment might well compromise the honesty of the account – a point reiterated by Green et al. (2014), who also point out that the portfolio becomes assessment rather than developmentally driven, thus reducing authenticity and the educational value of the learning activity.

McMullan (2006) found that students expressed this concern that they could not be truly honest and critical in their writing if anyone in authority or power was likely to see the portfolio. This creates a paradox. The portfolio is a means to develop knowledge and practice that requires honesty with oneself, but as an assessment and learning tool it also requires facilitation by a mentor. However, the very fact that the mentor is also a tutor and assessor places them in a position of authority and power, which in turn leads the student to censor their own writing in order to avoid criticism and the exposure of practices and private thoughts (Gannon et al. 2001; Dolan et al. 2004; McMullan 2006; Timmins and Dunne 2009; Green et al. 2014).

This may have significant implications for registered nurses who are undergoing the revalidation process, who while happy to discuss their PDR may not be so comfortable reflecting or allowing access to personal information with a confirmer who may be their manager. This is a prime example of where a person in authority has access to private thoughts which may not be authentic because the registrant may feel the need to write for their audience, potentially fearful of being honest as it may result in repercussions. In order to achieve honesty the relationship between confirmer and registrant should be trusting, mutually respectful and supportive. This will ensure that the revalidation process and the development of the nurse is authentic.

PRINCIPLES FOR PRACTICE

- Portfolios enable the practitioner to illuminate practice and should be honest in their analysis.
- Avoid writing for an audience – write for yourself.

CONFIDENTIALITY

REFLECTION POINTS

- Who has access to your portfolio?
- Where is the information stored?
- How do you ensure the confidentiality of your portfolio?

One possible solution to this problem is to offer the writer a promise of confidentiality by restricting the readership of the portfolio to a few selected internal markers. If writers are not assured of confidentiality regarding the portfolio's contents, then it becomes flawed as an assessment tool (Dolan et al. 2004;

McMullan 2006; Green et al. 2014). Summative assessment could lead to a reduced sense of ownership and compromise its use as a developmental tool. We have seen that the knowledge that the work will be viewed by a number of assessors can stifle thinking and writing as the author begins to analyze which information should be disclosed to specific people and which remains hidden from scrutiny. The spectre of censorship is apparent at this juncture. Censorship leads to impoverished reflective writing as key elements are omitted for fear of exposing poor practice and other ethical concerns. However, although a confidential approach might perhaps increase the likelihood of an honest account, Johns (1999) pointed out that, even when writing for no one's eyes except our own, there is a still a (sometimes subconscious) tendency to elaborate on or refrain from the truth in order to protect our own self-esteem.

However, the issue of confidentiality has to be considered not only from the writer's perspective but also from that of the people being written about (Green et al. 2014). The NMC Code of Conduct (2015a, Section 5) states:

> As a nurse or midwife, you owe duty of confidentiality to all those who are receiving care ... you must respect a person's right to privacy in all aspects of their care.

It may be argued that the use of reflective writing and its presentation within the portfolio compromises this standard as soon as the portfolio is submitted for examination or scrutiny by a third party. Despite making material anonymous, patient information and that of working colleagues is presented for assessment without their knowledge or consent. Such issues need to be addressed in order to maintain the integrity of working relationships with colleagues and patients, who should retain consent over the disclosure of information involving their practice, particularly where poor practice is highlighted (Timmins and Dunne 2009). The evidence shows that practitioners are reluctant to disclose or write about poor practice, preferring to reflect on positive incidents of care. Thus practitioners have to consider carefully what they are prepared to make public and what they wish to keep private (Bowers and Jinks 2004; Endacott et al. 2004; Joyce 2005).

The world of children's nursing is small and confined, and therefore incidents, locations and patients themselves may be easily recognizable despite the best attempts to conceal identities. As a result, the practitioner is presented with a conundrum: they need to reflect to learn from the incident, a private activity; yet they are also expected to produce written reflections to demonstrate learning and the development of practice, a public activity. This could lead to the development of parallel portfolios to avoid compromising confidentiality, and in turn result in two separate arenas of learning. 'Real' learning could be restricted to the private portfolio, whereas the public portfolio might result in 'public learning' led by the assessment process, which then becomes an intellectual activity rather than a scrutiny of the key personal and practice-led issues (Scholes et al. 2004; Nairn et al. 2006; Green et al. 2014).

PRINCIPLES FOR PRACTICE

- Confidentiality must be maintained and must not be compromised in the reflective writing.
- Access to the portfolio must be controlled by the learner.

STAKEHOLDER INTEREST AND CONTROL OF LEARNING THROUGH PORTFOLIO USE

REFLECTION POINTS

- Who or what shapes your learning – your needs, the patient's needs, the organization's needs?
- Is this reflected in your portfolio?

We have seen that portfolios should be personal and concerned with the personal learning which the children's nurse needs to undertake. However, there is an issue of social control and monitoring of learning by the stakeholder who funds the CPD. Nurses are under an obligation to constantly refine their developmental learning, critical thinking and delivery of care commensurate with their experience and level of expertise (NMC 2015a, 2015b). However, as the NHS evolves, nurses may find themselves undertaking education and training which is shaped by the organization rather than their own professional needs and the needs of the children and families in their care. The learning may be shaped by the need to revalidate and be confirmed in order to continue as a registrant, local organizational policy and the need to standardize roles, particularly at advanced levels (Bowers and Jinks 2004; Department of Health 2008a; Welsh Assembly Government 2009; NMC 2015b). The document *A High Quality Workforce* (Department of Health 2008b) sets out to improve access to funding for education to support diverse educational experiences designed to promote CPD. It has been suggested that nurses now have the opportunity to hold their employers accountable if they do not deliver or invest in their education (Tweddell 2008). This demands a strong personal and political voice as well as a sense of 'personal advocacy' that continued professional and personal development will have an impact on the delivery of care.

However, this can be a reciprocal arrangement, with employers also holding staff accountable to ensure that learning is occurring and practice is being enhanced. Indeed, the PDR or annual appraisal which incorporates key performance indicators, personal objectives, assessment of development, or the Knowledge and Skill Framework (KSF) (Department of Health 2004b) proposes to do exactly this via personal reviews which assess how an individual applies his or her knowledge and skills in practice (see below). The portfolio may be used as a means to assess and monitor this learning from both the employee's and employer's perspective. If the funding is provided, then the employer may feel obliged to ensure 'value for money', monitoring the quality of the learning and development by accessing the portfolio, especially if the educational programme is provided in-house. This would replicate to some degree what currently happens within educational settings, where the mentor, facilitator or lecturer accesses and assesses the portfolio for the learning which has occurred, with its inherent problems concerning confidentiality, honesty and other ethical issues (Garrett and Jackson 2006; Garrett et al. 2013; Green et al. 2014).

Indeed, it could be argued that such a use of portfolios may be seen as a means by which to monitor practice and the quality of the care delivered. If we postulate that nursing care, nursing practice and competence are to be based on a robust and rigorous evidence base, then it is logical that the employer will require evidence that this is occurring on a personal as well as a collegiate level. This would seem to suggest social control of learning, which is an insidious process that would stifle the creativity and dynamism inherent in children's nursing practice. It would also stifle the creativity and diversity to be found in the personal portfolio (Bowers and Jinks 2004; Endacott et al. 2004; Byrne et al. 2007; Jasper and Mooney 2013; Jasper and Rosser 2013).

Conversely, the portfolio may be used to demonstrate career development, critical thinking skills, evidence-based practice and professional maturity at the annual professional review. The KSF underpins Agenda for Change and, as the Department of Health (2004b) notes,

> defines and describes the knowledge and skills which NHS staff need to apply in their work in order to deliver quality services. It provides a single, consistent, comprehensive and explicit framework on which to base review and development for all staff. (Section 1.1, p. 3)

The KSF, which is incorporated into the annual appraisal or PDR, aims to facilitate the development of services which meet the needs of the public through investing in staff development. This is to be achieved by supporting individual members of staff and teams to learn and develop throughout their careers so that they can work effectively. The KSF states that all staff should have access to the same structured opportunities for learning, development and review (Department of Health 2004b). It is a broad, generic framework which focuses on the application of knowledge and skills to practice; it does not articulate the specific knowledge or skills that are required to undertake the role. It proposes that specific standards and competencies would need to be developed. The review process focuses on how the individual applies his or her knowledge and skills to their post, developing a personal development plan, engaging in learning and development, and evaluating and reflecting on the application of the learning to practice (Department of Health 2004b). The KSF sets gateways for development and career progression. Thus the use of the portfolio in the PDR or appraisal is invaluable within this situation in which individual learning and development can be clearly shown and in which the maturation of the professional over time could be demonstrated to support their career aspirations and role development. This is particularly effective within the current economic climate, when financially it may not be practical to release staff from busy units onto 'expensive' courses. The portfolio is a vehicle by which children and young people's nurses can demonstrate their professional learning and development not only to satisfy the requirements for ongoing registration but also to illustrate the completion of their developmental objectives at their professional review as part of their ongoing career development (NMC 2015b). This is also beneficial to the employer, who can verify whether nurses are developing appropriately and whether their investment in educating staff is returned. The KSF focuses on what is done rather than on what staff know and can bring to the role personally. The caveat to this should be that there must be a holistic approach to the delivery of care and professional development and not one based solely on the acquisition of skills and competencies. This would lead to a reductionist approach at a time when children and young people's nursing and nursing generally are striving to exhibit a holistic approach to service development and care delivery to children and families (Storey and Haigh 2002). The revalidation process can go some way toward ensuring a more holistic approach as the evidence required includes reflection, participatory learning and discussions about clinical practice, all of which can be tailored and focused onto the specific skills, knowledge, practices and nursing care of children, young people and their families (NMC 2015b).

PRINCIPLES FOR PRACTICE

- Portfolios can be used to demonstrate current and future learning needs and the impact on practice and care delivery.
- Portfolios demonstrate evidence of ongoing CPD to the employer, mentor, tutor and NMC.
- Portfolios can demonstrate competence and progression of learning, knowledge and skills to meet requirements of the KSF.

VALIDITY AND RELIABILITY

Despite the increasingly central role of the portfolio in education and practice the issues and debates concerning reliability and validity recur and have yet to be resolved. These issues constitute a threat particularly when portfolios are being used as a method of course assessment (Gannon et al. 2001; Hill 2012; Green et al. 2014). Hill suggests that if the portfolio is to be used as in summative evaluation, then further quantitative and qualitative work is required around its validity. Currently there is a lack of evidence supporting its use as a summative evaluation tool (Hill 2012).

The question of the validity and reliability of portfolios, and thus of their use and utility, is to some extent dependent on how we define a portfolio. If a portfolio is seen purely as a collection of factual information and evidence, then it is a fairly straightforward process to establish its validity and reliability through the use of a set standardized criteria. However, measuring the extent to which learning and reflection has taken place is rather more complex and complicated. Green et al. (2014) point out that portfolios favour those with developed writing and reflective skills. Thus they ask, 'What is being assessed?' It can be suggested that on a purely factual analysis the portfolio may be assessed for writing skills, reflective ability and data collection skills using a rubric. Nevertheless these skills plus the writer's growth and development are highly individual and may defy assessment using standardized criteria. It can also be suggested that the use of the portfolio as a summative assessment tool contradicts its ethos. In short, if it is claimed that the portfolio is about individual growth and development, then the use of a standardized criterion contradicts the individualism promoted by the portfolio.

However, it also depends on what is understood by validity and reliability in the context of portfolio assessment (Gannon et al. 2001; Webb et al. 2003; Green et al. 2014). Quantitative definitions from nursing research have been used which although a method of assessment 'proven to be reliable and valid in the traditional, numerical sense' (Polit and Beck 2014) might not be valued by those from the qualitative tradition. Hill (2012) discusses the development of evaluation tools to address the concerns of validity and reliability. She discusses the tools and how quantitative data do provide credence to the portfolio. However, the portfolio assessment requires trained assessors who have attended a specific, intensive orientation programme and also have 3 years experience with a mentor. She suggests this ensures that there is consistency in the assessors' approaches and judgments. Rossetti et al. (2012) outline similar practices in their work on portfolios. Although questions must revolve around practicality and the exclusive and elitist nature of the assessment process, it may be argued that this is also a strength as the small number of assessors increase inter-marker reliability and consistency. Qualitative approaches, when applied to the assessment of portfolios, translate into the need for a wide variety of sources and types of evidence that learning has taken place, a clear criterion for what constitutes a pass at different academic levels, and the need for consensus based on 'tripartite meetings' between the student, representatives from practice and representatives from the academic setting (Hill 2012; Green et al. 2014).

However, when portfolios are used as a means of informal continual professional or practice development, or even when they are used as a formative rather than a summative course assignment, the issues are somewhat different. For example, if the purpose of the portfolio is exclusively as a tool for enhancing personal learning from and for practice, then issues about internal and external generalizability or transferability are no longer of concern, along with the debate about who has a right or an obligation to view the portfolio. Furthermore, questions of credibility, dependability and confirmability, which all relate to whether 'data sources are identified and described accurately' (Webb et al. 2003), take on a somewhat different complexion. It may be argued, for example, that as much self-discovery and exploration of practice can occur through writing an account of a fictional event than from something that actually happened (see, for example, Rolfe 2005). The question to be asked of a portfolio kept for personal developmental reasons might be 'what has been learned from this writing?' rather than 'how can we ensure the validity and reliability of the portfolio entries?' Once the focus shifts from the *content* of the portfolio to the *process* of writing it, then we could reasonably argue that the only person capable of providing an answer to the question is the writer himself or herself, and it must be done with honesty.

Further work is therefore required if portfolio use is to be appropriate and ultimately useful in practitioners' development. Portfolio use requires further research if its future is to be assured (McMullan 2006; Timmins and Dunne 2009; Hill 2012; Green et al. 2014).

KEY POINTS

- Validity and reliability are recurring issues in assessing the portfolio quality.
- Quantitative assessment of validity and reliability may not be appropriate.
- Qualitative measures may be more appropriate as they capture the richness of the portfolio entries.

MOVING FORWARD: USE OF PORTFOLIOS IN CHILDREN'S NURSING

We have seen that there are a number of issues that still need to be addressed in relation to the use of portfolios in nursing generally, and children and young people's nursing in particular. However, we have also suggested that portfolios can be a very powerful means of developing the learning and practice of individual nurses and the profession in general. We will now turn our attention to some of the positive uses of portfolios and explore some recent innovations in portfolio development.

There is a shortage of literature relating to the use of portfolios in children and young people's nursing. The available research relates very generally to nursing across all fields of practice, and thus principles have to be extrapolated in order to illuminate their use within children and young people's nursing practice and education. The claims made for portfolios relate to the demonstration of personal knowledge, developmental learning and competence which can be related directly to the development of practice, knowledge and critical thinking within children's nursing. Children and young people's nursing has its own specific body of knowledge and competencies associated with caring for a diverse group of children, young people and families from birth to 18 years of age and up to the early 20s (Casey 1993; NMC 2004; Children and Young People's Health Outcomes Forum 2012; Royal College of Nursing [RCN] 2012b, 2013). As identified throughout this book, children and young people's nursing covers a vast range of care situations, from caring for the well child in the community (school nurses and health visitors), to sick children with complex needs who require continuing care at home or in hospice settings, to acutely ill children cared for in the community, to the sick child and young person requiring acute care within the diverse settings in hospital (Casey 1993; Department of Health 2004a; Welsh Assembly Government 2005; Smith and Coleman 2010). Children and young people's nurses, like all nurses, have a professional obligation to remain updated, to develop practice and to develop critical thinking skills to analyze the evidence upon which care is based (Welsh Assembly Government 2004; NMC 2015a, 2015b). The portfolio enables the practitioner to demonstrate the specific knowledge, skills and attitudes required to work with children and young people in diverse settings while engaging in reflective practice to maintain learning, develop insight and promote the development of the practice of children and young people's nursing (Welsh Assembly Government 2004; RCN 2012b, 2013; NMC 2015b).

PORTFOLIOS AND CAREER DEVELOPMENT

REFLECTION POINTS

- Think about your career – Where do you see yourself in 5 years time?
- How will you demonstrate your competence to follow that career pathway?
- Will you collect evidence or use a portfolio (effectively) with reflective writing to demonstrate progression of learning, thinking and suitability for the career pathway?

Accessing specific child-oriented courses may be difficult for many reasons. The number of specific courses may be limited and based away from the workplace at a centre of learning, requiring prolonged periods of time away from practice, thus depleting staffing numbers. Because of the specialist nature of practice and the requirement for children and young people's nurses to hold specific qualifications (Department of Health 1991; RCN 2003; NMC 2004, 2010) arranging cover may be difficult, despite the NMC's requirement that all graduate nurses should be able to meet the essential needs of all client groups (NMC 2010). Ultimately, children and young people have a right to access and be nursed by appropriately qualified children and young people's nurses, but there is concern if the only courses available to them are generic in nature. It is at this point that the portfolio proves invaluable as a tool to demonstrate the specific knowledge and practice focus that children and young people's nurses possess. The portfolio enables children's nurses to structure their learning either formally (course led) or as part of their CPD requirements for revalidation and registration purposes, and to illustrate clearly the development of their practice and the application of children and young people's nursing knowledge to children and young people's practice (Welsh Assembly Government 2004; NMC 2015a, 2015b). The portfolio allows flexibility to meet the demands of the children and young people's nurses' situation academically and professionally. This flexibility meets the needs of practitioners working within diverse areas and allows for the portfolio to be eclectic in nature to reflect the often complex multidisciplinary care situations that children's nurses work in. It enables children and young people's nurses to explore their own professional values and ethics when working with children, young people and their families, and also enables them to explore issues such as multidisciplinarity, which requires integrated working, collegiate relationships and a deep appreciation of all practitioner roles, which implies that professional boundaries need to be flexible and open (Department of Health 2004a, 2004b; Welsh Assembly Government 2005; NMC 2015a, 2015b).

This also has implications for the career development of children and young people's nurses. The *Post Registration Career Framework for Nurses in Wales* (Welsh Assembly Government 2009) and *Towards a Framework for Post-Registration Nursing Careers* (Department of Health 2008a) have specified the need for distinct career pathways through which nurses may progress. This will require educational initiatives to meet the demands of the children and young people's nurses as they progress through the levels and create career pathways commensurate with their professional reviews. This is an optimum time to engage with portfolios to demonstrate development of learning, competency and critical thinking as each children and young people's nurse meets the personal objectives set within the review (Department of Health 2004b, 2008a; Welsh Assembly Government 2005, 2009; Jasper and Mooney 2013). The frameworks demand that educational opportunities are provided and that these initiatives are flexible enough to meet the ever-changing healthcare situation. The individual practitioner's aspirations must also be accounted for within these initiatives, as some may wish to remain generalist children and young people's nurses while others may progress toward specialist areas and then on to advanced practice and beyond (Department of Health 2004b, 2008a; Welsh Assembly Government 2009). The frameworks, if implemented, clearly steer the development of a focused and robust career pathway within children and young people's nursing. Thus education must be flexible and rigorous enough to meet the practitioners' needs (Centre for the Development of Health Care Policy and Practice 2008). This is particularly pertinent at a time when children and young people's nurses are developing their expertise as they progress toward specialist and advanced nursing roles. The portfolio can clearly demonstrate the acquisition of new knowledge and new skills which are specific to children and young people's nursing. This is accompanied by charting both professional and personal development as the practitioner demonstrates their ability to meet the core competencies of the roles.

Portfolios are an excellent medium for children and young people's nurses to develop their critical thinking and competencies and to engage in reflective writing to consolidate and demonstrate their learning and development. They provide the perfect way to illustrate and talk about the specific and specialist knowledge and competencies required to work with children, young people and families. They also provide a way to explore the care of children and young people with whom the children and young people's nurse may have had little previous experience. For example, this is pertinent to the care of children and young people with mental health problems who are encountered in settings and via routes not traditionally associated with mental health problems (Department for Children, Schools and Families and Department of Health 2008, 2009, 2010; RCN 2014a, 2014b). Nurses are reluctant to engage with these children and young people as they feel they lack knowledge to underpin practice, confidence and skills (as discussed in previous chapters). They feel overwhelmed by the number and complexity of problems of the children and young people they care for (Wilson et al. 2007; Buckley 2010; RCN 2014a, 2014b). The portfolio is perfect for detailing the learning journey at this point. It provides a flexible medium for practitioners to acquire knowledge and to reflect on their personal issues and professional responsibilities, while exploring the wider clinical perspective in relation to multidisciplinary liaison and working practices. Thus the portfolio provides an excellent opportunity for personal learning objectives and opportunities to be identified and for the children and young people's nurse to study, reflect and develop competency in the care of this client group (Department for Children, Schools and Families and Department of Health 2008; Department of Health 2009; Welsh Assembly Government 2009; NMC 2015b).

The portfolio should demonstrate a maturity in its composition as the nurse's career progresses and his or her learning matures. The presentation of the portfolio should mirror this progression, providing an authentic evaluation of the personal and professional domains of practice until, at the advanced practitioner level, the cake mix model is evident and the criteria for assessment are clearly mapped to enable the clarity and maturity of thinking and practice to be apparent (Jasper and Fulton 2005; Hill 2012; Garrett et al. 2013; Jasper and Rosser 2013; Green et al. 2014).

PRINCIPLES FOR PRACTICE

- Portfolios can be used by children and young people's nurses to map and support their career development in their chosen specialty.
- Portfolios can enable children and young people's nurses to reflect on and analyze their practice in relation to children and young people with whom they have limited experience.
- Portfolios can be used to articulate the special and specific knowledge required by children and young people's nurses.

REFLECTION POINTS

- Is the portfolio a tool for learning or can it be used in a wider context to discuss nursing issues?
- What is happening politically in your field of practice?
- Could the use of a portfolio be beneficial in demonstrating your area of expertise?

Politically, the portfolio provides a voice for children and young people's nursing to demonstrate the value and importance of its special and specific domain of practice and the rights of the child and family to be cared for by appropriately educated, knowledgeable, skilled professional children and young people's nurses. Despite copious reports and recommendations spanning 50 years which state this point succinctly, the generalist agenda remains a threat (Ministry of Health 1959; Department of Health 1991, 2004a, 2008a; Davies 2008, 2010). The NMC (2009) reviewed and held a consultation on the pre-registration nursing education programme, curriculum and competencies following the publication of policy which highlighted the rapidly changing delivery of healthcare and the requirement for nursing to meet these challenges (Department of Health 2004a, 2006, 2008b; Welsh Assembly Government 2009). This consultation has resulted in the publication of the *Standards for Pre-Registration Nursing Education* (NMC 2010). The ethos of the standards is that all nurses should possess generic and specific competencies so that all nurses have some skills in caring for the essential needs of all client groups (NMC 2010). This is reiterated by the Shape of Caring Review (RCN 2012a, Health Education England 2015), which discusses the need for a nurse who is flexible and can deliver person-centred care within a range of settings. An overview of educational progression is presented which suggests that the current curriculum be replaced with 2 years of whole person core training and 1 year of field-specific education. This would be followed by a year of preceptorship within the specific field of nursing (Health Education England 2015). This has serious consequences for the care of children, young people and their families who may be cared for by nurses who are less skilled and competent in delivering the specific nursing care they require because of the focus on generic skills across a range of settings. Such an approach fails to recognize that children and young people require specific care delivered by children and young people's nurses who hold the requisite skills and knowledge to ensure high-quality, safe and effective care is a priority.

It may be argued that this represents a poorly disguised move toward genericism which children and young people's nurses must resist. Certainly, economically and managerially, a generically competent workforce is cheaper, flexible and more easily moved around hospital settings to cover staff shortfalls. However, this can be refuted on the grounds that it is not safe, and that it conflicts with the ethos of children and young people's nursing and the right to access appropriate and safe healthcare. More importantly, it contravenes the rights of children and young people to be valued as a specific and special client group (Department of Health 2004a; Welsh Assembly Government 2005; RCN 2012b). Subsequently it is not safe or effective to disband children and young people's nursing as a specialist field, and research is available to demonstrate that children's nurses are cost-effective and that when children and young people are nursed by appropriately qualified nurses, the clinical outcomes are better and the hospital stay shorter (Welsh Assembly Government 2005; Department of Health 2004a; RCN 2012b, 2013). This is also true of other clinical situations in which experienced qualified children and young people's nurses have a direct impact on the quality of care and recovery of the children, e.g. community children's nursing (Royal College of Nursing and Children's Community Nursing Forum 2000).

Portfolios can offer a voice for children and young people's nurses to resist the dangerous rise of genericism both personally and professionally. The personal portfolio can be used as a vehicle to demonstrate not only personal learning and development but also the political and interdisciplinary issues affecting the delivery of care to children, young people and their families (Jasper and Mooney 2013; Jasper and Rosser 2013; Byrne et al. 2007). Professionally, the portfolio can again be used to demonstrate the need for specialist nurses to care for this special group of patients and can be done using personal and departmental portfolios. This is applicable for all levels of children and young people's nurses but can be particularly effective in developing the critical thinking and integration of research and practice at the advanced practice level. Portfolios could highlight areas for scholarly discussion, resulting in research, policy production and publication (Welsh Assembly Government 2004; Rassin et al. 2006; Jasper and Mooney 2013; Jasper and Rosser 2013).

PRINCIPLES FOR PRACTICE

- Portfolios enable children and young people's nurses to demonstrate their value as a distinct branch of the family of nursing.
- Portfolios can be used to argue and refute the move toward generic approaches to nursing.
- Portfolios give a voice to children and young people's nurses to articulate the key issues which affect children and young people's nursing.

DEPARTMENTAL/TEAM PORTFOLIOS

REFLECTION POINTS

- Once you have read the section below, think about your ward/department/team.
- How would you encourage practitioners to contribute to a ward/team/departmental portfolio?
- What would be the aims of such a portfolio in your workplace?
- What would you include in a ward/departmental/team portfolio?

Rassin et al. (2006) argue that, although personal portfolios have personal benefits, the use of the portfolio could be broadened to a departmental or team level. They suggest that a departmental portfolio can be used as a managerial and evaluation tool of all activities in the department. They hypothesize that it provides insight into the team's development and achievements over time and can thus identity future goals and provide evidence of good clinical governance (Department of Health 2006, 2008a; Rassin et al. 2006; Welsh Assembly Government 2009; Rossetti et al. 2012). It can also be concluded from this that research could be identified and pursued, thus giving the team the opportunity to research and develop its own practice initiatives.

Departmental portfolios can be used as a collective tool to gather data, educate, evaluate functions of the department, consolidate staff knowledge and aspirations and also provide evidence of good practice. They can highlight areas where practice, research, service development, staff development and others require further work. The portfolio would provide opportunities for staff to reflect and self-evaluate their practice (Rassin et al. 2006; Rossetti et al. 2012). This would provide a prime initiative to develop a portfolio which contains clear, convincing reflections on the practice of children and young people's nursing, demonstrating the required practice knowledge and competencies and providing ongoing evaluation of the development of the nursing and multidisciplinary team in terms of care delivery, research opportunities and the evidence base underpinning personal and professional practice.

A departmental portfolio would provide educational opportunities and insights into the value of this specialty. Extrapolating the issues raised within educational research, it can be clearly seen that the use of a departmental portfolio would highlight the scholarship of children and young people's nursing practice with regard to practice development, critical thinking skills, reflective skills and the use of evidence to underpin actual practice (McClellan Reece et al. 2001; Corry and Timmins 2009). The departmental portfolio would build into a body of evidence to illustrate the currency and value of children and young people's nursing not just within discrete departments but also wherever children and young people are nursed and require the input of a children and young people's nurse on a 'consultancy' basis (Department of Health 1991, 2004a; Welsh Assembly Government 2005). This would act as a political voice for children and young people's nursing, children's nurses and the multidisciplinary team in putting forward convincing arguments for the value of their specialty and providing evidence refuting the move toward genericism.

PRINCIPLES FOR PRACTICE

Departmental portfolios provide a platform to:

- Illuminate the knowledge, skills, intricacies and nuances of children and young people's nursing
- Demonstrate scholarship within the children and young people's nursing team
- Educate those who are not children and young people's nurses and other professionals about the needs of children, young people and their families and the value of children and young people's nurses in terms of knowledge, research, policy and scholarship

E-PORTFOLIOS

CASE STUDY

Jayne is a children and young people's nurse who also works as a link nurse with the diabetic advanced nurse practitioner (ANP). Jayne has a deep interest in this area of practice and wishes to undertake a master's degree in advanced clinical practice so that when the current ANP retires in 2 years Jayne will able to apply for the role. Jayne is working at a hospital 50 miles from the university and cannot obtain regular study leave to attend the course. The university wishes to facilitate learning and assess practitioners in a more innovative way.

REFLECTION POINT

Think about how this might be done to satisfy the academic and practice components of the course and meet Jayne's learning needs.

With the rise in access to, and the popularity of, electronic learning resources it is only logical that the move should be made from paper-based portfolios to electronic portfolios. Policy initiatives and practitioners' views point the way toward more work-based assessments which need to be flexible, responsive to need and accessible while stimulating and promoting learning and critical thinking (Department of Health 2006, 2008a; Centre for the Development of Health Care Policy and Practice 2008; Welsh Assembly Government 2009). This has implications for practitioners who, as healthcare delivery evolves in innovative ways, may find they are working in settings which are remote from traditional learning centres (Lawson et al. 2004). The use of an e-portfolio enables the practitioner to access educational programmes and submit work electronically.

One of the criticisms levelled at the use of the traditional portfolio was that after a period of time it became impractical to transport as it was bulky. Also, as more courses are being assessed via the portfolio, so storage of the artefacts becomes problematic (Bowers and Jinks 2004; Bogossian et al. 2009; Timmins and Dunne 2009). E-portfolios would appear to solve these issues. They are portable, easily accessible and, in conjunction with Internet access, provide a rich, valuable learning experience. They also enable freedom of network and mobile access, data storage and backup (thus avoiding loss, etc.) hyperlinks and use of multimedia artefacts. They are more interactive, as the facilitator also has access to add comments and engage in a dialogue via the portfolio (Garrett and Jackson 2006; Garrett et al. 2013; Green et al. 2014; Andrews and Cole 2015). Andrews and Cole (2015) discuss how the use of e-portfolios in their nursing course enables a progressive digital education. This involves digital competency, becoming familiar with the software; digital usage, writing in the journal and developing artefacts; and digital transformation, examples of reflection, competencies and capabilities. All of these are brought together into a portfolio. They suggest that students are more aware of their strengths and weaknesses and can demonstrate higher levels of self-assessment and metacognitive skills. The research suggests that the artefacts themselves are enhanced due to the variety available to the author, e.g. video, audio input and pictures. These can be manipulated to suit the portfolio and the audience. Thus the portfolio can be reworked with new artefacts or existing ones manipulated to suit a future employer or a different assessor. The artefacts can also be added almost contemporaneously to ensure accuracy of recall and authenticity (Karsten 2012; Green et al. 2014). It can be argued that to some degree this meets the concerns about confidentiality and privacy raised earlier in conjunction with traditional paper-based portfolios, since the risk of an unwanted or uninvited audience is greatly reduced. Safety of the data is ensured providing the appropriate security software is installed and monitored (Garrett and Jackson 2006; Bogossian et al. 2009; Andrews and Cole 2015).

It is suggested that the ability to capture and report on nursing activities will exist almost in real time. Access to an online portfolio will enable the children and young people's nurse to capture professional development and competence activities shortly after the event and thus reduce activity that is not accounted for or degradation of information because of memory loss or distortion (Garrett and Jackson 2006; Bogossian et al. 2009; Green et al. 2014; Andrews and Coles 2015). Garrett and Jackson (2006) found that those students who were given mobile devices (portable digital assistants [PDAs]) enjoyed using them as they could access information quickly and make notes on critical incidents and record images. This could then be uploaded to the main portfolio on their computer. However, their expected use in the clinical area did not materialize as the students felt they were too busy and that writing reflectively was time-consuming. The reality was that the students wanted a more open format to the portfolio which was structured to capture specific information and to use desktop computers to write the more complex involved reflective pieces (Dornan et al. 2002; Garret and Jackson 2006; Andrews and Cole 2015). The aim of keeping events and writing concurrently was not met as students completed their reflective writing at a later time, resulting in the portfolio being completed within the same timescale as for the paper-based portfolio (Garrett and Jackson 2006; Bogossian et al. 2009).

Bogossian et al. (2009), in a small study, gave three students a tablet PC to take into practice with the aim of maintaining an e-portfolio concurrent with events. They found that similar issues recurred. Either time constraints and the busyness of the ward made it difficult to record the students' incidents and learning experiences or the students found it difficult to find space to use their devices without disturbing anyone. The students were also reluctant to use the PC at the bedside in front of patients. Thus students recorded their thoughts on paper and then transferred them to the PC later. The PC was used not just to record incidents but also to communicate with educational staff and other students, for teaching purposes and to access web-based information as well as storage of documents (Berglund et al. 2007; Bogossian et al. 2009; Green et al. 2014; Andrews and Cole 2015). There appeared to be an eclectic use of the device, which motivated completion of the portfolio. Concerns centred on security of both the information recorded and the device itself. Students needed to be vigilant in locking the screen to prevent unauthorized access to information and the physical security was an issue regarding loss or theft. Thus students completed work at home ostensibly because it was quieter and calmer; however, this made the portfolio remote from clinical practice, which defeated the aim of its use in practice.

Thus the use of e-portfolios would appear to be an interesting development. There are some caveats to this. Managerially and culturally there may need to be a shift in how e-portfolios and PDAs are regarded. New technology being used at the bedside is unfamiliar to practitioners, and users of such technology found that they were being judged in a negative light for using the e-portfolio or PDA (Dion 2006; Garret and Jackson 2006; Bogossian et al. 2009).

Although there are practical constraints in using them while working with patients, as the research has shown, their use for development and learning is apparent. The portfolio can be used to create a dialogue with the facilitator, who can enable the reflective process and stimulate the development of critical thinking skills as an ongoing process which is in agreement with the practice situation (Lawson et al. 2004; Garrett and Jackson 2006; Bogossian et al. 2009; Garrett et al. 2013; Andrews and Cole 2015).

The e-portfolio has advantages in that reflective writing is confidential between the facilitator and the student, adding to the privacy and trust that needs to be engendered in the process, thus possibly leading to a more honest approach to writing. However, when multiple assessors are used Garrett et al. (2013) found students were uneasy about who had access to their work. Despite access being restricted the perception was their work was accessible to more than one assessor and they wanted only their current work to be available. This contradicts the ethos of the developmental aspect of the portfolio; plus the confidentiality of the student also needs to be respected (Garrett et al. 2013; Green et al. 2013). The other advantages lie in being able to access the portfolio online at a time suitable to the writer in a location which is appropriate and not being constrained (Lawson et al. 2004; Mason et al. 2004; Andrews and Cole 2015). This is particularly important with distance learning, when children and young people's nurses may be some distance from their tutor. Also, with online courses gaining popularity for a variety of reasons, the online portfolio becomes an excellent means of assessing knowledge, practice issues, critical thinking and reflective writing in order to ascertain how the evidence which underpins practice is conceptualized and utilized in care delivery (Lawson et al. 2004; Mason et al. 2004; Andrews and Cole 2015).

The e-portfolio would appear to provide a secure, flexible environment in which to write, reflect and gather information, thus building a live document which captures and develops the ability to write in a cohesive integrated manner as the children's nurse progresses through his or her education and learning experiences, either within the constraints of a formal education process or as a means of ensuring personal professional development both to develop practice and to ensure continued registration. E-portfolios go well together with the notion of adult learning, which underpins the ethos of the portfolio. E-portfolios enable self-directed learning which recognizes the skill, the experiences and the person who is active and dynamic and their learning (Knowles 1990; Andrews and Cole 2015).

PRINCIPLES FOR PRACTICE

- E-portfolios are a dynamic, interactive medium for capturing experiences and learning from them at the same time.
- E-portfolios widen access to opportunities for education, reflection and critical writing.
- E-portfolios meet the concerns regarding confidentiality.
- E-portfolios allow the use of varied artefacts and multimedia.

CONCLUSION

Portfolios have become increasingly popular as a means of assessing learning and development both professionally and within educational programmes, where it is believed the portfolio allows learners the freedom to explore and reflect upon their knowledge base, knowledge acquisition and the application to practice. Indeed, a substantial number of courses now use portfolios as assessment tools because they are so flexible, dynamic and individual. Although portfolios have been perceived as a solution for developing personal and professional learning, which it is proposed develops and refines practice, it can be clearly seen that a number of tensions exist. The portfolio was originally a private enterprise designed to enable practitioners to reflect on their learning, development and practice, but in the United Kingdom it has become a statutory requirement for either formative or summative assessment.

The construction and development of a portfolio is suggested to be an individual, personal, flexible process which relies on a level of competence that learners may not have despite exhibiting higher levels of critical thinking and analysis in other areas. Also, issues around confidentiality and honesty need to be addressed, as it is possible for the learner to feel exposed and intimidated when writing for a 'public' audience, i.e. mentor or tutor, possibly leading to the adoption of a censorious writing style. Rigour is also an issue as a debate has taken place around ensuring the reliability and validity of the portfolio in terms of its capacity to assess learning, critical thinking and analytical ability as well as the transference into and refinement of knowledge in practice.

However, the available evidence demonstrates that practitioners do value an alternative method of assessing their learning and the opportunity to reflect on their practice. Portfolios provide an opportunity to reflect on how competencies are achieved in practice, whether they are academic requirements or requirements of the KSF, as well as facilitating analysis of the complex knowledge required to deliver high-quality care. They are a valuable adjunct in career progression as they demonstrate the maturation and development of the practitioner.

Portfolios in all their forms would appear to be an adjunct to the practice of children and young people's nursing to illustrate and support the contention that children and young people's nursing is a specialist area of practice and that ongoing education is vital for its development both personally and professionally. Children's nurses can use portfolios to demonstrate the specific knowledge, competencies and skills required to deliver high-quality care to children, young people and their families, thus providing a response to the rise of the generic argument. This can be achieved through the use of personal portfolios or developing departmental portfolios which demonstrate the knowledge and expertise of the children and young people's nursing team. This provides a valuable resource for teaching and can give a political voice to children's nurses to put forward arguments related to their specialist field of practice.

Although portfolios are seen as a positive innovation with much to offer the learner in terms of flexibility underpinned by adult learning principles, the research has focused on the use of portfolios by learners, mentors and academics. The research base is developing in relation to the claims that portfolios facilitate learning and critical thinking as well as positively influencing competence and the quality of care delivered. There needs to be further robust research into this area to substantiate these claims and to clearly demonstrate that portfolios as a learning tool do influence the quality of care delivered if the portfolio is to survive as both an assessment and development tool within nursing.

SUMMARY OF PRINCIPLES FOR PRACTICE

- Children and young people's nurses need to develop a clear understanding of the purpose and structure of the portfolio for their practice.
- Children and young people's nurses need to articulate and showcase the specific body of knowledge and clinical expertise required to care for children, young people and their families.
- Children and young people's nurses must be clear that they are writing for themselves and not a perceived audience in order to develop practice knowledge.
- Children and young people's nurses need to use portfolios as a powerful tool to identify learning and professional development in order to meet the demands of the Knowledge and Skills Framework and advance nurses' careers.
- Children and young people's nursing teams can use portfolios to demonstrate expertise, innovation, research and development in clinical practice, which can inform and be used as a consultative tool.

REFERENCES

Andrews T, Cole C (2015) Two steps forward, one back: the intricacies of engaging with e-portfolios in nursing undergraduate education. *Nurse Education Today* **35**(4): 568–72.

Berglund M, Nilsson C, Révay R, et al. (2007) Nurses' and nurse students' demands of functions and usability in a PDA. *International Journal of Medical Informatics* **76**(7): 530–7.

Bogossian FE, Kellett SEM, Mason B (2009) The use of tablet PCs to access an electronic portfolio in the clinical setting: a pilot study using undergraduate nursing students. *Nurse Education Today* **29**: 246–53.

Bowers SJ, Jinks AM (2004) Issues surrounding professional portfolio development for nurses. *British Journal of Nursing* **13**(3): 155–9.

Buckley S (2010) Caring for those with mental health conditions on a children's ward. *British Journal of Nursing* **19**(19): 226–30.

Byrne M, Delarose T, King CA, et al. (2007) Continued professional competence and portfolios. *Journal of Trauma Nursing* **14**: 24–31.

Casey A (1993) Development and use of the partnership model of nursing care. In Glasper A, Tucker A (eds.) *Advances in child health nursing.* London: Scutari Press.

Centre for the Development of Health Care Policy and Practice (2008) *Towards a framework for post-registration nursing careers: report of the outcomes from the national consultation*. Leeds: CDHPP, University of Leeds.

Children and Young People's Health Outcomes Forum (2012) *Children and young people's health outcomes strategy: report of the Children and Young People's Health Outcomes Forum*. London: DH. Available at https://www.gov.uk/government/uploads/system/uploads/attachment_data/file/216852/CYP-report.pdf.

Corry M, Timmins F (2009) The use of teaching portfolios to promote excellence and scholarship in nurse education. *Nurse Education in Practice* 9: 388–92.

Davies R (2008) Children's nursing and future directions: learning from 'memorable events'. *Nurse Education Today* 28(7): 814–21.

Davies R (2010) Marking the fiftieth anniversary of the Platt Report: from exclusion to toleration and parental participation in the care of the hospitalised child. *Journal of Child Health Care* 14(1): 6–23.

Department for Children, Schools and Families and Department of Health (2008) *Children and young people in mind: the final report of the national CAMHS review*. London: DCSF/DH.

Department for Children, Schools and Families and Department of Health (2009) *Healthy lives, brighter futures: the strategy for children and young people's health*. London: DCSF/DH.

Department for Children, Schools and Families and Department of Health (2010) *Keeping children and young people in mind: full government response to the CAMHS review*. London: DCSF/DH.

Department of Health (1991) *The welfare of children and young people in hospital*. London: DH.

Department of Health (2004a) *The National Service Framework for Children, Young People and Maternity Services*. London: DH.

Department of Health (2004b) *The NHS Knowledge and Skills Framework (NHS KSF) and the development review process*. London: DH. Available at http://webarchive.nationalarchives.gov.uk/20130107105354/http://www.dh.gov.uk/prod_consum_dh/groups/dh_digitalassets/@dh/@en/documents/digitalasset/dh_4090861.pdf.

Department of Health (2006) *Modernising nursing careers: setting the direction*. London: DH.

Department of Health (2008a) *Towards a framework for post-registration nursing careers: consultation response report*. London: DH.

Department of Health (2008b) *A high quality workforce: NHS next stage review*. London: DH. Available at http://webarchive.nationalarchives.gov.uk/20130107105354/http:/www.dh.gov.uk/en/Publicationsandstatistics/Publications/PublicationsPolicyAndGuidance/DH_085840.

Department of Health (2009) *New horizons: a shared vision for mental health*. London: HM Government.

Dion K (2006) Nursing portfolios: drivers, challenges and benefits. *Deans Notes* 27(4).

Dolan G, Fairbairn G, Harris S (2004) Is our student portfolio valued? *Nurse Education Today* 24: 4–13.

Dornan T, Carroll C, Parboosingh J (2002) An electronic learning portfolio for reflective continuing professional development. *Medical Education* 36: 767–9.

Endacott R, Gray MA, Jasper MA, et al. (2004) Using portfolios in the assessment of learning and competence: the impact of four models. *Nurse Education in Practice* 4: 250–7.

Gannon FT, Draper PR, Watson R (2001) Putting portfolios in their place. *Nurse Education Today* 21: 534–40.

Garrett BM, Jackson C (2006) A mobile clinical portfolio for nursing and medical students using personal digital assistants. *Nurse Education Today* 26: 647–54.

Garrett BM, McPhee M, Jackson C (2013) Evaluation of an eportfolio for the assessment of clinical competence in a baccalaureate program. *Nurse Education Today* 33: 1207–13.

Gerrish K (1993) An evaluation of a portfolio as an assessment tool for teaching practice placements. *Nurse Education Today* 13: 172–9.

Green J, Wyllie A, Jackson D (2014) Electronic portfolios in nursing education: a review of the literature. *Nurse Education in Practice* 14: 4–8.

Health Education England (2015) *Raising the bar: Shape of Caring Review: A review of the future of education and training of registered nurses and care assistants*. London: HEE/NMC.

Hill TL (2012) The portfolio as a summative assessment for the nursing student. *Teaching and Learning in Nursing* 7: 140–5.

Hull C, Redfern L (1996) *Profiles and portfolios*. Basingstoke: Macmillan.

Hull C, Redfern L, Shuttleworth A (2005) *Profiles and portfolios*, 2nd ed. Basingstoke: Palgrave Macmillan.

Jasper M, Mooney G (2013) The context of professional development. In Jasper M, Mooney G, Rosser M (eds.) *Vital notes for nurses: professional development, reflection and decision making in nursing and health care*, 2nd ed., Chapter 1, pp. 6–40, Chichester: Wiley.

Jasper M, Rosser M (2013) Work based learning and portfolios. In Jasper M, Mooney G, Rosser M (eds.) *Vital notes for nurses: professional development, reflection and decision making in nursing and health care*, 2nd ed., Chapter 5, pp. 136–167, Chichester: Wiley.

Jasper MA, Fulton J (2005) Marking criteria for assessing practice based portfolios at master's level. *Nurse Education Today* **25**: 377–89.

Johns C (1999) Reflection as empowerment? *Nursing Inquiry* **6**: 241–9.

Joyce P (2005) A framework for portfolio development in postgraduate nursing practice. *Journal of Clinical Nursing* **14**: 456–63.

Karsten K, (2012) Using E-portfolio to demonstrate competence in associate degree nursing students. *Teaching and Learning in Nursing* **7**: 23–6.

Kicken W, Brand-Gruwel S, van Merrienboer J, Slot W (2009) Design and evaluation of a development portfolio: how to improve students' self directed learning skills. *Instructional Science* **37**(5): 453–73.

Knowles M (1990) *The adult learner: a neglected species*, 4th ed. Houston: Gulf Publishing.

Lawson M, Nestel D, Jolly B (2004) An e-portfolio in health professional education. *Medical Education* **38**: 569–70.

Mason R, Pegler C, Weller C (2004) E-portfolios: an assessment tool for online courses. *British Journal of Educational Technology* **35**(6): 717–27.

McClellan Reece S, Pearce C, Devereaux Melillo K, Beaudry M (2001) The faculty portfolio: documenting the scholarship of teaching. *Journal of Professional Nursing* **17**(4): 180–6.

McColgan K (2008) The value of portfolio building and the registered nurse: a review of the literature. *Journal of Perioperative Practice* **18**(2): 64–9.

McMullan M (2006) Students' perceptions on the use of portfolios in pre-registration nursing education: a questionnaire survey. *International Journal of Nursing* **43**: 333–43.

McMullan M, Endacott R, Gray MA, et al. (2003) Portfolios and assessment of competence: a review of the literature. *Journal of Advanced Nursing* **41**: 283–94.

Ministry of Health (1959) *The welfare of children in hospital*. Platt Report. London: HMSO.

Nairn S, O'Brien E, Traynor V, Williams G, et al. (2006) Student nurses' knowledge, skills and attitudes towards the use of portfolios in a school of nursing. *Journal of Clinical Nursing* **15**: 1509–20.

Neades BL (2003) Professional portfolios: all you need to know and were afraid to ask. *Accident and Emergency Nursing* **11**: 49–55.

Nursing and Midwifery Council (2004) *Standards of competence for registered nurses*. London: NMC.

Nursing and Midwifery Council (2008) *The prep handbook*. London: NMC. Available at http://www.nmc-uk. org/Educators/Standards-for-education/The-Prep-handbook/.

Nursing and Midwifery Council (2009) *Review of pre-registration nursing education – phase 2*. London: NMC. Available at http://www.health.herts.ac.uk/immunology/MentorshipUpdate/N.

Nursing and Midwifery Council (2010) *Standards for pre-registration nursing education*. London: NMC. Available at https://www.nmc.org.uk/globalassets/sitedocuments/standards/nmc-standards-for-pre-registration-nursing-education.pdf.

Nursing and Midwifery Council (2015a) *The code: professional standards of practice and behaviour for nurses and midwives:* London: NMC. Available at http://www.nmc-uk.org/Documents/Standards/nmcTheCode StandardsofConductPerformanceAndEthicsForNursesAndMidwives_TextVersion.pdf.

Nursing and Midwifery Council (2015b) *How to revalidate with the NMC: requirements for renewing your registration*. London: NMC. Available at http://www.nmc.org.uk/globalassets/sitedocuments/revalidation/how-to-revalidate-print-friendly-version.pdf.

Polit DF, Beck CT (2014) *Essential of Nursing research: appraising evidence for nursing practice,* 8th ed. Wolters Kluwer/Lippincott, Williams and Wilkins.

Rassin M, Silner D, Ehrenfeld M (2006) Departmental portfolio in nursing: an advanced instrument. *Nurse Education in Practice* **6**: 55–60.

Rolfe G (2005) The deconstructing angel: nursing, reflection and evidence-based practice. *Nursing Inquiry* **12**: 78–86.

Rossetti J, Oldenburg N, Fisher Robertson J, Coyer S, Koren ME, Peters B, Uhlken C Musker K (2012) Creating a culture of evidence in nursing education using student portfolios. *International Journal of Nursing Education Scholarship* **9**(1).

Royal College of Nursing (2012a) *Quality with compassion: the future of nursing education.* Report of the Willis Commission. London: RCN.

Royal College of Nursing (2012b) *RCN competencies: core competencies for nursing children and young people*. London: RCN.

Royal College of Nursing (2013) *Defining safe staffing levels for children and young people's services: RCN standards for clinical professionals and service managers*. London: RCN. Available at www.rcn.org.uk/-/media/royal-college-of-nursing/documents/.

Royal College of Nursing (2014a) Children and young people's mental health – every nurse's business. Available at http://www.rcn.org.uk/professional-development/publications/pub-004587.

Royal College of Nursing (2014b) *Mental health in children and young people: an RCN toolkit for nurses who are not mental health specialists*. London: RCN.

Royal College of Nursing and Children's Community Nursing Forum (2000) *Promoting effective teamworking for children and their families*. London: RCN and Community Children's Nursing Forum.

Scholes J, Webb C, Gray M, et al. (2004) Making portfolios work in practice. *Journal of Advanced Nursing* **46**(6): 595–603.

Smith L, Coleman C (2010) *Family centred healthcare: concept, theory and practice*. Basingstoke: Palgrave Macmillan.

Snadden D, Thomas ML (1998) Portfolios learning in general practice vocational training – does it work? *Medical Education* **32**: 401–6.

Storey L, Haigh C (2002) Portfolios in professional practice. *Nurse Education in Practice* **22**: 44–8.

Timmins F, Dunne PJ (2009) An exploration of the current use and benefit of nursing student portfolios. *Nurse Education Today* **29**: 330–41.

Tweddell L (2008) Building a quality workforce fit for the future of nursing. *Nursing Times* **104**(27): 10.

Webb C, Endacott R, Gray MA, et al. (2003) Evaluating portfolio assessment systems: what are the appropriate criteria? *Nurse Education Today* **23**: 600–9.

Welsh Assembly Government (2004) *Realising the potential: a strategic framework for nursing, midwifery and health visiting in Wales into the 21st century*. Briefing paper 7. *Nurturing the future: a framework for realising the potential of children's nurses in Wales*. Cardiff: WAG.

Welsh Assembly Government (2005) *National Service Framework for Children, Young People and Maternity Services in Wales*. Cardiff: WAG.

Welsh Assembly Government (2009) *Post registration career framework for nurses in Wales*. Cardiff: WAG.

Williams GA, Park JR, Traynor V, Nairn S, O'Brien E, Chapple M, Johnson S (2008) Lecturers' and students' perceptions of portfolios in an English school of nursing. *Journal of Clinical Nursing* **18**: 1113–22.

Wilson P, Furnivall J, Barbour RS, et al. (2007) The work of the health visitor and school nurse with children with psychological and behavioural problems. *Journal of Advanced Nursing* **61**(4): 445–55.

Index